HEALTH SERVICES
RESEARCH METHODS

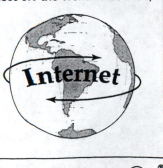

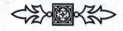

HEALTH SERVICES
RESEARCH METHODS

Leiyu Shi, Dr.P.H., MBA, MPA

Department of Health Administration
School of Public Health
University of South Carolina
Columbia, South Carolina

Delmar Publishers

I(T)P® International Thomson Publishing

Albany • Bonn • Boston • Cincinnati • Detroit • London • Madrid
Melbourne • Mexico City • New York • Pacific Grove • Paris • San Francisco
Singapore • Tokyo • Toronto • Washington

NOTICE TO THE READER

Cover Design: Carol D. Keohane

Delmar Staff:

Publisher: William Brottmiller
Assistant Editor: Hilary A. Schrauf
Senior Project Editor: Judith Boyd Nelson

Production Coordinator: James Zayicek
Art and Design Coordinator: Carol D. Keohane

COPYRIGHT © 1997
Delmar is a division of Thomson Learning. The Thomson Learning logo is a registered trademark used herein under license.

Printed in the United States of America
7 8 9 10 XXX 05 04 03

For more information, contact Delmar, 3 Columbia Circle, PO Box 15015, Albany, NY 12212-0515;
or find us on the World Wide Web at http://www.delmar.com

International Division List

Japan:
Thomson Learning
Palaceside Building 5F
1-1-1 Hitotsubashi, Chiyoda-ku
Tokyo 100 0003 Japan
Tel: 813 5218 6544
Fax: 813 5218 6551

Australia/New Zealand:
Nelson/Thomson Learning
102 Dodds Street
South Melbourne, Victoria 3205
Australia
Tel: 61 39 685 4111
Fax: 61 39 685 4199

UK/Europe/Middle East:
Thomson Learning
Berkshire House
168-173 High Holborn
London
WC1V 7AA United Kingdom
Tel: 44 171 497 1422
Fax: 44 171 497 1426

Latin America:
Thomson Learning
Seneca, 53
Colonia Polanco
11560 Mexico D.F. Mexico
Tel: 525-281-2906
Fax: 525-281-2656

Canada:
Nelson/Thomson Learning
1120 Birchmount Road
Scarborough, Ontario
Canada M1K 5G4
Tel: 416-752-9100
Fax: 416-752-8102

Asia:
Thomson Learning
60 Albert Street, #15-01
Albert Complex
Singapore 189969
Tel: 65 336 6411
Fax: 65 336 7411

Library of Congress Cataloging-in-Publication Data
Shi, Leiyu.
   Health services research methods / Leiyu Shi.
      p. cm. — (Delmar series in health services administration)
   Includes bibliographical references and index.
   ISBN 0-8273-7133-0
   1. Medical care—Research—Methodology. 2. Public health—
   Research—Methodology. I. Title. II. Series.
   [DNLM: 1. Health Services Research—methods. 2. Research Design.
3. Data Collection—methods. 4. Statistics—methods. W 84.3 S555h 1997]
RA425.S515 1997
362.1'072—dc20
DNLM/DLC   96-16768
for Library of Congress   CIP

INTRODUCTION
TO THE SERIES

This Series in Health Services is now in its second decade of providing top quality teaching materials to the health administration/public health field. Each year has witnessed further strengthening of the market position of each of the principal books in the Series, also reflecting the continued excellence of the products. Each author, book editor, and contributor to the Series has helped build what is widely recognized as the top textbook and issue collection of books available in this field today.

But we have achieved only a beginning. Everyone involved in the Series is committed to further expansion of the scope, technical excellence, and usability of the Series. Our goal is to do more for you, the reader. We will add new books in important areas, seek out more excellent authors, and increase the physical attributes of the book to make them easier for you to use.

We thank everyone, the authors and users in particular, who have made this Series so successful and so widely used. And we promise that this second decade will be dedicated to further expansion of the Series and to enhancement of the books it contains to provide still greater value to you, our constituency.

Stephen J. Williams
Series Editor

DELMAR SERIES IN HEALTH SERVICES ADMINISTRATION

CONTENTS

FOREWORD

T his volume is, as far as I know, the first book-length effort to codify the methods of health services research. It therefore deserves notice as an important milestone in the evolution of this new intellectual endeavor, quite aside from the many intrinsic merits of Dr. Leiyu Shi's *Health Services Research Methods*.

Passing an important milestone provides an occasion both for looking back and for trying to see into the future. The appearance of the first textbook in health services research, then, suggests two themes for this foreword:

- the somewhat anomalous rise of this recent multidisciplinary enterprise;
- the significance of the advent of the first textbook for the future evolution of health services research.

Health services research differs from the typical pattern of empirical research traditions in the twentieth century. Generally speaking, the emphasis in natural science on acute analysis and the development of better scientific equipment has resulted in successive advances in reductionism. Thus, periodically a given level of phenomena is subjected to explanation in terms of smaller components of matter or the action of more fundamental forces than previously. Each such wave of reductionism in some sense "dissolves" the observed phenomena into units that appear to be more "true" but also more esoteric. It also often fragments the established tradition of inquiry into new microdisciplines. Yet in the "Postscript 1969" to *The Structure of Scientific Revolutions*, historian T. S. Kuhn points out that modern physics, which became the model natural science in this century, was created by the merger of communities of "natural philosophers" and mathematicians in the nineteenth century.[1]

Health services research, in contrast, has developed into a recognized discipline by merging health-related methods and results from a number of the traditional disciplines of inquiry, ranging from sociology and political science or policy analysis and economics through epidemiology to nursing, medicine, and pharmacology. Many commentators would even add that bioethicists (and, therefore, applied philosophers such as those at Georgetown University's Kennedy Institute of Ethics and the Hastings Center) have an important contribution to make.[2] Unlike the paradigms of twentieth-century science, health services research does not generally put in question the putative object of its

[1] Thomas S. Kuhn, *The Structure of Scientific Revolutions*, 2nd edition enlarged (Chicago: University of Chicago Press, 1970), p. 179.

[2] See, for example, Daniel Wikler, "What Has Bioethics to Offer Health Policy," *Milbank Quarterly* 69:2 (1991), pp. 233–251.

study, because it does not involve a radically reductionist methodology. Indeed, health services research is in part *defined* by its field of interest rather than by a method, although methods—and agreement about methods among researchers—is as central to the creation of this discipline as to any other unique discipline. Health services research is also an enterprise that is aimed at improving health services: it therefore seeks practical rather than theoretical wisdom.

In his first chapter, Dr. Shi states this view in an apt definition:

> As an applied multidisciplinary field, health services research can be defined as scientific inquiry to produce knowledge about the resources, provision, organizing, financing, and policies of health services at the population level. . . . Since no conceptual framework from a single discipline takes into account all aspects of a health services problem or is inherently superior to others, a cohesive mixture of various academic disciplines that encompass a great variety of perspectives is often required to carry out health services research successfully. Health services research may be considered as the application of the biomedical, social, and other scientific disciplines to the study of how to deliver health services to groups of people.

Progress in understanding health services, then, has come only as those of us schooled in various of the traditional academic disciplines relinquish strict adherence to the sectarian methods and shibboleths that informed our doctoral training and enter into dialogue together over a substantive field of health care.

The phrase "health services research" began to be widely used in the 1960s, and the field was developing rapidly by 1981, when the Association for Health Services Research was formed.[3] Pioneers who attended the organization's annual meetings in the early years speak glowingly of the intellectual excitement of those relatively small gatherings, where the leading researchers from different disciplines who had organized the association shared their research. The Reagan administration's threat to cut funding for health services research provided the impetus for establishing the association. Ironically, the success of the Reagan and Bush administrations in creating national payment systems for Medicare (using diagnosis-related groups and the resource-based relative value scale) brought health services research to the center of the business of the national government for the first time. This development, which is surely not an outcome that those conservative officials desired, is in some respects parallel to the process by which the Manhattan project in the Second World War irretrievably enmeshed government policy in a natural science (physics).

---

[3] The historian Daniel M. Fox, president of the Milbank Memorial Fund, has made important contributions to our understanding of the development of the field of health services research. See his "The Development of Priorities for Health Services Research: The National Center, 1974–76," *Milbank Memorial Fund Quarterly* 54:3 (1976), pp. 237–248; "Health Policy and the Politics of Research in the United States," *Journal of Health Politics, Policy and Law* 15:3 (1990), pp. 481–499; and "The *Milbank Quarterly* and Health Services Research, 1977–1990," *Milbank Quarterly* 69:2 (1991), pp. 185–197.

The late 1970s and first half of the 1980s was also the most intense period of activity for the RAND Corporations's Health Insurance Experiment (HIE), which was led by economist Joseph Newhouse. HIE was a large-scale experiment to observe the behavioral and health consequences of different configurations of health insurance. With government funding that was estimated in 1987 at more than 127 million in then current dollars, HIE was arguably the social scientist's opportunity to do "big science" like the physicists with their superconducting supercollider or the biologists involved in the human genome project.[4] At a more general level, many researchers in this period responded to the perceived need for research to help policymakers choose between regulatory and market reform (or "procompetition") strategies for controlling health care costs and fostering access to health care.

With the publication of its first textbook, health services research has now acquired yet another of the accounterments of an established discipline. In *Structure of Scientific Revolutions*, Kuhn uses the notion of a "textbook" both literally to refer to specific volumes and metaphorically to mean the exemplary models and training materials that inculcate common ways of doing intellectual business, thereby generating and maintaining a particular scientific community. It is from such texts that new generations of scientists learn the paradigms that govern normal science. Although textbooks are often disparaged in the culture of universities, occasionally a specific textbook in the first sense is recognized for its contribution in forming or reforming a discipline. Campbell and Stanley's *Experimental and Quasi-Experimental Designs for Research*, Paul Samuelson's many editions of his introduction to economics, Beauchamp and Childress' *Principles of Biomedical Ethics*, and Sabine's *History of Political Theory* come to mind as works that have made such contributions. It just might be the case that health services research is ripe for a textbook that will communicate its emerging "paradigm"—loosely, its operating norms and mores.

In closing, it is worth considering whether the emergence of a synergistic field of study that brings together insights and methods from a number of the traditional disciplines, resists undue reductionism, and acknowledges openly its ameliorationist motivation might be the harbinger of analogous developments in other scientific fields.

If other new forms of inquiry with characteristics like those of health services research become widespread, it will be necessary to devise new organizational vehicles for accomplishing research and education. At least for the social sciences, the formally demarcated disciplines that generated the departmental structures of traditional universities in North America are largely historical vestiges of once lively and coherent intellectual traditions or of long-forgotten administrative compromises. Many of the faculty within

---

[4] William P. Brandon, "A Large-Scale Social Science Experiment in Health Finance: Findings, Significance, and Value," *Journal of Health Politics, Policy and Law* 20:4 (1995), pp. 1051–1061. The HIE findings were published in more than 330 journal articles and RAND reports and in a summary volume, Joseph P. Newhouse, et al., *Free for All? Lessons from the RAND Health Insurance Experiment* (Cambridge, MA: Harvard University Press, 1993).

these traditional departments, especially junior faculty, seem eager to break out of the administrative straightjackets. To call academic departments the "sinkhole of interdisciplinary research" (as this commentator once thoughtlessly did) is both intemperate and impolitic. Nonetheless, the needs of multidisciplinary research will force universities to make more appropriate administrative arrangements during the next quarter century. If appropriate organizational structures to support new intellectual enterprises do not develop in universities, health services research will increasingly be dominated by think tanks and consultants. The universities and the society will both be poorer if the new style of multidisciplinary inquiry epitomized by health services research cannot flourish in traditional academic settings.

William P. Brandon
University of North Carolina—Charlotte

PREFACE

Health services research is a rapidly expanding field of inquiry. Typically health services researchers conduct investigations within different fields: health policy, health systems research, health outcomes research, clinical epidemiology, technology assessment, clinical decision analysis, operations research, health economics, medical sociology, medical anthropology, to name a few. An important impetus to the rapid development of health services research is the breathtaking advance of the medical enterprises. The growing costs of the medical care systems and the increasing role of government in financing health institutions and services, and in paying for medical education, require the generation of information about the effectiveness, efficiency, and appropriateness of these enterprises. As health care costs continue to escalate and as the nation approaches health care reform, there will be an increasing demand for health services research.

Despite the extensive literature related to health services research, few textbooks existed that examined the field of health services research and systematically described the design, methodology, and analysis commonly used in health services research. As a student and later a professor in health services research, I was continually nagged by the lack of a relevant textbook on health services research. The research methods books I have encountered are primarily written by sociologists with little health care applications. Students frequently complain about the lack of relevance of those textbooks. In the course of teaching "Health Services Research Methods" in the past six years, I have developed the current textbook that integrates health services research applications in the presentation of research methods and analysis.

There are a number of features of this book. First, the book intends to be a practical guide for those interested in health services research. Steps will be delineated and illustrated clearly in the text, tables, and figures. Second, health services research examples are used throughout. Third, the book integrates research design with analysis. While this is not a statistical textbook, commonly used statistics are discussed in terms of their use for different levels of analysis and the nature of the variables. Fourth, the book also provides resources for students and researchers of health services. For example, the book includes current health services research journals, funding sources (public and private), and data sources.

The book is organized into 15 chapters. Chapter 1 lays the groundwork for the chapters that follow by describing the scientific foundations of health services research. Chapter 2 examines the conceptualization of health services research by summarizing major health services research topics. Chapter 3 describes the preparation for health services research including identifying relevant data sources, exploring potential funding sources, developing a research plan or proposal, and getting prepared organizationally and administratively to carry out the research. Chapters 4 through 9 summarize and illustrate the various types of health services research methods including research review, meta-analysis, secondary analysis, research analysis of administrative records, qualitative research, case study, experiment, survey research, longitudinal study, and evaluation research. Chapter 10 looks at research design options. Chapter 11 summarizes sampling procedures in health services research. Chapter 12 presents measurement issues in health services research. Chapter 13 delineates major data collection methods. Chapter 14 focuses on representative statistical analyses carried out in health services research. Chapter 15 explores ways of publicizing research findings.

The major audiences of this book include doctoral- and master-level students in health services administration programs. Students from nursing administration and clinical nursing programs can also benefit from this book. These programs may be offered by schools of public health, medical schools, schools of nursing, schools of business administration, schools of public administration or public policy. Students in other disciplines with an interest in health services research are also potential targets. For doctoral programs, a two-semester sequence could be set aside for the research methods course. The course focus may be given to enhance the following areas: knowledge regarding health services research topics and conceptualization; research methodology with emphasis on design; survey research including design, sampling, questionnaire preparation, measurement, interview, pretest, and coding; and statistical analysis with emphasis on the choice of appropriate statistical methods. Sufficient emphasis should be given to the integrated nature of various stages of health services research. If only one semester can be allocated, as in most master's level programs, the emphasis should be given to the conceptual understanding of research stage with particular focus on conceptualization, methods, design, and survey measurement. The remaining content areas of the book may be integrated with other courses (e.g., statistics, health policy).

In addition to students, health services practitioners and researchers can also benefit from the book. They include those working in public health agencies, nonprofit health services organizations, insurance companies, and the like. My private consulting experience in these sectors shows that many of them are involved in health services research and frustrated by the lack of a relevant guidebook.

The preparation of this book, both at the initial and later phase, has been greatly aided by a number of devoted reviewers who themselves are active health services researchers. The author wishes to thank Dr. William P. Brandon for writing the foreword and reviewing the earlier chapters of the book, and Drs. James R. Ciesla and Doulgas A. Singh for reviewing the entire manuscripts and offering numerous valuable suggestions and corrections. Similar thanks and gratitudes are extended to all those who have reviewed either the proposal or selected chapters of the manuscripts and provided comments and feedback. Their time and effort spent in reviewing the manuscripts are warmly and graciously appreciated and acknowledged. The author is also grateful to Delmar Publishers and series editor Stephen Williams for encouraging the development and publishing of this book. The direct assistance provided by Delmar staff William Burgower, Hilary Schrauf, and Debra Flis are much appreciated, as are the efforts of Judith Boyd Nelson, Tim Conners, Carol Keohane, and James Zayicek. All suggestions concerning any aspects of this first edition of the book are welcome and will be acknowledged and incorporated in future editions.

Leiyu Shi

ABOUT THE AUTHOR

Leiyu Shi is currently an associate professor of health services research and chair of the Department of Health Administration, School of Public Health, University of South Carolina. He obtained a doctorate in health services research and administration from the University of California, Berkeley. He also has an MBA and an MPA degree. Dr. Shi has extensive research and publication experience in the area of health services research. He is a coauthor of the book *Physician Recruitment and Retention: A Guide for Rural Medical Group Practice* and author of about 40 publications on evaluation research, primary care, and rural health.

CHAPTER

1

Scientific Foundations of Health Services Research

LEARNING OBJECTIVES

- To understand and describe the major characteristics of scientific inquiry.
- To understand and describe the process of generating scientific theory.
- To understand and describe the major types of relationship between variables.
- To understand and describe the major characteristics of health services research.
- To understand and describe the process of health services research.

Chapter 1 lays the groundwork for the chapters that follow. By providing an overview of the scientific foundations of health services research, the chapter serves as a framework on which specific aspects of health services research are based. The nature of scientific inquiry is discussed, followed by a description of health services research. Since social scientists have made significant contributions to the development of health services research, the discussion of scientific inquiry centers on social science research. The chapter concludes with a summary of the stages of health services research, based on the major components of scientific inquiry. After completing this chapter, readers should be ready to examine some of the more concrete aspects of health services research related to the delineated stages.

THE NATURE OF SCIENTIFIC INQUIRY

The origin of the word *science* is the Latin word *scientia*, which indicates "knowledge." The major purpose of **scientific inquiry** is to create knowledge that clarifies a particular aspect of the world around us (Kaplan, 1964). The fundamental assumption of scientific inquiry is that life is not totally chaotic or random but has logical and persistent patterns of regularity (Sjoberg and Nett, 1968). This assumption, labeled **positivism**, is responsible for the two major pillars of scientific inquiry: **scientific theory** and **empiricism.** Scientific theory is related to the logical aspect of science and is used as a framework to guide the understanding and explanation of patterns of regularity in life (DiRenzo, 1967). Empiricism is the approach used in scientific inquiry to discover the patterns of regularity in life (Hempel, 1965, 1967). Scientific inquiry relies on or derives from data that can be observed under specifiable conditions (Selltiz, Wrightsman, and Cook, 1976). A scientific understanding of the world must be logical and correspond with what we observe. Since empirical evidence is assumed to exist independent of researchers, it is important that researchers maintain **objectivity** in their observations, uninfluenced by their personal feelings, conjectures, or preferences. Research methods, properly used, strengthen the objectivity of the observational aspect of the research. Statistical methods offer a device for comparing what is logically expected with what is actually observed. This textbook deals primarily with research methods—demonstrating how to conduct empirical health services research. The remainder of this section takes a closer look at these important characteristics of scientific inquiry, namely, positivism, scientific theory, empiricism, and objectivity.

Positivism

All sciences, physical, natural, social, or health, are based on the fundamental assumption that there exists a persistent pattern or regularity in what is being studied. This assumption is sometimes challenged, particularly in the study of social phenomena as demonstrated by Bailey (1994). Wilhelm Dilthey (1988), a nineteenth-century sociologist, took the extreme position that humans had free will, and thus no one could generalize about their actions. He believed that scientists can only study unique events, not make generalizations.

The opposite view was upheld by Emile Durkheim (1974), who believed that social phenomena, just like physical phenomena, are orderly and generalizable. Social scientists could study and explain social phenomena just as well as physical scientists study and explain physical phenomena. Durkheim's study of suicide rates in European countries was an example. His work on suicide began in 1888, and his monumental book *Le Suicide* was published in 1897 (see Lester, 1994). Durkheim (1951) noted that although suicide rates changed over time, they were consistently and inversely correlated with the degree of social integration. This finding was later termed "Durkheim's law of suicide."

However, most social scientists favor an intermediate approach as espoused by Max Weber. According to Weber (1949), social phenomena are the product of both social laws and human volitional action. The fact that humans have free will does not mean that their actions are random and totally unpredictable. Rather, human actions are guided by rational decision making and can be predicted by understanding the rationale behind the actions.

Although many social scientists agree that social phenomena are orderly enough to be explained and predicted, they also believe that not all social phenomena can be explained or predicted with complete accuracy. This is because existing theories, methods of data collection, and current techniques of data analysis are not sufficiently developed to explain social phenomena (Bailey, 1994). In addition, social phenomena may be changing over time. Similarly, but to a lesser extent, not all physical phenomena can be explained or predicted with complete accuracy. For example, most observers agree that the space program is backed by sophisticated scientific theory and sound engineering application. The explosion of the spaceship *Challenger*, however, showed that physical science can also experience failure.

The fact that there are exceptions to regularity is insufficient evidence to overthrow the assumption that regularity exists in both physical and social phenomena, because scientific inquiry is concerned with the study of patterns rather than exceptions. The pattern that, given the same educational level, men earn more money than women overall is not problematic when a particular woman earns more than a particular man. The trend that women live longer than men overall is not violated when a particular man lives longer than a particular woman. Social scientists primarily study social patterns rather than individual exceptions. Regularities and patterns are probabilistic and do not need to be manifested in every observation.

It is also important to know that a particular pattern may not always persist (Skinner, 1953). In other words, regularity is not certainty. Scientific "truth" is based on observable evidence, but such evidence is always open to change through possible contradiction by new evidence. Thus, at some point a scientific proposition is accepted because it describes or interprets a recurring, observable event. But just because an event has occurred on several occasions is no guarantee that it will always recur. Scientific knowledge represents the best understanding that we have been able to produce thus far by means of current empirical evidence.

Scientific Theory

Scientific inquiry generally works within the framework of scientific theories. Scientific theories are used to derive research hypotheses, plan research, make observations, and explain generalizations and patterns of regularity in life (Zetterberg, 1954). Theories are based on overwhelming evidence, used as explanations or predictions of phenomena, and are potentially testable (McCain and Segal, 1977). The creation of theories is typically based on considerable supporting evidence. Theories are then used to provide a systematic explanation and to make predictions for a particular phenomenon. A statement that does not seek to explain or predict something is not a theory. Theories must also be potentially testable. A statement that is too vague to be understandable is not an adequate theory.

In searching for theories, scientists generally do not start out with a completely clean slate. Rather, they are influenced by the **paradigms** of their disciplines. A paradigm is normative in that it reflects a general perspective, a fundamental model or scheme that breaks down the complexity of reality and organizes our views. As such, paradigms are deeply embedded in the socialization of researchers and tell them what is important, legitimate, and reasonable (Patton, 1990, pp. 37–39). Often, a paradigm doesn't readily provide answers to research questions, but it tells researchers where to look for answers and provides them with concepts that are the building blocks of theories.

For example, many theories have been suggested to account for the fact that females in the United States and in other modern industrialized societies have higher rates of morbidity than males but live longer than males. One biomedical explanation of this posits a fundamental physiological difference that causes women to experience more morbidity than men but to live longer for reasons not yet clearly understood. A sociological suggestion is that the different roles men and women play in society expose them to different sources of illness or disability. A psychological explanation is that perhaps men and women do not differ in their underlying rates of morbidity. Rather, they have differential perceptions of and tolerance for morbidity, as well as different ways of expressing their feelings about that morbidity. Our social systems might have processed them differently so that it appeared, when we count up hospital visits and the like, that women have greater morbidity rates.

Since it is possible to have several theories that explain a given empirical regularity and make similar predictions, the confirmation of a prediction does not confirm that only one theory is correct (Hempel, 1967). Scientific inquiry is directed toward testing and choosing from alternative theories. One theory is generally judged to be superior to other competing theories if it: (1) involves the fewest number of statements and assumptions, (2) explains the broadest range of phenomena, and (3) predicts most accurately (Singleton, Straits, and Straits, 1993, p. 24). In short, scientific theories should be efficient, comprehensive, and accurate.

There is an intimate connection between theory and research. Theory provides guidance for research. Research, in turn, verifies, modifies, or reconstructs theory. This interactive process between theory and research contributes to the enrichment and development of scientific theories. Specifically, there are two components within this process: the **deductive process,** which emphasizes theory as guidance for research, and the **inductive process,** which stresses research as impetus for theory (Salmon, 1967, 1973). In the deductive process, hypotheses are derived from existing theories to provide guidance for further research. Indeed, scientific research is guided by accumulated scientific knowledge. In the inductive process, existing theories are corroborated or modified, and new theories are developed from research findings. The resulting corroborated, modified, or reconstructed theories guide future research along similar fields of inquiry.

Empiricism

The most critical characteristic of scientific inquiry is that it is based on empiricism. Empirical evidence is the only means scientists use to corroborate, modify, or construct theories. Whether a question can be studied scientifically depends on whether it can be subjected to verifiable observations (Singleton, Straits, and Straits, 1993). That is, it must be possible for the scientist to make observations that can answer the question.

The empirical requirement of scientific inquiry has several ramifications. First, it means that nonempirical ways of acquiring knowledge cannot produce scientific evidence. Examples of nonempirical means include appeals to authority, tradition, common sense or intuition, and so on.

In general, scientists do not generalize about the world based on what an authority or expert says. An authority or expert may be knowledgeable about the subject matter, but his opinion alone cannot serve as scientific evidence to prove or refute a hypothesis. However, this does not mean experts cannot be studied in research. A representative sample of experts can be surveyed regarding their perceptions of issues of research interest.

Tradition refers to inherited culture made up of firmly accepted knowledge about the workings of the world (Babbie, 1992). These are the things that "everyone knows." An example is to consult a doctor when one is sick. The advantage of tradition is that one is spared of the task of starting from scratch in searching for understanding. The disadvantage is that tradition limits us from seeking a fresh and different understanding of something that everyone already knows. Tradition is not always correct. Maybe better diet and exercise are more important to one's health than relying on medical treatment.

Common sense cannot be regarded as scientific evidence. Common sense tends to be unconditional, uncomplicated, and nonsituational, and it does not require systematic testing. It limits people's reliance to the familiar and implies that seeing is believing, although the reverse is often true. When one believes in something, one is more likely to see (notice) it.

Second, empiricism in science also implies that researchers focus on problems and issues that can be observed. Observations may be direct, as in field studies, or indirect, as in surveys and interviews that primarily rely on the empirical experience of research subjects. These observations are then used to form *constructs,* an intangible or nonconcrete characteristic or quality on which individuals or populations differ. Examples of constructs are patient satisfaction with a physician's office visit, or the American people's impression of the health care system. Constructs are often the building blocks of scientific theories.

Third, empiricism means scientific inquiry cannot settle debates on values or beliefs. Scientific inquiry has to do with what is, not what should be. This means that philosophical questions about righteousness, essence, or morality are beyond the realm of science. For example, the value judgment that people should not use birth control is an opinion, not a testable statement. Science cannot determine whether a market-controlled health care system (or "lassez-faire" system) is better or worse than a government-controlled and -financed system (or "single-payer" system) except in terms of some set of agreed-on criteria. We could only determine scientifically whether the "lassez-faire" or "single-payer" system better supports access to care and/or cost containment if we could agree on some measures of access and cost containment, and our conclusion would have no general meaning beyond the measures agreed upon.

The fact that scientific inquiry cannot settle values or beliefs does not mean it is not influenced by them. Rather, personal values and beliefs frequently influence the process of research. Indeed, the challenge for scientists, particularly in the social sciences, is to maintain objectivity and openness in their scientific inquiry.

Objectivity

Scientists, like most people, have their own values and often make value judgments. Having values and making value judgments in and of themselves are not problematic. But, in terms of research, individual values may affect the validity of the inquiry and make the findings biased. The problem with value judgments in research is that they are not only essentially untestable but may also make a researcher prejudiced in undertaking research. Although difficult, researchers should strive to suppress values and conduct "value-free" research in order to minimize bias in their findings. They are perfectly free to hold and express their values in a nonresearch environment.

Even though researchers may hold back their personal values while conducting research, they are likely to be influenced by their scientific disciplines or paradigms. Different paradigms tend to espouse different values. They affect the types and scope of problems to research, the methods adopted, and the ways to interpret the findings.

Biases may enter into the selection of problems for study and the preference for certain research strategies. Often, where and how one looks largely determine the answers one will find. Since it is very hard to think beyond one's established paradigm and difficult to suppress one's professional values, it is important that researchers state their professional values (i.e., the research paradigm) explicitly so that readers may judge for themselves the limitations of the research when considering other relevant paradigms. Perhaps the worst approach is to deny that one has a value position that has in fact influenced the research. Such a lack of openness will make it difficult for the reader to assess the validity of the research.

Sometimes, particularly in social sciences, maintaining objectivity is difficult through no fault of the researchers. If subjects know that they are being observed by researchers, they often will feel self-conscious and may alter their behavior, either consciously or unconsciously. This reactivity problem exists because social interaction with subjects is often part of the social science research process.

The reactive effect of research on the social phenomena being studied is known as the **Hawthorne effect,** derived from the study of workers assembling telephone relays in the Hawthorne Plant of the Western Electric Company in Chicago (Roethlisberger and Dickson, 1939). In studying the impact of varying working conditions on work performance among employees, researchers were surprised to note that productivity increased even when rest periods were eliminated. They later realized that it was a reactive effect. The attention from the researchers altered the very behavior (worker productivity) that the researchers wished to study.

Fortunately, scientists adopt numerous measures to enhance objectivity. During the research process, scientists use procedures to control for, minimize, or eliminate, as far as possible, sources of bias that may mislead their findings. Research findings are often open to a variety of interpretations. The concept of control is to use procedures (either by design or by statistical modeling) to exclude alternative explanations. For example, in medical research, a double-blind procedure is often used to assign patients to experiment or control groups. Patients in the control group use a placebo; neither patients nor doctors know which group patients belong to. This procedure is designed to rule out the possibility of doctors' and patients' expectations contributing to the effectiveness of a treatment. The Hawthorne effect may be reduced through an improved design (for example, by using more control groups including those whose subjects are not aware of the research, or by extending the study period since the reactive effect tends to be relatively short-lived). The use of control procedures to reduce biases is a common procedure researchers use to enhance objectivity.

Peer review is another measure to improve objectivity. When a group of scientists can independently agree on the results of a given observation, validity is enhanced. Replication is another measure that can be used. If it is possible for two or more independent researchers working under the same conditions to agree that they are observing the same event, validity is further enhanced. To meet the requirement of objectivity and openness in scientific inquiry, researchers provide detailed accounts of their study, delineating their methods of observation and analysis. Such a process enables other researchers to assess whether the researchers have maintained objectivity or to repeat the study themselves under similar conditions. These and many other measures to enhance objectivity will be discussed throughout this book.

THE PROCESS OF THEORY CONSTRUCTION

Since much of scientific inquiry follows the interactive process of theory verification and/or construction, and there are some important concepts embedded in the process, a more detailed discussion of this process (listed below) (Babbie, 1992, pp. 58–59; Dubin, 1969) is warranted.

The process of theory construction:

Step 1. Specify the topic
Step 2. Specify the assumptions
Step 3. Specify the range of phenomena
Step 4. Specify the major concepts and variables
Step 5. Specify the propositions, hypotheses, and relationships
Step 6. Specify the theory

Specify the Topic

The first step in theory verification and/or construction is to specify the research topic of interest. Existing theories and literature related to the topic should be identified and used as guidance for determining the nature and scope of the inquiry. Since knowledge is cumulative, the inherited body of information and understanding is the takeoff point for the development of more knowledge. The practice of reviewing the literature in research papers serves this purpose of identifying relevant theories and findings or the lack of both.

Specify the Assumptions

The second step in theory verification and/or construction is to specify the **assumptions** related to the research focus. Assumptions are suppositions that are not yet tested but are considered true. In general, assumptions should make sense to most people. When in doubt, researchers should test their assumptions rather than consider them true. For example, when the telephone interview is used as a data collection method, the assumption is that it can reach a representative sample of the population of interest. If this assumption is not necessarily true, as in studies of Medicaid recipients or indigent patients, then researchers need to conduct a pretest to verify whether the telephone is a proper channel to reach the study population prior to full-scale data collection.

Specify the Range of Phenomena

The third step in theory verification and/or construction is to specify the range of phenomena the current research and existing theories address. For example, will the research and theories apply to people of the world or only to Americans or only to young Americans? Research or theories are more useful the greater the range of phenomena they cover, although broader theories are more difficult to construct. For one thing, data have to be collected from a wider spectrum of the population.

Specify the Major Concepts and Variables

The fourth step in theory verification and/or construction is to specify the major **concepts** and **variables.** Concepts are mental images or perceptions (Bailey, 1994). They may be difficult to observe directly, such as equity or ethics, or they may have referents that are easily observable, such as a hospital or a clinic. A concept that has only a single, never-changing value is called a *constant.* A concept that has more than one measurable value is called a *variable.* A concept or variable may contain several categories, falling along a recognizable continuum. The variable "old-age," for example, is a continuum containing many different values or categories, such as ages 65–74, 75–84, or 85 and older. Usually the values or categories of a variable are designated quantitatively (i.e., signified by numbers, as in the case of age), but some variables have categories designated by word labels rather than by numbers. For example, gender is a variable whose categories are designated by the labels "male" and "female."

Variables may be classified as **independent** and/or **dependent.** Generally, a variable capable of effecting change in other variables is called an independent variable. A variable whose value is dependent upon one or more other variables, but which cannot itself affect the other variables, is called a dependent variable. The dependent variable is the variable we wish to explain, and the independent variable is the hypothesized explanation. In a causal relationship, the cause is an independent variable and the effect a dependent variable. For example, since smoking causes lung cancer, smoking is an independent variable and lung cancer a dependent variable.

Often we can recognize a variable as independent simply because it occurs before the other variable. For example, we may find a relationship between race and level of education. Race clearly comes before schooling and, therefore, must be an independent variable. Education level can in no way influence race, since race has already been determined at birth. When one variable does not clearly precede the other, it may be difficult to designate it as dependent or independent. An example is the relationship between health status and income. If a person has adequate income, he or she may have the financial resources to maintain good health status. Or when a person has good health status, he or she will have the opportunity to earn better income. The question is, Which comes first: good health status or adequate income? Perhaps each influences the other. The treatment of these variables will be discussed in the next step when we consider causal relationship.

Specify the Propositions, Hypotheses, and Relationships

The fifth step in theory verification and/or construction is to specify the propositions, hypotheses, and relationships among the variables. A **proposition** is a statement about one or more concepts or variables (Bailey, 1994). Just as concepts are the building blocks of propositions, propositions are the building blocks of theories. Depending upon their use in theory building, propositions have been given different names including hypotheses, empirical generalizations, constructs, axioms, postulates, and theorems.

A proposition that discusses a single variable is called a univariate proposition. An example is: "Forty million of the citizens in the United States do not have any type of health insurance." It is a univariate proposition because only one variable, "have any type of health insurance," is contained in the statement.

A bivariate proposition is one that relates two variables. An example is: "The lower the population density in a county, the lower the physician-to-population ratio in that county." It is a bivariate proposition because two variables, "population density" and "physician-to-population ratio," are contained in the statement.

A proposition relating more than two variables is called a multivariate proposition. An example is: "The lower the population density in a county, the lower the physician-to-population ratio and hospital-to-population ratio in that county." It is a multivariate proposition because three variables, "population density," "physician-to-population ratio," and "hospital-to-population ratio," are contained in the statement. A multivariate proposition can be written as two or more bivariate propositions. For example, (1) "the lower the population density in a county, the lower the physician-to-population ratio in that county" and (2) "the lower the population density in a county, the lower the hospital-to-population ratio in that county." This would allow for one portion of the original proposition to be rejected without rejecting the other portion, based on later statistical tests.

When a proposition is stated in a testable form (that we can in principle prove right or wrong through research) and predicts a particular relationship between two or more variables, it is called a **hypothesis.** Normative statements, or those that are opinions and value judgments, are not hypotheses. For example, the statement that every person should have access to health care is a normative statement. It is a value judgment that cannot be proved right or wrong.

This definition also excludes statements that are too abstract to be tested. Consider the statement that the poor do not have adequate access to health care. Although this is a valid proposition, we would not call it a testable hypothesis until the concepts of poor, adequacy, and health care are measured or defined on an empirical level. For example, we can define poor as those with income below the poverty line, adequacy as the U.S. average, and health care as number of physician office visits. We can then state, "Compared with the U.S. average, those with income below the poverty line have lower rates of physician office visits." This becomes a testable hypothesis.

Hypotheses may be generated from a number of sources. They may be deducted from a formal theory that summarizes the present state of knowledge about the research problem. This is the standard deductive process. Or they may be inspired by past research or by commonly held beliefs. Or they may be generated through direct analysis of data. The two latter approaches are used typically when there is an absence of relevant theories related to the topic of research. Regardless of how hypotheses are expressed, they should indicate at least the form of the relationship between variables. A hypothesis is an expected but yet unconfirmed relationship between two or more variables. An adequate hypothesis statement about two variables indicates which variable predicts or causes the other or how changes in one variable are related to changes in the other.

The properties of the relationship (Singleton, Straits, and Straits, 1993, pp. 78–80; Miller, 1991; Baily, 1994) between two variables include whether the relationship is positive or negative, the strength of the relationship, whether it is symmetrical or asymmetrical, whether the relationship is linear or curvilinear, whether the relationship is spurious or involves an intervening or suppressor variable, and which variable is an independent or dependent variable (as in a causal relationship).

Positive versus Negative Relationships

In a **positive** or *direct,* **relationship,** both variables vary in the same direction, that is, an increase in the value of one variable is accompanied by an increase in the value of the other variable. Similarly, a decrease in one variable is accompanied by a decrease in the other variable. For example, if an increase in one's income level is accompanied by an increase in health insurance coverage, the relationship is positive. In a **negative** or *inverse,* **relationship,** the variables vary in opposite directions. An increase (decrease) in one variable is accompanied by a decrease (increase) in the other variable. For example, if an increase in educational level is accompanied by a decrease in smoking, the relationship is inverse. A negative relationship does not imply that the variables are less strongly related than those in a positive relationship.

Strength of Relationships

The strength of the relationship reflects how much the variables are related. When two variables are unrelated, knowing the value of one does not tell us the value of the other. The more two variables are related, the more accurately we can predict the value of one variable based on the value of the other. Statistics can be used to measure the strength of a bivariate relationship.

Symmetrical versus Asymmetrical Relationships

In a **symmetrical relationship,** change in either variable is accompanied by change in the other variable. In an **asymmetrical relationship,** change in one variable is accompanied by change in the other, but not vice versa. For example, the relationship between poverty and health status may be considered symmetrical in that a poor person is more likely to have poorer health status, which in turn makes that person even poorer. The relationship between smoking and lung cancer would be asymmetrical because smoking could cause lung cancer, but lung cancer could not cause smoking.

Linear versus Nonlinear Relationship

In a **linear** (or *straight-line*) **relationship,** the two variables vary at the same rate regardless of whether the values of the variables are low, intermediate, or high. In a **nonlinear relationship** (e.g., curvilinear), the rate at which one variable changes in value is different for different values of the other variable. For example, the relationship between packs of cigarettes smoked and chances of getting lung cancer may be considered as linear in that the more cigarettes one smokes the greater is the chance of getting lung cancer. The relationship between education and income may be described as nonlinear. Higher education level leads to higher income, up to a point, when additional education has no marginal impact on income. In other words, going to school forever would not guarantee that one will become a millionaire.

Spurious, Intervening, Suppressor Relationship

When a correlation between two variables has been caused by a third or extraneous variable, rather than by their interrelationship, the relationship is called *spurious.* The variable that causes a **spurious relationship** is an antecedent variable, which is causally related to both the independent and dependent variables (see Figure 1–1).

An apparent relationship between two variables may be caused by an **intervening variable** that is between the independent and dependent variables. For example, as Figure 1–1 shows, variables X and Y may be highly correlated, but only because variable X causes a third variable, Z (the intervening variable), which in turn causes variable Y.

A **suppressor variable** suppresses or conceals the relationship between two variables because it is positively associated with one variable and negatively associated with the other (Bailey 1994). The true relationship between the two variables can be found out after controlling for the suppressor variable (i.e., include the suppressor variable in the analysis). For example, we might hypothesize a positive relationship between level of access and health status (the greater the access, the better the health status), conduct a

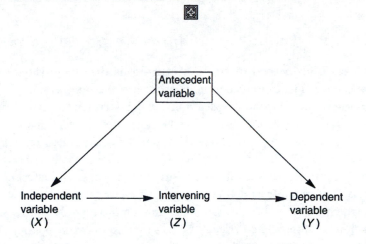

FIGURE 1–1 Types of variables: Antecedent, intervening, independent, and dependent.

study, but find no existing relationship. The relationship may be suppressed by the variable "age," which is inversely correlated with health status (the higher the age, the lower the health status) and positively correlated with access (the higher the age, the greater the access level). In other words, younger age tends to elevate health status but lower access level, whereas older age raises access level but reduces health status. The combined effect is likely to cancel out the relationship between access and health status. If access and health status are studied for each age group separately, the relationship between them will reappear.

Existing theories play a significant role in the identification of independent, dependent, spurious, and intervening variables. Theories also help researchers understand the complex relationships among variables and indicate the process that connects events. Research findings can then be used to validate, modify, or reconstruct existing theories.

Causal Relationship

When we say that two variables are related, we mean simply that they vary together, so that a change in one is accompanied by a change in the other and vice versa. Such variation is often referred to as concomitant variation or correlation. The discovery that there is a relationship between two variables does not ensure that the relationship is a causal one, that change in one variable causes change in the other variable.

There are three basic requisites to a **causal relationship:** statistical association, sequence of influence, and nonspuriousness. For one variable to be a cause of the other, the two variables must be statistically significantly related. However, a perfect association between variables is not required of a causal relationship, because a perfect association may be expected only under the theoretical condition that "all other things are held constant." In health services research, a phenomenon is typically caused by multiple factors, which may not be all identified. Causal relationships may also be affected by relatively imprecise measurements. Commonly, statistics are used to judge whether an association is strong enough to imply a meaningful causal relationship.

The second criterion needed to establish causality is that there should be a clear cause–effect sequence. The causal factor must occur first, before the effect. The temporal sequence is often one major way to determine which factor is the cause and which is the effect. That is, the one that occurs first is the cause and the one that occurs second is the effect. Causal relationship is easily determined for asymmetrical relationships, where the cause precedes the effect in time. Given the complexity of social science research, some definitions allow for the possibility that the cause and effect occur simultaneously. Thus, it is possible to define cause for symmetrical relationships, or mutual causation, in which variable A causes variable B and simultaneously B causes A, so that each factor is both a cause and an effect. The relationship between poverty and disease is one such example.

The third criterion of causality is nonspuriousness; that is, a change in one variable results in a change in another regardless of the actions of other variables. If two variables happen to be related to a common extraneous variable, then a statistical association can exist even if there is no inherent link between the two variables. Therefore, to infer a causal relationship from an observed correlation there should be good reason to believe that there are no "spurious" factors that could have created an accidental relationship between the variables. When an association or correlation between variables cannot be explained by an extraneous variable, the relationship is said to be nonspurious. To infer nonspuriousness the researcher ideally must show that the relationship is maintained when all extraneous variables are held constant. Circumstances seldom allow a researcher to control all variables. Therefore, the researcher tries to include as many relevant variables as possible in the analysis. For example, heavy alcohol consumption is strongly associated with cirrhosis of the liver. The causal link between heavy alcohol consumption and liver cirrhosis is strengthened by the fact that this rate remains the same when other variables, including gender, urban–rural residence, and socioeconomic status, are taken into account or controlled for.

Specify the Theory

The final step in theory verification and/or construction is to specify the theory as applied to a particular phenomenon under investigation. The theory may be a corroborated or revised existing theory or a newly constructed theory. Theory is the result of hypothesis testing that examines, based on empirical evidence, the anticipated relationships among variables. The formal description of a theory consists of the definitions of related concepts, the assumptions used, and a set of interrelated propositions logically formed to explain the specific topic under investigation (McCain and Segal, 1977).

The theory-research process described is somewhat idealistic. Researchers use this process to guide and measure their research activities even though they cannot always live up to the ideal due to some realities of scientific research.

The first reality is that theoretical knowledge is not yet well developed in many areas of social science research (Singleton, Straits, and Straits, 1993). Frequently, unanticipated findings occur that cannot be interpreted meaningfully in light of current theories. The terms theory and hypothesis are often used interchangeably. Theory may have a loose meaning and refer to speculative ideas used to explain phenomena. The course of inquiry may be irregular rather than follow a smooth path from theory to hypothesis to observation and to generalization. Reports of research process may be merely the result of hindsight.

Sometimes theories are created based on observation rather than on deduction from existing theories. These theories are referred to as **grounded theories.** Glaser (1992) and Strauss (1990) summarized the process of developing grounded theory as: (1) entering the field or proceeding with research without a hypothesis, (2) describing what one observes in the field, and (3) explaining why it happens on the basis of observation. These explanations become the theory, which is generated directly from observation.

The second reality is that it is often very difficult to establish causality in social science research. One reason is due to the limitations of existing theories, which may not be sufficient to identify the proper causes. Another reason is that the identified causes cannot be properly controlled. Further, since much of the data in social sciences are gathered via the survey and interview method, we often cannot tell the temporal sequence of the factors of interest. Hence, we cannot be certain of the cause(s) and effect(s) and may have to treat the relationship as symmetrical without implying causality.

The third reality is that applied social science research such as health services research has developed from practical needs and problem solving. The imperatives of theory development are often less critical than the need to solve problems that arise in the real world. Where useful, researchers draw from the theoretical perspectives of social science disciplines but do not aim to develop theories. Often they begin with a real-life problem, formulate a hypothesis about a suspected relationship, investigate the relationship, and revise the hypothesis as necessary.

HEALTH SERVICES RESEARCH

As an applied multidisciplinary field, **health services research** can be defined as scientific inquiry to produce knowledge about the **resources,** provisions, organizing, **financing,** and policies of health services at the population level (White, 1992, pp. xvii–xxiv; Frenk, 1993; Institute of Medicine, 1979) (see Figure 1–2). The development of health services research has been significantly influenced by the enhancing role of the federal government as a major financier, provider, regulator, and planner of health services since the 1960s (Choi and Greenberg, 1982; Mechanic, 1973). The increasing involvement of the federal government in health services (e.g., Medicare and Medicaid)

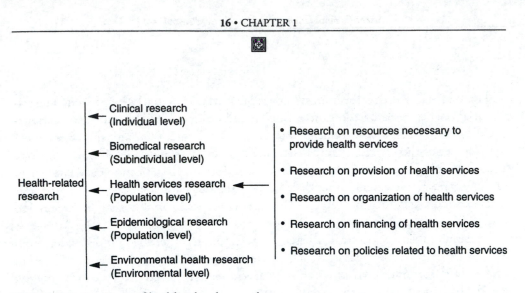

FIGURE 1–2   Types of health related research.

and the rapid increase of health care expenditure contribute to the increasing need for information and research related to the quality, availability, and cost of health services delivery (Gaus and Simpson, 1995). The establishment of the National Center for Health Services Research (NCHSR) and the increasing reliance on request for proposal (RFP) approach to grant letting in contrast to investigator-oriented approach have ensured that health services research is problem-oriented and focuses on desired policy issues. The creation of the Agency for Health Care Policy and Research in 1989 doubled the funding base for health services research to nearly $100 million and added statutory authority for outcomes research, guideline development, and research dissemination to the work of the NCHSR (Gaus and Simpson, 1995). Social and biomedical scientists have also contributed to the development of health services research through the application of applied social science research to problem solving and public decision making (Bice, 1980).

Health services research includes two major levels. The first may be called organization-level research, which focuses on the micro- and intraorganizational levels of health services, including research on health resources, provisions, organizing, and financing. The second may be called policy-level research, which focuses on the macro- and interorganizational levels of health services. Its purpose is to investigate the social, political, and economic determinants, design, implementation, and consequences of health policies related to the specific forms of health resources, provisions, organizing, and financing adopted by the organized social response. Chapter 2 will summarize current focuses of health services research. The following describes the four major characteristics of health services research: scientific, interdisciplinary, population-based, and applied.

Scientific

Health services research is scientific inquiry. Practitioners of health services research are primarily social scientists. The philosophical foundations of social science disciplines go beyond subject matters and provide guidance to health services researchers. The scientific principles of positivism, theory, empiricism, and objectivity apply to health services research as well. Health services researchers believe that there are regularities in the delivery of health services. Scientific theories, many from the social sciences, provide guidance for health services research, which in turn contribute to the development of social scientific theories related to the health phenomena. The major research process ordinarily associated with empirical research, including problem conceptualization and formulation, measurement and data collection, and analysis and interpretation, are also necessary components of the process of health services research. Maintaining objectivity is crucial for health services researchers, given the complexity and personal nature of health services and the diverse interest groups involved.

The application of scientific principles in health services research, as in social science disciplines, is not without constraints. The complexity of problems addressed in health services and their variations in time and place complicate analytic research efforts in health services research. Because health services research takes place in particular locations and periods and is focused on different levels of generality, particular studies cannot satisfy the needs and interests of all potential audiences. Findings from a study done in a particular health care institution, city, or state often may not be generalizable to other settings because of circumstances that are peculiar to the site in which the study was done. For the same reasons, data from national studies often do not apply to local situations, and vice versa.

Health services research is also constrained by the state of the art of the theories and methods of disciplines that contribute to health services research. Since much of health services research is based on the theories and methods of social sciences, its ability to explain events is limited by the level of development of those sciences. There is still considerable debate about the validity of fundamental social science concepts when applied to health services research. The uncertainty is compounded by the concerns of much of health services research with such elusive and judgmental issues as the general health status of populations, quality of care, access to care, and economic value of life, to name just a few.

The limitations of available data for research also contribute to the difficulty. Data for health services research are drawn principally from population surveys, records and documents, and direct observation. Each of these methods admits various biases that militate against clear-cut description and analysis. Answers to seemingly straightforward questions may not be found from existing data sources, and special studies conducted to determine these answers are often expensive and time-consuming. For example, the annual series of national health care expenditure estimates produced by the Health Care Financing Administration provides valuable information on the amount and categories of public and private expenditures for health care (Levit, Lazenby, Cowan, and Letsch, 1991). Similarly, the series of publications from the National Health Survey conducted by the National Center for Health Statistics (1993) yields national estimates of the prevalence of illness and the use of health services. However, those studies are expensive and their publication or electronic dissemination typically falls behind by many years. Furthermore, the protection of privacy afforded individuals and institutions by law, and the economic and political advantages that accrue to some from concealing certain types of information, frequently lead to incomplete data that limit the validity of analyses.

The classic experimental design remains the ideal foundation on which to conduct scientific research. Due to the difficulty of establishing truly experimental situations, studies in health services research are primarily based on nonexperimental or quasi-experimental designs. Thus, it is difficult to draw strong conclusions regarding cause and effect. Often, ethical concerns prevent investigators from controlling events and circumstances that are extraneous to the principal research problems, introducing bias into results. Since patients cannot be forced to participate in experiment or control, self-selection is often used to recruit study subjects. Differences between participants and non-participants could obscure study findings. Ethical behavior also includes not deceiving subjects or putting them in dangerous and uncomfortable positions. Practical problems such as time and resource constraints may also limit the options available to researchers. These difficulties inherent in health services research account to a large extent for the seeming inconclusiveness of much of the research, and underscore the need for an inter-disciplinary approach to health services research.

Interdisciplinary

Health services research is **interdisciplinary.** Health services include biological and social factors. Since no **conceptual framework** from a single discipline takes into account all aspects of a health services problem or is inherently superior to others, a cohesive mixture of various academic disciplines that encompass a great variety of perspectives is often required to carry out health services research successfully. Health services research may be considered as the application of biomedical, social, and other scientific disciplines to the study of how to deliver health services to groups of people.

The first required disciplines are those of biomedical sciences. Input from biomedical sciences is important for several reasons. First, there is a biological dimension of human populations, which is expressed, in the distribution of genetic characteristics, herd immunity, and the interaction of humans with other populations, such as microorganisms (Frenk, 1993, p. 476). To achieve a proper understanding of any health condition in a population (a particular disease, for example), we must understand the biological processes that underlie the condition. Biological sciences contribute to the understanding of human populations through the study of biological determinants, risk factors, and consequences of health processes in populations, as well as the use of methods and techniques derived from the biological sciences to characterize such phenomena (Institute of Medicine, 1979). Examples of such applications include health surveys that require laboratory tests to measure the prevalence or incidence of a given condition, and toxicological analysis of environmental risks. Second, medical sciences also contribute to health services research in important ways. For example, the normative clinical standards of care as accepted by the medical professions have to be taken into account before any assessment of health services can be made. Practice patterns of individual doctors must be known before data can be aggregated coherently.

Social science disciplines contribute significantly to health services research (Choi and Greenberg, 1982; Bice, 1980). First, since human populations are organized in societies, social sciences are indispensable for a full understanding of health services in populations. Second, similar to health services research, social science disciplines are more likely to focus on groups rather than individuals. Third, many health services researchers were trained in social science disciplines, including sociology (e.g., medical sociology), economics (e.g., health economics), law (e.g., health law), psychology (e.g., clinical psychology), and political science (e.g., health policy). Their research is influenced by the conceptual frameworks, theories, and methods espoused by their respective disciplines.

Health services researchers benefit from demography (i.e., the study of population) in two important ways. First, the facts about population size, composition, rates, and so on are needed for good health planning. Planners need data about current and projected population to estimate needs for health services and potential use of those services. National health legislation has had a direct impact on demographers' work. Because of increasing emphasis on local and regional health planning, demographers are producing more data with local-level detail and are developing estimation techniques for small populations. Second, health researchers and planners with some training in demography can use techniques generally employed in this discipline to compute rates, map population distribution, and the like. For example, using data on hospital patients and estimates of population size, local heath professionals can compute hospital discharge rates for their local geographic or service areas. Thus, demographers provide important descriptive information for health services researchers and planners, and they have developed methods that health workers can use to describe populations.

In addition to biomedical and social sciences, positive contributions to health services research have also come from the quantitative sciences, including mathematics, statistics, operations research, and computer sciences. Advances in computerized multivariate analyses, for example, have enhanced modeling capabilities and opened up possibilities to research on certain types of questions that previously could not be addressed.

Behavioral sciences are crucial to the understanding of health services. Behavioral research draws upon knowledge from epidemiological studies that identify behavioral determinants of illness, such as diet and smoking habits, and examines their social and psychological components. The interests of behavioral and health services research come together in studies of effects of lifestyles on the utilization of health services and in research on the influence of health services on individuals' health-related habits.

The influence of the physical sciences should also be considered, particularly in the study of problems that have an environmental component. Research findings pertaining to the environmental causes of health problems are important in health services research, because they give insight into the kinds of health problems that prompt people to seek medical care (Institute of Medicine, 1979).

Administrative sciences, which themselves are an amalgam of the social and quantitative sciences, have made significant contributions to the study of health services through the refinement of a body of knowledge related to organization theory, decision theory, information theory, and financial analysis. Nor can the impact of educational sciences be ignored. Effective educational programs are usually directed toward groups of people, health services institutions, and health professionals.

The fact that many biomedical and social science disciplines are involved in health services research does not mean interdisciplinary research has been achieved. Interdisciplinary research requires the integration of different disciplines in the study of a particular phenomenon. Too often, much health services research is carried out within a single disciplinary boundary by economists, sociologists, psychologists, or administrators. The logical and practical necessities that set the limits of analytic studies encourage investigators, working from different theoretical perspectives, to focus on selected aspects of problems and to disregard others. A conventional belief is that the development of science necessarily implies a growing specialization and fragmentation of the objects of study and the consolidation of independent disciplines (e.g., medical sociology, health economics). For instance, research relating to the impact of the prospective payment systems would employ the theories and methods of economics to assess its effects on hospital cost containment, while ignoring its effects on patients and community, typically studied with the perspectives and approaches of sociology or political science. Obviously, health services phenomena are not divided into the same categories as the researchers' disciplines but have complex and comprehensive characteristics that pose an essential challenge to scientific knowledge.

The fragmentation of knowledge as a basis for organizing research has a restrictive impact on problem solving and decision making. In applied fields, decision makers face complex problems that do not recognize the arbitrary boundaries imposed by scientific subspecialization or disciplinary fragmentation. The comprehensive information needed to solve complex problems cannot be obtained if studies are narrowly conceived and knowledge is generated in small pieces that are difficult to aggregate. Research results become less definitive, and their implementation often difficult. The challenge for health services research is to break with isolation and disciplinary fragmentation and integrate the theoretical perspectives and methods across scientific disciplines around comprehensive problems, thus achieving significant advances in knowledge.

The conceptual framework of biomedical research has its own limitations when applied to health services research. No explicit attention is given to matters other than therapeutic interventions and disease processes. Indeed, a major assumption of the **randomized clinical trial** is that all factors that may influence an organism and be associated with the intervention under investigation are controlled by randomization. To the extent that this assumption is tenable, the randomized clinical trial can assess the effects (e.g., safety and efficacy) of therapeutic interventions on an individual's disease without the disturbing influences of extraneous matters, such as the characteristics of physicians and hospitals. In practice, however, relatively few such studies are carried out. Consequently, most information about the efficacy of medical procedures is derived from studies done in practice settings where the conditions of the randomized clinical trial cannot be achieved.

Population-Based

Health services research focuses on populations rather than individuals. As Figure 1–2 indicates, the focus on population differentiates health services research from other health-related research. For example, **clinical research** focuses primarily on studying the efficacy of the preventive, diagnostic, and therapeutic services applied to the individual patients (Institute of Medicine, 1979). **Biomedical research** is primarily concerned with the conditions, processes, and mechanisms of health and illness at the subindividual level (Frenk, 1993). **Environmental health research** concentrates on services that attempt to promote the health of populations by treating their environments rather than by treating specific individuals.

Like health services research, **epidemiological research** focuses on the population level by studying the frequency, distribution, and determinants of health and diseases (Donabedian, 1976). The explanatory factors related to health and diseases are drawn principally from individuals' physical, biological, and social environments and their lifestyle and behavioral patterns.

> Epidemiological research may be classified according to the point of departure for analysis. On the one hand, it is possible to start with a set of determinants to study their various consequences; this is the case of environmental, occupational, genetic, and social epidemiology. On the other hand, research may begin by examining some specific health condition (e.g., positive health, infectious diseases, chronic and degenerative ailments, injury) to investigate its multiple determinants. (Frenk, 1993, p. 473)

The results of epidemiological research provide the conceptual foundation for health services research. Studies employing epidemiological methods to assess the impacts of particular health interventions on general health status or other outcomes would be classified as health services research (Institute of Medicine, 1979).

There are, however, other fields, such as bioepidemiology, clinical epidemiology, decision analysis, and technology assessment, that, similar to health services research, deal with connections and interfaces among the major types of health-related research. Indeed, the future development of health-related research will depend on its ability to build bridges across different levels of research. Such integration across research levels, as well as across scientific disciplines as discussed above, will contribute toward achieving a full understanding of the broad field of health, rather than a fragmented piece.

Applied

Health services research is an **applied** field. It is almost always defined by its practical, problem-solving orientation and is determined as much by what one wants to do, is paid to do, and can do as by the needs of theory development. Its priorities are established by societal questions and problems about health services. Studies in health services research are frequently occasioned by existing problems related to specific populations identified by societal groups and decision makers. "Research in the field of health services has generally stemmed not from curiosity, but from a need to have facts on which to base organization, administration, and legislation and this search for facts has been frankly for public policy purposes, to provide a factual basis for a given policy" (Anderson, 1985; p. 237).

Knowledge generated through health services research can be applied to the study of specific populations, such as children, pregnant women, the poor, elderly, and migrants; particular problems, such as AIDS and mental or dental health; and specific programs, such as community, environmental, occupational, and international health. The products of health services research are often assessed primarily in terms of their usefulness to people with decision-making responsibilities, whether clinicians, administrators of health care institutions or government programs, or officials charged with formulating national health care policy. Indeed, the institutionalization of health services research within the nation's major universities and research institutions (e.g., Rand) and the sharp increase in health services research activities over the past two decades have been primarily due to the increased funding from the federal government as a result of its expanded roles in health care delivery, financing, planning, and regulation, and its desire for relevant research for guidance and evaluation.

The belief that studies in health services research should have direct implications for action and problem solving does not mean that theories and general knowledge should be ignored. Producing research results of direct utility to the client is important but not all-inclusive to health services research. If health services researchers restrict themselves to resolving problems for specific clients but do not concern themselves with accumulating evidence and building theories, then ultimately the problem-solving process will be based on techniques not easily generalizable from one situation to another. For each problem to be solved, techniques have to be worked out from scratch. In the long run, health services research will be inefficiently conducted and costly to the clients for lack of established methodology and theories. Without collective norm and standard, it would also be difficult to judge the quality of research and the soundness of analyses and corresponding recommendations or to teach the conduct of health services research. The challenge to health services researchers is to balance the two competing demands of their efforts: the problem-solving, practical orientation demanded by users and sponsors of research, and the professional standards of theory developing set by their scientific disciplines and enforced by their peers. Available theories and methodology provide the framework within which health services researchers try to model practical problems of health care in ways that will produce insights that can be used to improve the system. The following section summarizes the major components of scientific inquiry as applied in health services research.

THE PROCESS OF HEALTH SERVICES RESEARCH

Scientific knowledge is verifiable. If a study is repeated with a different sample of the population, a second confirmation of the findings, called *replication,* will lend further support to the research finding. To make verification possible, the researcher should design his or her study in acceptable ways and clearly communicate the process of conducting research.

The word *process* refers a series of activities that bring about an end result or product (Singleton, Straits, and Straits, 1993). In scientific inquiry, typically the product itself, knowledge, is never "finished" but constantly refined to fit new evidences. The end of one investigation often marks the beginning of another. The most characteristic feature of the scientific process is its never-ending cyclical nature. We always accept each finding tentatively, knowing that it may be proved wrong in further investigations.

The traditional model of science consists of three major elements: theory, operationalization, and observation (Babbie, 1992; Singleton, Straits, and Straits, 1993). Researchers begin with an interest in some aspect of the world. They then develop a theoretical understanding of the relevant concepts. The theoretical considerations result in a general hypothesis, or an expectation about the way things ought to be in the world if the theoretical expectations are correct. The notation $Y = f(X)$ indicates that Y (e.g., health status) is a function of (is in some way caused by) X (e.g., socioeconomic status). At that level, however, X and Y have general rather than specific meanings.

In the **operationalization** process, general concepts are converted to specific indicators or variables, and the procedures to identify and concretely measure the variables are delineated. This operationalization process results in the formation of a testable hypothesis. For example, heath status may be operationalized as the number of doctor visits and hospitalization days per year, and socioeconomic status as a combination of income, education, and occupation measures.

The final step in the traditional model of science is observation, examining the world and recording what is seen or heard based on identified measurements. For example, the number of doctor visits and hospitalization days are counted, and data measuring income, education, and occupation, as well as other relevant control variables, are collected and analyzed. The results of the analysis are used to test the research hypothesis.

This deductive approach is often referred to as the traditional model of science. The inductive approach starts with a set of observations. Then, a pattern that best represents or summarizes the observations is sought. A tentative explanation about the pattern of the relationship between the variables of interest is suggested. This tentative suggestion helps generate further expectations about what should be observed in the real world. Thus, the deductive phase starts with theory and conducts observations guided by theory, whereas the inductive phase starts with observations and works toward developing a theory. Both deduction and induction are routes to the construction of scientific theories.

The following are the specific stages of health services research, based on the scientific model of theory, operationalization, and observation. Table 1–1 relates each of the stages to specific chapters of the book that provide detailed coverage of the major elements contained in each stage. Even though the sequencing of the stages is not fixed and practicing health services researchers often skip over one or more stages and sometimes move backward as well as forward, each of the stages is dependent upon the others and some have to be conducted before others. For example, one cannot analyze data before one has collected the data. One cannot formulate an adequate hypothesis without an understanding of the related subject matter. The researcher needs to have adequate knowledge of the earlier stages before he or she can perform the latter tasks. A researcher can do irreparable harm to the study by performing one of the early steps inadequately—for example, by writing an untestable hypothesis or by securing an inadequate sample. Research, then, is a system of interdependent related stages.

Conceptualization

The conceptualization stage of the research process requires the researcher to understand the general purpose of the research, determine the specific research topic, identify relevant theories and literature related to the topic, specify the meaning of the concepts and variables to be studied, and formulate general hypotheses or research questions.

Groundwork

The groundwork stage of the research process requires the researcher to identify relevant data sources, explore potential funding sources, develop a research plan or proposal (to obtain funding), and get prepared organizationally and administratively to carry out the research.

Research Methods

The researcher then needs to choose the specific type(s) of research method(s) for the particular study. By "method" we simply mean the general strategy to study the topic of interest. Many research methods are available for health services researchers, including research review (including meta analysis), secondary analysis (including research analysis of administrative records), qualitative research (including case study), experiment, survey research (including longitudinal study), and evaluation research. Each of those

TABLE 1–1 Stages of health services research

Stage of research	*Chapter of coverage*
Conceptualization	Chapter 2
Groundwork	Chapter 3
Research Methods	Chapters 4–9
Research Design	Chapter 10
Sampling	Chapter 11
Measurement	Chapter 12
Data Collection	Chapter 13
Data Processing	Chapter 13
Data Analysis	Chapter 14
Application	Chapter 15

methods has strengths and weaknesses that determine its suitability for a given problem. Often the best strategy is a combination of different approaches.

Research Design

Once the research problem has been clearly formulated, the researcher then develops an overall plan or framework for investigation. Research design addresses the planning of scientific inquiry—anticipating the subsequent stages of the research project, including the choice of research method(s) (the previous stage), unit of analysis, the variables to be measured, data collection, and analysis strategy. Thinking through and planning for the critical stages of research in advance could prevent important omissions and reduce serious errors. However, not all problems can be foreseen, especially in exploratory and qualitative research, and later changes are often necessary.

Sampling

In the sampling stage of the research process, the researcher must be clear about the population of interest for a study, which may be defined as the group about which we want to be able to draw conclusions. Since we are almost never able to study all the members of the population that interest us, we must sample subjects for study. In addition to the unit of analysis, the researcher must decide upon the appropriate sample size and sampling procedures.

Measurement

The measurement, or operationalization stage, involves devising measures that link particular concepts to empirically observable events or variables. The validity and reliability of measurement should be ascertained. Since survey research is frequently used, health services researchers should be knowledgeable about the general guidelines and specific techniques in writing survey questionnaire instruments.

Data Collection

The data collection stage of the research process entails the collection of empirical data. The type of research method selected often influences the choice of the method of observation. The two commonly used direct data collection methods are interview (telephone or face-to-face) and questionnaire survey. The relative advantages and disadvantages of these and other possibilities should be taken into account in selecting the observation method(s).

Data Processing

Generally it is difficult to analyze and interpret data in their raw format. Before analyzing the data, the researcher needs to transform or process the data into a format suitable for analysis. In the case of a survey, the "raw" observations are typically in the form of questionnaires with responses checked or answers written in blank spaces. The data-processing phase for a survey typically involves coding or classifying responses and converting the information into a computer-readable format.

Data Analysis

The data analysis stage of the research process employs statistical procedures to manipulate the processed data for the purpose of drawing conclusions that reflect on the hypotheses or research questions related to the study. Researchers need to be knowledgeable about the choice of commonly used descriptive and analytic statistical procedures. Such knowledge is important to facilitate independent research and improve the design of research and measurements.

Application

The final stage of the research process emphasizes the interpretation and use of the research findings. The researcher may communicate the findings to the sponsor(s) through a specially prepared report, or publish the results in scientific journals. The results may also be communicated through the media, delivered in professional conferences, or prepared as a monograph or a book. The contributions to scientific theories and policy formulation are often the greatest enjoyment the researcher obtains from his or her painstaking efforts. Finally, the researcher should provide suggestions for further research on the subject and outline the shortcomings that could be overcome in future studies.

SUMMARY

The aim of scientific inquiry is to produce and enhance knowledge. The assumption is that there is a logical pattern in life that can be studied, and scientific theory can be produced to explain this logical pattern. The approach to conduct scientific inquiry is through empiricism, using empirical evidence to corroborate, modify, or construct scientific theories. Since empirical evidence exists independent of researchers, it is crucial that investigators maintain their objectivity in searching for and explaining empirical evidence, uninfluenced by their personal beliefs and biases.

Health services research and scientific inquiry have much in common. Both believe in social regularity and the importance of theories in explaining such regularity. Both are empirically oriented and stress the importance of objectivity in collecting and interpreting empirical evidence. The practical orientation of health services research comes from its emphasis on solving problems and producing knowledge useful to users and sponsors of research. Health services research may be considered as a social scientific inquiry designed to gain a better understanding of certain aspects of health services resources, provisions, organizing, financing, and policies. Its process follows that of scientific inquiry and includes conceptualization, preparation or groundwork, design (consisting of choice of research method, sampling, measurement, data collection, processing, and analysis), and the application of research findings.

Key Terms

scientific inquiry	positivism
scientific theory	empiricism
objectivity	paradigm
deductive process	inductive process
constructs	assumption
Hawthorne effect	epidemiological research
concept	variable
clinical research	environmental health research
independent variable	dependent variable
randomized clinical trial	biomedical research
proposition	hypothesis
positive relationship	negative relationship
spurious relationship	causal relationship

symmetrical relationship   asymmetrical relationship
grounded theory   interdisciplinary
linear relationship   nonlinear relationship
applied   operationalization
intervening variable   suppressor variable
health services research   resources
financing   conceptual framework

Review Questions

1. What are the major characteristics of scientific inquiry?

2. What is the purpose of scientific theory?

3. What is the relation between theory and research?

4. Can research be "value-free"? Why or why not?

5. What is the process of generating scientific theory?

6. Identify the major types of relationship between variables.

7. What conditions are necessary to establish a causal relationship?

8. What is grounded theory?

9. What are the major characteristics of health services research?

10. How are the principles of scientific inquiry reflected in health services research?

11. What is the interdisciplinary nature of health services research?

12. What is the distinction between health services research and other health-related research such as clinical research, biomedical research, environmental health research, and epidemiological research?

13. Why do we consider health services research as applied research?

14. What is the distinction between inductive and deductive research?

15. How does the process of health services research reflect the characteristics of scientific inquiry?

REFERENCES

Anderson, O. W. (1985). *Health Services in the United States.* Ann Arbor, MI: Health Administration Press.

Babbie, E. (1992). *The Practice of Social Research.* Belmont, CA: Wadsworth Publishing Co.

Bailey, K. D. (1994). *Methods of Social Research*. 4th ed. New York: Free Press.

Bice, T. (1980). Social science and health services research: Contribution to public policy. *Milbank Memorial Fund Quarterly* 56(Spring), 173–200.

Choi, T., and Greenberg, J. N. (1982). *Social Science Approaches to Health Services Research*. Ann Arbor, MI: Health Administration Press.

Dilthey, W. (1988). *Introduction to the Human Sciences: An Attempt to Lay a Foundation for the Study of Society and History*. Detroit: Wayne State University.

DiRenzo, G. J. (Ed.). (1967). *Concepts, Theory, and Explanation in the Behavioral Sciences*. New York: Random House.

Donabedian, A. (1976). *Aspects of Medical Care Administration: Specifying Requirements for Health Care*. Cambridge, MA: Harvard University Press.

Dubin, R. (1969). *Theory Building: A Practical Guide to the Construction and Testing of Theoretical Models*. New York: Free Press.

Durkheim, D. (1951). *Suicide: A Study in Sociology*. Glencoe, IL: Free Press.

Durkheim, D. (1974). *Sociology and Philosophy*. New York: Free Press.

Frenk, J. (1993). The new public health. *Annual Review of Public Health*, 14, 469–90.

Gaus, C. R., and Simpson, L. (1995). Reinventing health services research. *Inquiry*, 32, 130–134.

Glaser, B. G. (1992). *Emergence vs. Forcing: Basics of Grounded Theory Analysis*. Mill Valley, CA: Sociology Press.

Glaser, M. (1972). *The Research Adventure: Promise and Problems of Fieldwork*. New York: Random House.

Hempel, C. G. (1965). *Aspects of Scientific Explanation and Other Essays in the Philosophy of Science*. New York: Free Press.

Hempel, C. G. (1967). Scientific explanation. In S. Morgenbesser (Ed.), *Philosophy of Science Today*. New York: Basic Books.

Institute of Medicine. (1979). *Health Services Research*. Washington, DC: National Academy of Sciences.

Kaplan, A. (1964). *The Conduct of Inquiry*. San Francisco: Chandler.

Lester, D. (1994). *Emile Durkhem Le Suicide One Hundred Years Later*. Philadelphia: The Charles Press.

Levit, K. R., Lazenby, H. C., Cowan, C. A., and Letsch, S. W. (1991). National health expenditures, 1990. *Health Care Financing Review*, 13, 29–54.

McCain, G., and Segal, E. M. (1977). *The Game of Science*. 3rd ed. Belmont, CA: Brooks/Cole.

Mechanic, D. (1973). *Politics, Medicine and Social Science*. New York: Wiley.

Miller, D. C. (1991). *Handbook of Research Design and Social Measurement*. Newbury Park, CA: Sage.

National Center for Health Statistics. (1993). *Health United States, 1992*. Hyattsville, MD: Public Health Service.

Patton, M. Q. (1990). *Qualitative Evaluation and Research Methods*. Newbury Park, CA: Sage.

Roethlisberger, F. J., and Dickson, W .J. (1939). *Management and the Worker: An Account of a Research Program Conducted by the Western Electric Co. Hawthorne Works, Chicago.* Cambridge, MA: Harvard University Press.

Salmon, W. C. (1967). *The Foundation of Scientific Inference.* Pittsburgh: University of Pittsburgh Press.

Salmon, W. C. (1973). *Logic.* 2nd ed. Englewood Cliffs, NJ: Prentice-Hall.

Selltiz, C., Wrightsman, L. S., and Cook, S. W. (1976). *Research Methods in Social Relations.* 3rd ed. New York: Holt, Rinehart, and Winston.

Singleton, R. A., Straits, B. C., and Straits, M. M. (1993). *Approaches to Social Research.* New York: Oxford University Press.

Sjoberg, G., and Nett, R. (1968). *A Methodology for the Social Researcher.* New York: Harper and Row.

Skinner, B. F. (1953). *Science and Human Behavior.* Toronto: Macmillan.

Strauss, A. L. (1990). *Basics of Qualitative Research: Grounded Theory Procedures and Techniques.* Newbury Park, CA: Sage.

Weber, M. (1949). *The Methodology of the Social Sciences.* Glencoe, IL: Free Press.

White, K. L. (1992). *Health Services Research: An Anthology.* Washington, DC: Pan American Health Organization.

Zetterberg, H. L. (1954). *On Theory and Verification in Sociology.* New York: Tressler.

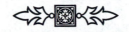

CHAPTER

2

Conceptualizing Health Services Research

LEARNING OBJECTIVES

- To understand and describe the major steps in the conceptualization stage of health services research.
- To identify the determinants of health.
- To become familiar with the general subject areas of health services research.

Before collecting and analyzing data, the researcher needs to know what data to collect and analyze. The process of finding out what data need to be collected and analyzed is called conceptualization. The first part of this chapter takes a close look at the major steps in the conceptualization stage. Then, to illustrate conceptualization in health services research, the second part of the chapter provides a summary of the major content areas in health services research.

THE CONCEPTUALIZATION STAGE

Conceptualization is the process of specifying and refining abstract concepts into concrete terms. As stated in the previous chapter, in the conceptualization stage of the research process, researchers need to understand the general purpose of their investigation, determine the specific research topic, identify relevant theories and literature related to the topic, specify the meaning of the concepts and variables to be studied, and formulate general hypotheses or research questions.

Research Purpose

Like other scientific inquiry, health services research serves many purposes. Three of the general purposes are exploration, description, and explanation (Singleton, Straits, and Straits, 1993, pp. 91–93; Babbie, 1992). A given study can have more than one of these purposes. **Exploratory research** is usually conducted when relatively little is known about the phenomenon under study; that is, the subject of study is itself relatively new and unstudied. The researcher explores the topic in order to become familiar with it and to gain ideas and knowledge about it. Exploratory research often results in generating meaningful hypotheses about the causal relationships among variables or in identifying a more precise research problem for investigation. Thus, exploratory study is not conducted to test hypotheses or provide satisfactory answers to research questions. Rather, it hints at the answers and gives insights into the research methods that could provide more definitive answers. The reason exploratory study is seldom definitive in itself is its lack of representation. An example of exploratory health services research is the study of the impact of **diagnosis-related groups (DRGs)** on particular interchanges between providers and consumers, such as discussions between doctor and patient about a hospital discharge that may be premature.

Exploratory study may also be conducted when the researcher is examining a new interest. In other words, the subject has been studied by others but not the researcher. The investigation is exploratory to the researcher. A third situation in which an exploratory study may be conducted is in testing the feasibility of a new methodology. The subject may have been studied before, but the researcher is interested in applying a new methodology to the subject this time. The results of the study will provide guidance for larger-scale, more complexly designed studies.

Descriptive research is conducted to describe some phenomenon. Descriptive studies summarize the characteristics of particular individuals, groups, organizations, communities, events, or situations as completely, precisely, and accurately as possible, with the ultimate purpose of formulating these descriptions into conceptual categories. The nature of the description, however, differs from exploratory research. A descriptive study is much more structured, carefully conceived, deliberate, systematic, accurate, and precise. It provides detailed numerical descriptions of relatively few dimensions of a well-defined subject. Descriptive research can be an independent research endeavor or, as is more commonly the case, part of a causal research project.

Examples of descriptive health services research include the series on national trends in public health statistics prepared by the National Center for Health Statistics (1993) and published in *Health, United States.* The series covers four major subject areas: health status and its determinants, utilization of health resources, health care resources, and health care expenditures. The National Center for Health Statistics also periodically publishes findings from national health surveys that provide useful national estimates of the prevalence of illness and the utilization of health services. Another example is the series of estimates of national health care expenditures produced by the Health Care Financing Administration that provides valuable information on the amount and categories of public and private expenditures for health care (Letsch, Lazenby, Lent, and Cowan, 1992). Data from these types of descriptive studies identify trends and variations that raise theoretical and policy questions that invite further analysis to reveal their correlates and causes, which is the objective of explanatory research.

Explanatory research, also called *analytic* or *causal research,* attempts to seek answers to research hypotheses or problems. It may be conducted to explain factors associated with a particular phenomenon, answer cause–effect questions, or make projections into the future. While exploratory research is concerned with questions of "what" and descriptive research with questions of "how," explanatory research answers questions of "why" or "what will be." Explanatory research differs from descriptive research in the scope of the description. Whereas descriptive research seeks information about isolated variables, explanatory research examines the relationships among these variables. Explanatory research is inherently more difficult than descriptive research.

An example of explanatory health services research is the study of the relationship among health insurance coverage, utilization of services, and health status. Since all these factors influence each other, a descriptive study is unlikely to uncover the true relationship. For example, those with poorer health status may choose more complete health insurance coverage for total expenses or high-cost procedures and may also utilize more services. Those who believe their health is better will choose "shallow" coverage that does not cover high-cost procedures. In this case, greater utilization is associated with poorer health status, and both utilization and health status are associated with greater insurance coverage. An explanatory study conducted to address the complex relationship among insurance coverage, utilization, and health status is the Health Insurance Experiment conducted by a research team of the RAND Corporation (Newhouse, Manning, and Morris 1981; Brook, Ware, and Roger, 1983; OTA, 1992). The research used an experimental design in which individual households were randomly assigned to insurance plans with different financial incentives. One purpose of the experiment was to examine the impact of levels of cost sharing among privately insured patients on levels of utilization. The study indicates that for persons with average income and health, health outcomes were neither significantly improved when care was free nor adversely affected by requirements of cost sharing. However, vision, dental, and oral health improved for individuals receiving free care.

The differences in research objectives can lead to differences in research designs. For example, exploratory research typically uses qualitative research methods such as case studies, focus groups, or guided interviews. These methods are often used because, when exploring a topic about which one has little knowledge, the researcher has few guidelines to help determine the relevant variables and whom to study. Descriptive research frequently employs survey research methods. Information is gathered from a set of cases carefully selected to enable the researcher to make estimates of the precision and generalizability of the findings. Explanatory research, on the other hand, is more likely to be associated with experimental research designs that randomly select and assign subjects into different experiment and control groups. However, in health services research, experimental designs tend to be very expensive and are often impossible because of the difficulty in getting subjects to agree to random assignment. Explanatory research relies heavily on multivariate analyses and model-building techniques based on sound theoretical framework. Table 2–1 summarizes the major differences among exploratory, descriptive, and explanatory research.

Research Topic

Health services research typically starts with a question or problem that can be answered or solved through empirical investigation. Formulating a research question or problem is often a difficult process. Experienced and novice researchers alike often spend considerable amounts of time narrowing down the topic. The choice of a research topic is influenced by a number of factors including whether the research aims at addressing a social problem; testing or constructing a scientific theory; the researcher's personal interests, ability, and resources available; and professional reward.

Health services researchers typically engage in research projects of an applied nature. The focus and development of health services research are intimately related to interest in basic social problems related to health services. This has been a major source of research topics. Indeed, many people today are attracted to health services research because of its perceived relevance to social problems, its problem-solving focus, and its likely impact on policy. *Policy* entails decision making at various levels, from health ser-

TABLE 2–1   Differences among exploratory, descriptive, and explanatory research

	Exploratory Research	*Descriptive Research*	*Explanatory Research*
Purpose	gain familiarity, insight, ideas; conduct new area of research; test new method	describe characteristics of units under study	test hypothesis, answer cause–effect research questions; make projections
Questions to answer	"what"	"how"	"why," "what will be"
Sequence	initial	follow-up	last
Rigor in study design	little	enhanced	great
Theoretical guidance	little	some	required
Knowledge about subject matter	little	somewhat	a lot
Research methods	qualitative (case study, field observation, focus group)	survey research	experiment or other case-control designs; longitudinal research
Sample size	small	large	medium or large
Number of variables examined simultaneously	univariate	univariate, bivariate	multivariate
Statistical analysis	little	descriptive statistics	multivariate statistics
Expenses	inexpensive	reasonable to expensive	expensive
Representativeness of findings	no	yes	yes

vices facilities, such as whether to use nurse practitioners and physician assistants as substitutes for physicians, to state legislation over **Certificate of Need (CON)** regulation to congressional action related to **Medicare** and **Medicaid** reimbursement. Results of policy-relevant research may be valuable to decision makers in planning future courses of action.

Although not as frequent, health services research may be conducted to test or construct scientific theories. Many health services researchers are trained in social science disciplines that have the goal of advancing knowledge. Their disciplinary framework provides direction in topic selection, research focus, and study design. They draw upon social science theories in health services research and, in the process, modify existing theories or develop new ones.

Researchers' personal interests and experience can play a significant role in the selection of topic. The completion of a research project usually entails overcoming numerous obstacles, both anticipated and unanticipated. A genuine commitment is critical to the successful completion of a research project. Researchers are more likely to be committed to a project in which they have a personal interest.

Researchers' ability and the resources available to them are also important determinants of topic selection. Their research skill affects all important phases of the research process, including study conceptualization. Ideally, the research focus should reflect the background and training of researchers. The resources available to the researchers are practical considerations. For example, an important concern for any research project is funding. Do researchers have sufficient funding for the study? The availability of relevant data also dictates whether a topic can be studied adequately. Many researchers select their topic based on available data. Research using secondary data avoids many of the problems associated with data collection and greatly speeds up the progress. The drawback is that the research is confined by the variables already collected. Other important resources include time, computer, and support personnel. The availability of these resources plays a significant role in topic selection.

Professional award and recognition also influence the choice of a research topic. Researchers may pursue topics regarded as "hot" or prestigious in their disciplines. The goal may be to publish in premier scholarly journals or advance their careers in terms of tenure and promotion. In this climate where securing funding is almost more important than conducting research, researchers may have to follow the directions of funders whether they are federal agencies or private foundations.

The selection of a research topic is typically influenced by several of the above-mentioned factors. In other words, those factors are not mutually exclusive. A research project may have problem solving as its primary objective while simultaneously addressing a theoretical question. The same research may be influenced by the availability of funding and other resource constraints. It may also coincide with the researcher's personal interests and values, as well as the personal and professional rewards.

Theories and Literature

Having identified or formed a general idea of the research topic, researchers proceed to conduct a thorough review of the current literature related to the topic. Chapter 4 delineates the process of conducting literature review. Literature review is necessary because researchers' personal experiences, however extensive, are limited compared with the cumulative scientific knowledge. Research conducted after extensive review of the literature is more likely to be built on previous studies and contribute toward the further development of scientific knowledge. Appendix 1 summarizes many journals, arranged in alphabetical order, that publish health services research papers.

Literature review serves a number of purposes. First of all, literature review helps narrow down the topic. Research begins with a question or problem. Often, the question or problem is so vague or broad in scope that it provides little direction for research. Literature review makes researchers aware of the state of the art and the extent of research

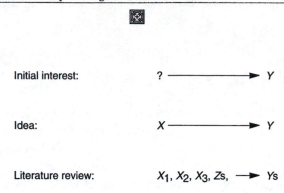

FIGURE 2–1 Identify relevant variables via literature review.

on the topic as well as current limitations. Researchers can then focus on those areas yet to be researched or with conflicting results.

Besides helping narrow and refine the topic, literature review may help identify theories related to the topic of interest. Theories provide guidance in the formulation of hypotheses to be tested through research. The ensuing research results will then have theoretical significance. In searching for relevant theories, researchers need not confine themselves only to the thinking of their paradigms. When proponents of different paradigms insist that only their view is correct, researchers cannot communicate effectively with each other. Rather, researchers should be open to the perspectives of different paradigms that have studied the topic. Taking into account alternative paradigms and theories stimulates research and generates more thorough findings.

Literature review helps identify relevant as well as control variables to be included in the analysis. Figure 2–1 illustrates this process. The initial topic of interest is represented by the variable Y. We are interested in finding out what causes Y. We identify the variable X as a potential cause of Y based on our experiences or the evidences we observe. But since our experiences are limited, it is very likely we have not considered all the potential causes of Y. A literature review will help identify, not only the potential causes (variable Xs), but also the factors (variable Zs) that need to be accounted for. Further, literature review suggests different dimensions of our topic (variable Ys). Thus, literature review enables us to operationalize our abstract concepts, a prerequisite for empirical research.

Literature review also suggests pertinent research design, procedures, and analysis methods by indicating how other researchers have addressed the topic. Researchers may use a previous investigator's method or even replicate an earlier study. Or, they can revise the research design. Just as researchers need to have an open mind for alternative theories, they need to be open to different methods. The development of health services research and the pursuit of knowledge will suffer if researchers only recognize the paradigms of their own disciplines. The tendency to promote one method at the expense of others can prevent researchers from seeing the essential complementarity of various methods.

Concepts and Variables

After the relevant literature has been reviewed, researchers have identified the concepts of interest and gained a better understanding of the research topic. Since concepts are mental images (conceptions), they need to be specified in understandable **terms.** Terms are names representing a collection of apparently related phenomena and serve the purpose of filing and communication (Babbie, 1992). Terms are specified to communicate what is meant by a particular concept. Since each concept is typically derived from many observations and experiences, one concept usually consists of several dimensions or layers of meanings. **Dimension** is a specifiable aspect of a concept. Each dimension contains only one aspect of a concept. Conceptualization is the process through which we specify the meaning of particular terms to represent the various dimensions of a concept. All terms must be defined in detail based on current literature and the unique situation of the research project. A typology may be developed where terms are carefully organized in a meaningful way as guided by theories and literature. Identifying the different dimensions of a concept and specifying the terms associated with these dimensions enable researchers to gain a more thorough and focused understanding of the research topic.

Concepts are defined on two levels: nominal and operational. A **nominal definition** serves as the working definition for the project and captures the major dimensions as agreed upon by the scientific community and reflected in the literature. Sometimes, however, there might be disagreement or lack of consensus as to the dimensions a particular concept should include. In these situations, the researchers' nominal definition serves to rule out other possible dimensions of the concept. Nominal definition is not specific as to how a concept is to be observed. Different researchers may use different ways of observation based on the nominal definition.

To be specific as to how a concept should be actually observed, researchers assign an **operational definition,** the second level of concept specification. An operational definition specifies a unique way of observation. It indicates what specific variables are to be observed, how they are observed, and how these observations are then interpreted. A variable must have two or more different values. Each dimension of a concept may be represented by several variables. Operational definition lays out all the "operations" or steps to be undertaken to measure a concept. Operational definition follows nominal definition and makes each of the specified dimensions more concrete and observable. Assigning an operational definition of a concept is often the product of the operationalization stage of the research process, discussed in Chapter 12 (Babbi, 1992). Like nominal definition, operational definition is a working definition of the concept as used in the research project (Babbi, 1992). Researchers may disagree in terms of the proper nominal and operational definitions to be used, but they can still interpret research findings based on these definitions.

Let us use the concept of socioeconomic status (SES) to illustrate these two levels of specification. Suppose we are interested in examining the relationship between socioeconomic status and health status. To reach a nominal definition, we may represent SES with three major dimensions or indicators: income, occupation, and educational attainment. This definition does not include many other possible dimensions of SES: savings, investment, property, inheritance, lifestyle, reputation, neighborhood, dependents, and so on. Nominal definition points out the direction for observation but operational definition is necessary to indicate how to make the observation. In this example, we may decide to ask the research subjects two questions about income (1. What is your total family income, including salary, pension, bonus, and interests, during the past twelve months? 2. What is your personal income during the past twelve months?), one question about occupation (1. What is your current occupation?), and two questions about education (1. What is your highest level of education? 2. How many years of formal education have you completed?). These five questions represent a working definition of SES. Others might disagree with the conceptualization (in terms of the nominal dimensions specified) and operationalization (in terms of the variables included) but can interpret the research results unambiguously, based on the definition of the term SES.

Research Hypotheses or Questions

The final step in the conceptualization stage is the formulation of research hypotheses or questions that describe the variables and the units to be studied. The major difference between research hypotheses and questions is that hypotheses specify the relationships among variables whereas questions do not. Hypotheses are usually related to a body of theory. Thus, **theoretical research** (sometimes called *basic* or *pure research*) generally involves testing hypotheses developed from theories that are intellectually interesting to the researcher. The findings might also have application to social problems, although this is not required. Research questions are typically associated with social problems at present. **Applied research** that focuses on current social problems generally specifies its purpose through research questions. Applied research may also use hypotheses statements. The choice is made based on current knowledge about the relationship among the variables of interest. Hypotheses may be formulated if current knowledge (from theories and evidences) indicates anticipated directions of the relationship among the variables of interest. When the relationship is unknown, research questions are posed in lieu of hypotheses.

The hypothesized relationship between the variables of interest determines how they are labeled. In a causal relationship, the variable presumed to cause changes is labeled as the independent variable. The variable presumed to change as a result of the intervention is labeled as the dependent variable. Other variables on which research subjects may differ and that might also affect the dependent variable are treated as control variables that are also included in the analysis. As a way of clarifying the hypothesis, researchers can draw a diagram of the presumed relationship among the variables (Grady and Wallston, 1988).

The formulation of research hypotheses or questions shares some common characteristics (Goode and Hatt, 1962). First of all, research hypotheses or questions must be conceptually clear. The concepts should be clearly defined and the nominal definition should be commonly accepted in the scientific world. Before achieving a definition, a researcher may want to share his or her definition, based on the literature review, with other researchers in the field. It is possible to neglect a portion of the literature that explores another important dimension of the concept. Peer consultation helps reduce such omissions.

Second, research hypotheses or questions must be statements of fact susceptible to empirical investigation—that is, statements that can be proven right or wrong through research. This requirement means researchers should exclude concepts that express attitudes, feelings, and values.

Third, research hypotheses or questions must be specific and narrowly defined to allow actual testing. Nominal definition alone is not sufficient. Operational specification of the relevant variables is also needed. Although formulation of research hypotheses or questions is primarily part of the conceptualization process, it also relies on operationalization. Research hypotheses or questions that only rely on nominal definition are general hypotheses or questions. Only those based on both nominal and operational definitions can be actually observed and tested. To make the hypotheses or questions sufficiently specific, researchers often break a general hypothesis or question (measuring a concept) into subhypotheses or subquestions (different dimensions of a concept).

Fourth, research hypotheses or questions must be practical. Many things we want to know about are not feasible. We cannot randomly assign people to a health status or illness. Many conditions and diseases are relatively rare and not enough patients exist to generate sufficient sample size. In addition to patients, researchers also need full support from institutions and providers to conduct any investigation.

Fifth, research hypotheses or questions must be suitable to available techniques and research methods. Researchers ignorant of the available techniques including research design and analysis are in a disadvantaged position to formulate usable hypotheses or questions. To make sure that hypotheses or questions can be tested with available techniques, researchers need to be aware of those techniques (or have consultants available to them). Literature review helps identify the techniques used and their strengths and limitations. Often, a topic can be approached with various methods and data analyzed in different ways. A competent researcher needs to know the most commonly used methods and techniques.

Finally, hypotheses are probabilistic in nature and may not be confirmed with certainty. We use the terms *tends to* or *more likely* to indicate this probabilistic nature. The reason is that the measures used to test hypotheses are usually not perfectly accurate and not all relevant variables can be identified or controlled.

The following statements, adapted from Singleton and his associates' (1993, pp. 87–91) excellent summary of research hypotheses, represent the most common forms of hypotheses.

Conditional Statements

Conditional statements (e.g., "if-then" statements) indicate that if one condition or situation is true, then another will also be true. An example would be: "If a person has a high level of income, then she will have a high level of health insurance." In a conditional statement, the condition following "if" is the cause, and the condition following "then" is the effect.

Continuous Statements

Continuous statements (e.g., the more X, the more Y) indicate that increases in one variable (X) are associated with increases (or decreases) in another variable (Y). Although continuous statements generally imply X causes Y, it also can mean Y causes X or that X and Y cause each other. Researchers should explicitly state the causal relationship in their discussion of the hypothesis. An example of continuous statement is: as income increases, health insurance coverage increases; or, expressed in slightly different form, the higher the level of income, the greater the insurance coverage.

Difference Statements

Difference statements indicate that one variable differs in terms of the categories of another variable. For example, when infant mortality is one variable and race is another (with African American and white as its two categories), we can use the difference statement to state the hypothesis: "Infant mortality rate is higher among African Americans than among whites." Whether "continuous" or "difference" statements are used to express a hypothesis will depend on whether the variables in the hypothesis are quantitative or dichotomous. If both variables could be quantified (such as income and extent of insurance coverage), then the relationship could be stated in the continuous form. If either variable could not be quantified (such as race), then the relationship would need to be stated in the difference form. Like continuous statements, difference statements are ambiguous about the causal connection between variables. Although the dichotomous variable is typically the cause, researchers still need to make explicit the causal connection between variables.

Mathematical Statements

Mathematical statements have the form $Y = f(X)$, which means "Y is a function of X" (McGuigan, 1978, p. 53). Here, Y is the dependent variable and X the independent variable that is hypothesized to cause Y. An example of using mathematical formula is: "$Y = f(X_1, X_2, X_3)$, where Y is medical care utilization, X_1 is insurance coverage, X_2 is age, and X_3 is a measure of health status." Relatively few hypotheses are stated in mathematical terms because researchers often consider their measurement to be less precise than the mathematical formula implies.

THE FIELD OF HEALTH SERVICES

Health services may be defined as the total societal effort, whether private or public, to provide, organize, and finance services that promote the health status of individuals and the community. Health status is important because a state of good health is a basic prerequisite for performing the tasks and duties associated with the different roles that individuals assume at different phases of their lives. Even though it is health we are concerned with, many of the health-related theories tend to focus on diseases. The three general theories of disease causality are germ theory, lifestyle theory, and environmental theory.

Germ theory was widely accepted in the nineteenth century with the rise of bacteriology (Metchnikoff, 1939). The doctrine of the theory states that for every disease there is a specific cause for which we can look. Knowing that specific cause will help us identify the solution to that problem. Microorganism is the causal agent in germ theory, and is thought to be generally environment free, presumably because Pasteur and others could induce the disease in laboratory animals 100 percent of the time. In reality, the disease does not necessarily occur every time microorganism is present. For example, not everyone exposed to tuberculosis ended up getting it. Germ theory is very reductionistic. With germ theory the source of disease is predominantly at the individual level and the disease may be communicated from one person to another (the phenomenon is referred to as contagion). Strategies to address the disease focus on identification of those people with problems, and follow-up medical treatment. A common approach is to look at two groups of people, those with the disease and those without it, and try to reduce disease causality to that fundamental difference between the two groups of people. Much of biomedical research is based on germ theory. The traditional epidemiological triangle (i.e., agent, host, and environment) was also developed based on the single-cause single-effect framework of germ theory (Dever, 1984).

Lifestyle theory is perceived differently today from the way it was in 1800s. Lifestyle was seen as a religious, moral issue. People were thought to get diseases as retribution for the way they lived. (Does this sound familiar to the contemporary health problem of AIDS?) Today we would think about lifestyle in relation to chronic diseases versus infectious diseases. Lifestyle theory tends to be reductionistic because it tries to isolate specific behaviors (e.g., nutrition, diet, exercise, smoking, drinking) as causes of the problem and defines solutions in terms of changing those behaviors. Thus, problems are defined as related to individuals, and solutions are based on individual interventions. It is environment-sensitive, not environment-free as in germ theory or environment-dependent as in environmental theory. For example, cigarette smoking is considered to be related to, although not caused by, advertising.

Environmental theory has a much more general approach. The focus is not so much on infectious diseases as on general health and well-being. It is not reductionist. Rather, it states that health must be understood by looking at it in the larger context of the community. Traditional environmental approaches focused on poor sanitary conditions, which were connected to disease but not in a one-to-one relationship. Recent environmental approaches examine the impact of production and consumption, considered to be the source of many contemporary health problems in society. Since the nineteenth century, there has been increasing industrialization with societies becoming increasingly oriented toward goods, production, and consumption. Overcrowded cities and filth are some of the byproducts. Environmental theory sees health as a social issue, and solutions tend to be at the policy and regulatory levels. Systems interventions rather than medical interventions are emphasized.

Comprehensive theories of health determinants incorporate the major elements of the three general theories, namely germ, lifestyle (including nutrition), and environmental theories, along with medical care services, in assessing the determinants of health status of the population. As early as 1973 Barbara Starfield (1973) suggested that the study of health status should recognize four major determinants of health status: the genetic makeup of patients, their behavior, medical practice, and the environment. Figure 2–2 is a Venn diagram depicting the interrelations among these determinants. Health status is related to outcome and is determined by the interactions of individuals' genetic constitution, their behavior, the social and physical environment, as well as medical practices.

In 1974 Henric Blum (1981) proposed an "environment of health" model, later retitled the "Force Field and Well-being Paradigms of Health." Blum advocated that the four major inputs contributing to health status are environment, lifestyles, heredity, and medical care, and emphasized that these inputs have to be considered simultaneously when addressing the health status of a population.

Figure 2–3 diagrams Blum's model. Health or the well-being of individuals, situated in the center, is made up of the interaction of three components: the psychic or mental component, the somatic or physical component, and the social component. For example, the loss of a job may affect a person's social health through reduced social functioning, that person's mental health through greater level of stress, and that person's physical health through such ailments as a stomachache. The diagram shows four major wedges or force fields that affect health: environment, heredity, medical care services, and lifestyles. The width of the wedges reflects their relative significance. The major force field is environment, which encompasses the physical and socioeconomic dimensions. Even though major efforts and expenditures in the United States have been directed toward the delivery of medical care, medical care services have relatively little impact on

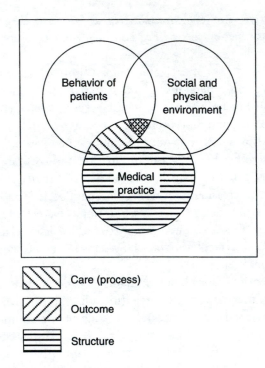

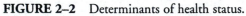

FIGURE 2–2   Determinants of health status.
From "Health Services Research: A Working Model," by B. Starfield, 1973, *The New England Journal of Medicine,* 289, p. 132. Reprinted with permission of the publisher.

health status. They are subdivided into three elements: curative (e.g., medical drugs, dental treatments, and medical professionals), restorative (e.g., hospital, nursing homes, and ambulatory services), and preventive (e.g., prenatal care, regular health checkups). The force fields are affected by even greater environmental factors of a nation, including population characteristics, natural resources, ecological balance, human satisfactions, and political and cultural systems.

Since the major purpose of health services is to improve the health status of the population, the measurement of health status will be examined along physical, mental, and social dimensions. The content areas of health services will then be delineated along with other determinants of health, namely, environment, lifestyles, and heredity.

Health Status

Health status measures reflect the needs and outcomes of health services for individuals and populations. As early as 1948 the World Health Organization (WHO) defined health as a "state of complete physical, mental, and social well-being and not merely the

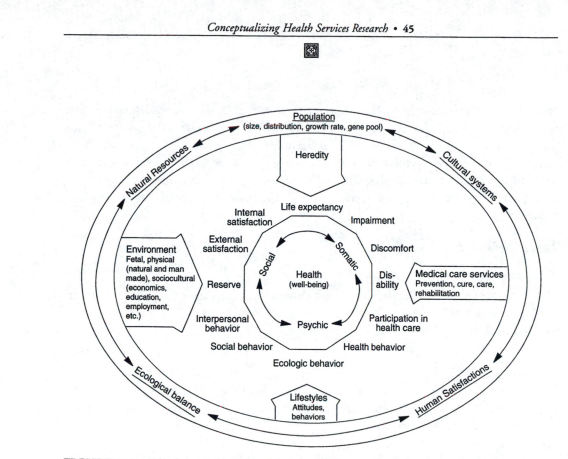

FIGURE 2–3   The force field and well-being paradigms of health.
From *Planning for Health,* by H. L. Blum, 1981, New York: Human Sciences Press. Adapted with permission of the author.

absence of disease or infirmity" (World Health Organization, 1948; Hanlon and Pickett, 1984). This definition recognizes that health is a crossroads where biological and social factors, individuals and community, and social and economic policies all converge (Frenk, 1993). In addition to its intrinsic value, health is a means for personal and collective advancement. It is not only an indicator of an individual's well-being, but a sign of success achieved by a society and its institutions of government in promoting well-being and human development.

While good or positive health is a major component of broad conceptual definitions of health, most commonly used indicators are actually measures of poor health (Wilson, 1984; Bergner, 1985; Dever, 1984; U.S. Department of Health and Human Services, 1987, 1990; Rice, 1991; Winkleby, Jatulis, Frank, and Fortmann, 1992; McGinnis and Foege, 1993; Feinstein, 1993). The major reason for this is that historically measurements of health status have been conceptually framed in terms of health problems such as disease, disability, and death. Granted, health problems are many and varied, but they all usually affect the length and/or quality of life. The length of life, or longevity, can be expressed in terms of average life expectancy, mortality rates, deaths due to specific causes, and other such indicators. **Quality of life** encompasses such life factors as independent functioning, family circumstances, finances, housing, and job satisfaction. The economic consequence of ill health is reflected in the term **burden of illness,** which refers to both direct and indirect economic costs associated with the use of health care resources and functional restrictions imposed by illness. The following describes commonly used measures related to the three major dimensions of health, physical health, mental health, and social well-being. A summary of these measures can be found in Table 2–2.

Physical Health Measures

Symptoms

Measures of symptoms reflect acute and chronic problems involving one or more of the body's functional systems. Examples of physical symptoms include toothache, sore throat with fever, and swollen ankles after waking up.

Mortality

Mortality-based measures are among the most often used indirect indicators of health. They include crude death rate, condition-specific death rates, infant mortality, and maternal mortality. Life expectancy at birth and remaining years of life at various ages are also commonly used measures.

Morbidity

Measures of morbidity include those measuring the incidence or prevalence of specific diseases. **Incidence** refers to the number of new cases of a disease in a defined population within a specified period of time. **Prevalence** refers to the number of instances of a given disease in a given population at a designated time (Last, 1981).

Most studies of health status make some attempt to measure morbidity or illness by determining whether or how many times the respondents were sick within a given time and by asking about the occurrence of certain diseases. Researchers are also interested in the conditions of illness. The estimates of acute conditions from ongoing surveys conducted by the U.S. government are based on reported conditions that had their onset

TABLE 2–2   Common health status indicators

Dimensions	Physical Health	Mental Health	Social Health
Measures	symptoms	symptoms	symptoms
	mortality	psychological state	social well-being
	morbidity	health perceptions	
	disability		
	use of health services		

within the two weeks prior to the interview (with the exception of certain conditions that are defined as chronic regardless of onset) and resulted in either medical attention or a day or more of restricted activity. Chronic conditions are generally those that have been present during the past year and have had a duration of at least three months.

Disability

Disability related to illness and injury consists of event-type and person-type indicators. Examples of event-type indicators are restricted activity days or "cutdown" days that are used to measure the impact of both acute and chronic illness, including bed days, work-loss days, and school-loss days. Person-type indicators are usually used to reflect the long-term impact of chronic conditions, including measures of limitation of mobility and functional activity. Examples of mobility limitation include confinement to bed, confinement to the house, and the need for help to get around inside or outside the house.

Activities of daily living (ADL) is often used to measure functional activity limitation of the elderly and the chronically ill. WHO defines functional status as "any restriction or lack of ability to perform an activity in the manner or within the range considered normal for a human being" (World Health Organization, 1980). ADL measures focus on the ability of a person to function independently or with assistance in activities such as bathing, dressing, toileting, transferring in and out of a bed or chair, continence, and feeding (Travis and McAuley, 1990). A set of measures somewhat related to ADL indicators are measures of functional capacity, including items such as ability to walk a quarter mile, walk up or down a flight of stairs, stand or sit for long periods, use fingers to grasp or handle, and lift or carry a moderately heavy or heavy object. These are called **instrumental activities of daily living (IADL)** that require a finer level of motor coordination than is necessary for the relatively gross activities covered in ADL scales (McDowell and Newell, 1987). IADL scales are used to measure less severe functional impairments and to distinguish between more subtle levels of functioning. The content of IADL scales stresses individual's functioning within her or his particular environment. When people are unable to perform numerous IADL activities (usually more than five) for an extended period of time, and they are not acutely ill, they are designated as handicapped.

Use of Health Services

While measures of health status have frequently been used to indicate the need for medical care, measures of the use of health services are often used as proxies for health, with implications for health status going in both directions, that is, high utilization as an indicator of poor health and lack of utilization as a presumption of poor health or at least a poor health practice. Specific indicators in this category include (1) number of doctor visits per person per year, (2) percentage of persons who have not seen a doctor within the past year, (3) interval between doctor visits, (4) short-stay hospital admission and discharge rate, and (5) short-stay hospital average length of stay.

Mental Health Measures

Symptoms

Mental health symptoms include psychophysiologic symptoms and psychological symptoms. Examples of psychophysiologic symptoms include low energy, headaches, and upset stomach. Examples of psychological symptoms include feeling nervous, depressed, and anxious. The major distinction between physical and psychophysiologic symptoms is that the latter are more likely to reflect an underlying psychological problem.

Self-Assessed Psychological State

Whereas physical functioning is reflected in behavioral performance, mental health involves feelings that cannot be observed. Thus, the assessment of general mental health requires measures of psychological state, that is, self-reports of the frequency and intensity of psychological distress, anxiety, depression, and psychological well-being.

General Health Perceptions

Self-ratings of health in general are among the most commonly used measures of health and well-being. Many studies have asked respondents about self-assessed health status, for example, "Would you say that your health in general is excellent, very good, good, fair or poor compared to people your age?" Measures of general health perceptions are sometimes criticized as subjective and unreliable. However, the subjectivity of the measure reflects an important aspect of health: personal feelings. It is a good predictor of patient-initiated physician visits, including both general medical and mental health visits. It is also highly correlated with many objective measures of health status.

Social Health Measures

The concept of social well-being extends beyond the individual to include the quantity and quality of social contacts and resources across distinct areas of life, including family, work, and community. Social health measures are often indicators of quality of life.

Symptoms

Symptoms of social health may be linked to health-related limitations in the performance of usual social role activities, including employment, schoolwork, and housework.

Social Well-Being

Social well-being includes two distinct categories of concepts, social contacts and social resources. Social contacts refer to the frequency of social activities a person undertakes within a specified time period. Examples include visits with family members, friends, and relatives, and participation in social events such as membership activities, professional conferences, and workshops. Social resources refer to the adequacy of interpersonal relationships and the extent that social contacts can be relied upon for support. Social contacts can be observed and, thus, represent the more objective of the two measures. However, one criticism of the social contact measure is its focus on events and activities without considering how they are qualitatively experienced. Unlike social contacts, social resources cannot be directly observed. They are best measured by asking the individuals directly. Questions include whether they can rely on their social contacts (e.g., friends, relatives) to provide needed support and company and whether they feel sufficiently cared for and loved.

Environment

Environment is defined as events external to the individual over which one has little or no control. It provides the context of health services provision, which consists of physical and social (including political, economic, cultural, psychological, and demographic) dimensions. These environmental conditions create risks that are a far greater threat to health than any present inadequacy of the medical care system.

Physical Dimension

In a physical environment, certain hazards show a close relationship to the use of energy (such as oil) by an expanding population. Per capita energy consumption is increasing concomitantly with the population and the standard of living. Thus, health hazards stemming from air, noise, and water pollution almost assuredly will also increase steadily. The resulting diseases and problems include hearing loss, infectious diseases, gastroenteritis, cancer, emphysema, and bronchitis. In limited cases, ionizing and ultraviolet radiation have serious health implications in terms of skin cancer and genetic mutation. These health problems will be reduced only by adopting strict environmental regulations, implementing standards and controls on the responsible agencies and industries, and educating the public about the risks involved. Collective action using government power can make great gains for the health of the public even as energy consumption increases. For example, the removal of lead from gasoline has meant that a generation of young Americans have grown up without the threat of lower levels of mental and physical functioning.

Social Dimension

A nation's political, economic, and cultural preferences exert significant influence on the health of its population. For example, a market-dominated country such as the United States is likely to favor a health care system that is procompetition and antigovernment. The U.S. cultural preference for individualism contributes to a health care system that is individualistic and disjointed rather than collective and organized.

At the individual level, **socioeconomic status (SES)** is an important social measure and a strong and consistent predictor of health status. The major components of SES include income, education, and occupational status. Individuals lower in SES suffer disproportionately from almost all diseases and show higher rates of mortality than those with higher SES. Countries that have universal health insurance (such as England) show the same SES-health gradient as that found in the United States (where such insurance is not provided), indicating that SES is an independent predictor of health status, after controlling for access to medical care. The potential pathways by which SES may influence health are through differential exposure to physical and social contexts, different knowledge of health conditions, adverse environmental conditions, such as exposure to pathogens and carcinogens at home and at work and to social conditions such as crime. Current U.S. medical policy may be moving toward the provision of health insurance to provide universal access to medical care. However, even if this goal is achieved, SES inequalities in health will persist.

The social dimension of environmental health also encompasses major factors involving behavior modification, psychological stress, perceptional problems, and interpersonal relationships. For example, crowding, isolation, accelerated rates of change, and social interchange may contribute to homicide, suicide, decisional stress, and environmental overstimulation.

Demographics also pose significant challenges to health care delivery. The increase of the elderly as a proportion of the total population and the aging of the elderly population are referred to as the "graying of America." Since the elderly population, particularly the oldest elderly (those age 85 and older), use a disproportionate share of health care resources, their increase indicates greater pressure on the health care system.

Lifestyles

The shift of the leading causes of death from infectious to chronic diseases such as heart disease, cancer, and injury indicates that **behavioral risk factors,** such as cigarette smoking, alcohol abuse, lack of exercise, unsafe driving, poor dietary habits, and uncontrolled hypertension, are increasingly predictive of higher risk for certain diseases and mortality. Behavioral risk factors are related to socioeconomic status. For example, the prevalence of smoking is greater for those with less education than for those with more education.

Lifestyles, or behavioral risk factors, can be divided into three categories: leisure activity risks, consumption risks, and employment participation and occupational risks (Dever, 1984). This division involves the aggregation of decisions by individuals affecting their health over which they have more or less control. Individuals have least control over employment and occupational factors, more control over consumption, and greatest control over leisure activity. Thus, the federal government has created regulatory agencies (e.g., OSHA) that force employers to maintain safe workplaces and practices. Leisure and consumption activities, in contrast, are relatively unregulated with the exception of efforts to control the use of illegal drugs and the purchase of tobacco and alcohol products by underaged youth.

Leisure Activity Risks

Some destructive behaviors are the result of leisure activity risks. Sexual promiscuity and unprotected sex can result in sexually transmitted diseases, including AIDS, syphilis, and gonorrhea. Lack of exercise is strongly associated with hypertension and coronary heart disease. It aggravates coronary heart disease, leads to obesity, and results in a lack of physical fitness.

Consumption Risks

Another kind of behavioral risk involves consumption patterns. These include (1) overeating (obesity); (2) cholesterol intake (heart disease); (3) alcohol consumption (motor vehicle accidents); (4) alcohol addiction (cirrhosis of the liver); (5) cigarette smoking (chronic obstructive pulmonary disease: chronic bronchitis and emphysema, lung cancer, and aggravating heart disease); (6) drug dependency (suicide, homicide, malnutrition, accidents, social withdrawal, and acute anxiety attacks); and (7) excessive glucose (sugar) intake (dental caries, obesity, and hyperglycemia).

Employment/Occupational Risks

Destructive lifestyles related to employment and occupational risks are usually difficult for individuals to control. Examples include dangerous occupations, unsafe workplaces, and stressful jobs. Work-related stress, anxiety, and tension can cause peptic ulcers and hypertension.

Heredity

The impact of heredity or human biology on health status is concerned with the basic biologic and organic makeup of individuals. For example, a person's genetic inheritance creates genetic disorders, congenital malformations, and mental retardation. The maturation and aging process is a contributing factor in arthritis, diabetes, atherosclerosis, and cancer. Obvious disorders of the skeletal, muscular, cardiovascular, endocrine, and digestive systems are subcomponents of complex internal systems.

Medical Care Services

Medical care services differ from other commodities in a number of important ways. First, the demand for medical care services stems from a demand for a more fundamental commodity, namely, health itself; the demand for medical care is therefore a derived demand.

The second complication is the so-called **agency relationship** (Sorkin, 1992). Because patients generally lack the technical knowledge to make the necessary decisions, they delegate this authority to their physicians with the hope that physicians will act for them as they would for themselves if they had the appropriate expertise. If physicians act solely in the interests of patients, the agency relationship would be virtually indistinguishable from normal consumer behavior. However, physicians' decisions will typically reflect, not only the preferences of their patients, but also their own self-interest, the pressures from professional colleagues and institutions, a sense of medical ethics, and a desire to make good use of available resources. One implication is that health care utilization may well depend on the organizational environment. For example, in an organizational setting where patients are prepaid, such as in a **health maintenance organization (HMO),** physicians may have the incentive to restrict the number of hospital admissions to less than what they would be if physicians were acting as "perfect" agents. Likewise, in hospitals where reimbursement is prospectively based, physicians may be pressured to restrict duration of stay. Organizational setting may therefore be one of the key variables in explaining medical care utilization.

The third complication concerns the nature of the price paid for health care. In most medical services, the money paid out-of-pocket at the point of usage is often significantly lower than the total eventual payment, largely due to insurance coverage. It is generally believed that the combination of comprehensive insurance for patients and fee-for-service payment for providers is what has driven the health care system to be the way it is at present—a voracious black hole for economic resources. Thus, the use of medical care services is related to how the services are financed.

Finally, medical care services are influenced by the environment in which services are provided, namely, the social, economic, demographic, technological, political, and cultural contexts surrounding the provision of health services. For example, among the major forces shaping the health care industry, the social reality of the growing number of uninsured is one of the major factors spearheading the current debate about health care reform. The economic picture of the country and the large federal deficit necessitate greater cost containment and fiscal accountability in addition to clinical accountability. Globalization of the economy results in the increasing prominence of big business, which is getting more involved in both the financing and delivery of medical services. The changing population composition—the growing proportion of the elderly—projects additional need for the professional labor supply. Technological growth and innovation contribute to medical care quality and expenditures at the same time. The distinctive American political culture tends to distrust power, particularly government power, and prefers voluntarism and self-rule in small homogeneous groups with limited purposes. This implicit American assumption that self-rule in small groups maximizes freedom may explain why there is no national health care system and why there are so many subsystems in the United States. However, many Americans do believe that health is a basic human right and access to medical care should be guaranteed. This belief in the social nature of health may explain the larger role of the government in health care relative to other sectors of the economy. Indeed the conflicts between market and social justice can account for many of the problems and contradictions surrounding the provision, organizing, and financing of health services. The principles of market and social justice are summarized in Table 2–3. Table 2–4 presents the major content areas of health services, including organizations, providers, types, the role of government, financing, and critical issues in health services. Appendix 2 provides a list of the major health services–related professional associations. For detailed discussion of these topics, please refer to the numerous books and articles on U.S. health care systems (e.g., Anderson and Newman, 1973; Aday and Anderson, 1974; Roemer, 1977; Weissert, 1978; Kaluzny, 1980; Last, 1981; Blum, 1981; Mechanic, 1983; Young, 1985; Donabedian, 1985; OTA, 1986; Eisenberg, 1985; McDowell and Newell, 1987; Caper, 1988; Preventive Services Task Force, 1989; Berwick, 1989; U.S. Department of Health and Human Services, 1990; Crandall, Deyer, and Duncan, 1990; U.S. General Accounting Office, 1991; Samuels and Shi, 1991; Porter and Witek, 1991; Office of Technology Assessment, 1991; Shortell and Reinhardt, 1992; Grob, 1992; McNeil, Pedersen, and Gatsonis, 1992; Iglehart, 1992; Bodenheimer, 1992; Sorkin, 1992; Blumenthal and Meyer, 1993; Samuels and Shi, 1993; Williams and Torrens, 1993; Stone, 1993; Weiner, 1993; Weiner and Lissovoy, 1993; Wennberg, Goodman, Nease, and Keller, 1993; Kindig and Yan, 1993; Schauffler and Rodriguez, 1993; Guadagnoli and McNeil, 1994; National Center for Health Statistics, 1995).

SUMMARY

Conceptualization is the first stage of health services research. It requires the researcher to understand the general purpose of research (i.e., exploration, description,

TABLE 2–3 Principles of market and social justice

Market Justice	*Social Justice*
• Individual responsibility for health	• Shared responsibility for health
• Self-determination of health	• Social determination of health
• Benefits related to individual efforts	• Certain benefits are assured
• Limited obligation to the collective	• Strong obligation to the collective
• Rugged individualism	• Community well-being supersedes that of individual
• Emphasis on individual behavior	• Emphasis on social conditions
• Limited government intervention	• Active government involvement

TABLE 2–4   Classification of major health service content areas

1. Organizations of Health Services

- System: system for the employed, insured; system for the unemployed, uninsured, and poor; system for active duty military personnel; system for retired, disabled veterans
- Hospitals: community (proprietary, nonprofit, multihospital system), government
- Hospital integration: vertical versus horizontal
- Nursing homes
- Mental health facilities
- Managed care approaches: HMO, PPO, IPA, EPA
- Ambulatory care facilities (clinics, outpatients, surgical centers, physician group practices, community and migrant health centers)
- Community-based programs: local and state health departments, home health agency, hospice programs
- Supportive organizations: government, business, regulatory organizations, insurance companies, educational institutions, professional associations, pharmaceutical and medical equipment suppliers
- Public health departments

2. Providers of Health Services

- Physicians (generalists, specialists, DOs)
- Dentists, nurses, pharmacists, therapists
- Nonphysician primary care providers: nurse practitioners, physician assistants, certified nurse midwives

3. Types of Health Services

- Preventive services: health promotion, disease prevention, health protection
- Primary care and community-oriented primary care
- Long-term care (home, community, institution)
- Mental health (inpatient facilities, residential treatment facilities, outpatient facilities, community-based services)
- Home care
- Hospice
- Dental care, vision care, foot care, drug dispensing
- Special segments: school health, prison health, Native American health, migrant health, AIDS patients

4. The Role of Government

- Medicare
- Medicaid

- Certificate of Need programs
- Veterans' Administration services
- State-, county-, and city-owned or operated general and special hospitals
- County and city health departments ambulatory care and public health services
- Health promotion/enhancement services (e.g., WIC)

5. Financing of Health Services

- Financing sources: private health insurance, out-of-pocket payment, government
- Financing objects: hospital care, physician services, nursing home care
- Methods of physician reimbursement: fee-for-service, capitation, salary, RBRVS
- Retrospective (cost-based versus prospective payment [DRGs])
- Public health financing: block grant versus categorical grant
- Health insurance terms: risk, moral hazard, adverse selection, deductible, co-payment, experience-rated, community-rated
- Health insurance types: voluntary (Blue Cross and Blue Shield, private, HMOs), social (Medicare, Workers' Compensation, CHAMPUS), welfare (Medicaid)
- Cost-containment approaches: cost sharing, utilization review, case management, selective contracting
- Financing reform: one-payer system, "laissez-faire" free-market approach, employer-based approach ("play or pay")

6. Critical Issues in Health Services

- Access to care
- Rural health, urban health
- Minority health
- Quality of care (structure, process, outcome, patient satisfaction)
- Ethics in health care

and explanation), determine the specific research topic (based on factors such as whether the research aims at addressing a social problem; testing or constructing a scientific theory; the researcher's personal interests, ability, and resources available; and professional reward), identify relevant theories and issues (through extensive review of the relevant scientific literature), specify the meaning of the concepts and variables to be studied (i.e., identify dimensions and define terms both nominally and operationally), and formulate general hypotheses (which specify the relationships among the variables to be studied) or research questions. Health, the major purpose of health services, may be conceptualized along three major dimensions: physical health, mental health, and social well-being. Its major determinants include factors related to the environment, lifestyles, and heredity, in addition to medical care services.

Key Terms

conceptualization

diagnosis-related groups (DRGs)

descriptive research

Medicare

dimension

nominal definition

theoretical research

health services

lifestyle theory

health status

burden of illness

prevalence

social well-being

social resources

socioeconomic status (SES)

behavioral risk factors

health maintenance organization (HMO)

exploratory research

Certificate of Need (CON)

explanatory research

Medicaid

term

operational definition

applied research

germ theory

environmental theory

quality of life

incidence

activities of daily living (ADL)

social contacts

environment

instrumental activities of daily living (IADL)

agency relationship

Review Questions

1. What are the major steps in the conceptualization stage of health services research?

2. Draw the distinctions among exploratory, descriptive, and explanatory or causal research. What conditions are most appropriate for each of the three major research purposes?

3. How do investigators identify research topics?

4. Why is literature review an integral part of research?

5. Draw the distinction between nominal and operational definitions of a concept under study. What are their respective roles in research?

6. What are the major characteristics of a research hypothesis? Identify some common ways of specifying research hypotheses.

7. What are the common indicators of health status?

8. Identify the determinants of health and explain how they affect health status.

9. Draw the distinctions between the following pairs of terms: incidence and prevalence; mobility limitation and functional limitation; ADL and IADL; social contact and social resources.

10. What are the behavioral risk factors that may contribute to diseases or poor health status?

11. What are the unique characteristics of medical care services compared with other market products or services?

REFERENCES

Aday, L. A., and Anderson, R. (1974). A framework for the study of access to medical care. *Health Services Research*, 9, 208–220.

Anderson, R., and Newman, J. (1973). Societal and individual determinants of medical care utilization in the United States. *Milbank Memorial Fund Quarterly*, 51, 95–124.

Babbie, E. (1992). *The Practice of Social Research*. Belmont, CA: Wadsworth Publishing Co.

Bergner, M. (1985). Measurement of health status. *Medical Care*, 23, 696–704.

Berwick, S. M. (1989). Health services research and quality of care. *Medical Care*, 27, 763–771.

Blum, H. L. (1981). *Planning for Health*. 2nd ed. New York: Human Sciences Press.

Blumenthal, D., and Meyer, G. S. (1993). Transforming the size and composition of the physician work force to meet the demands of health care reform. *New England Journal of Medicine*, 329, 1810–1814.

Bodenheimer, T. (1992). Private insurance reform in the 1990s: Can it solve the health care crisis? *International Journal of Health Services*, 22, 197–215.

Brook, R. H., Ware, J. E., and Roger, W. H. (1983). Does free care improve adults' health? Results from a randomized controlled trial. *New England of Medicine*, 309, 1426–1434.

Brown, L. (1991). The national politics of Oregon's rationing plan. *Health Affairs*, 10, 28–51.

Caper, P. (1988). Defining quality in medical care. *Health Affairs*, 8, 49–61.

Crandall, L. A., Dwyer, J. W., and Duncan, R. P. (1990). Recruitment and retention of rural physicians: Issues from the 1990s. *Journal Rural Health*, 6, 19–38.

Donabedian, A. (1985). Twenty years of research on the quality of medical care. *Evaluation and the Health Professions*, 8, 243–265.

Dever, A. (1984). *Epidemiology in Health Services Management*. Rockville, MD: Aspen.

Eisenberg, J. M. (1985). Physician utilization: The state of research about physician's practice patterns. *Medical Care*, 23, 461–483.

Feinstein, J. S. (1993). The relationship between socioeconomic status and health: A review of the literature. *The Milbank Quarterly*, 71, 279–322.

Frenk, J. (1993). The new public health. *Annual Review of Public Health*, 14, 469–490.

Goode, W. J., and Hatt, P. K. (1962). *Methods in Social Research*. New York: McGraw-Hill.

Grady, K. E., and Wallston, B. S. (1988). *Research in Health Care Settings*. Newbury Park, CA: Sage.

Grob, G. N. (1992). Mental health policy in America: Myths and realities. *Health Affairs*, 11, 7–22.

Guadagnoli, E., and McNeil, B. J. (1994). Outcomes research: Hope for the future or the latest rage? *Inquiry,* 31, 14–24.

Hanlon, G., and Pickett, J. (1984). *Public Health Administration and Practice.* New York: Times Mirror/Mosby.

Iglehart, J. K. (1992). The American health care system: Managed care. *New England Journal of Medicine,* 327, 742–747.

Kaluzny, A. D. (1980). *Health Services Organizations: A Guide to Research and Assessment.* Berkeley, CA: McCutchan.

Kaluzny, A. D., McLaughlin, C. P., and Simpson, K. (1992). Applying total quality management concepts to public health organizations. *Public Health Reports,* 107, 257–264.

Kindig, D., and Yan, G. (1993). Physician supply in rural areas with large minority populations. *Health Affairs,* Summer, 177–184.

Last, J. M. (1981). *A Dictionary of Epidemiology.* New York, Oxford, Toronto: Oxford University Press.

Letsch, S. W., Lazenby, H. C., Levit, K. R., and Cowan, C. A. (1992). National health expenditures, 1991. *Health Care Financing Review,* 14, 1–30.

Mechanic, D. (Ed.). (1983). *Handbook of Health, Health Care, and Health Professions.* New York: Free Press.

Metchnikoff, E. (1939). *The Founders of Modern Medicine: Pasteur, Kosh, Lister.* New York: Walden Publications.

McDowell, I., and Newell, C. (1987). *Measuring Health: A Guide to Rating Scales and Questionnaires.* New York, Oxford, Toronto: Oxford University Press.

McGinnis, J. M., and Foege, W. H. (1993). Actual causes of death in the United States. *JAMA,* 270, 2207–2212.

McGuigan, F. J. (1978). *Experimental Psychology: A Methodological Approach.* 3rd ed. Englewood Cliffs, NJ: Prentice-Hall.

McNeil, B. J., Pedersen, S. H., and Gatsonis, C. (1992). Current issues in profiling quality of care. *Inquiry,* 29, 298–307.

National Center for Health Statistics. (1993). *Health United States, 1992.* Hyattsville, MD: Public Health Service.

National Center for Health Statistics. (1995). *Health United States, 1994.* Hyattsville, MD: Public Health Service.

Newhouse, J. P., Manning, W. G., and Morris, C. N. (1981). Some interim results from a controlled trial of cost sharing in health insurance. *New England Journal of Medicine,* 305, 1501–1507.

Office of Technology Assessment (OTA). (1986). *Nurse Practitioners, Physician Assistants, and Certified Nurse Midwives: A Policy Analysis. (Health technology case study 37).* Washington, DC: U.S. Government Printing Office.

Office of Technology Assessment (OTA). (1991). *Health Care in Rural America.* (OTA-H-434). Washington, DC: U.S. Government Printing Office.

Office of Technology Assessment (OTA). (1992). *Does Health Insurance Make a Difference?—Background Paper.* (OTA-BP-H-99). Washington, DC: U.S. Government Printing Office, September.

Porter, M., and Witek, J. E. (1991). The nursing home industry: Past, present, and future. *Topics in Health Care Financing,* 17, 42–48.

Preventive Services Task Force. (1989). *Guide to Clinical Preventive Services: Report of the U.S. Preventive Services Task Force.* Baltimore: Williams and Wilkins.

Rice, D. P. (1991). Health status and national health priorities. *Western Journal of Medicine,* 154, 294–302.

Roemer, M. I. (1977). *Systems of Health Care.* New York: Springer.

Samuels, M. E., and Shi, L. (1991). *The Impact of Demographic Changes on the Needs for Selected Physician Specialties in the United States.* Rockville, MD: Bureau of Health Professions, U.S. Department of Health and Human Services, September.

Samuels, M. E., and Shi, L. (1993). *Physician Recruitment and Retention: A Guide for Rural Medical Group Practice.* Englewood, CO: Medical Group Management Association Press.

Schauffler, H. H., and Rodriguez, T. (1993). Managed care for preventive services: A review of policy options. *Medical Care Review,* 50, 153–198.

Shortell, S. M., and Reinhardt, U. E. (1992). *Improving Health Policy and Management: Nine Critical Research Issues for the 1990s.* Ann Arbor, MI: Health Administration Press.

Singleton, R. A., Straits, B. C., and Straits, M. M. (1993). *Approaches to Social Research.* New York: Oxford University Press.

Sorkin, A .L. (1992). *An Introduction to Health Economics.* New York: Lexinton Books.

Starfield, B. (1973). Health services research: A working model. *New England Journal of Medicine,* 289, 132–136.

Stone, D. A. (1993). The struggle for the soul of health insurance. *Journal of Health Politics, Policy and Law,* 18, 287–317.

Travis, S. S., and McAuley, W. J. (1990). Simple counts of the number of basic ADL dependencies for long-term care research and practice. *Health Services Research,* 24, 349–360.

U.S. Department of Health and Human Services (1987). *National Survey of Worksite Health Promotion Activities: A Summary.* Washington, DC: Office of Disease Prevention and Health Promotion.

U.S. Department of Health and Human Services (1990). *Healthy People 2000: National Health Promotion and Disease Prevention Objectives.* Washington, DC: Office of the Assistant Secretary for Health.

U.S. General Accounting Office (GAO). (1991). *Access to Health Care: States Respond to Growing Crisis.* (GAO/HRD-92-70). Washington, DC: U.S. Government Printing Office.

Weiner, J. P. (1993). The demand for physician services in a changing health care system: A synthesis. *Medical Care Review,* 50, 411–449.

Weiner, J. P., and Lissovoy, G. (1993). A taxonomy for managed care and health insurance plans. *Journal of Health Politics, Policy and Law,* 18, 75–103.

Weissert, W. (1978). *Long-Term Care: An Overview, Health United States, 1978.* (DHEW Publication No. 78-1232). Washington, DC: U.S. Government Printing Office.

Wennberg, J. E., Goodman, D. C., Nease, R. F., and Keller, R. B. (1993). Finding equilibrium in U.S. physician supply. *Health Affairs,* Summer, 89–103.

Williams, S. J., and Torrens, P. R. (Eds.). (1993). *Introduction to Health Services.* 4th ed. Albany, NY: Delmar Publishers.

Wilson, R. W. (1984). Interpreting trends in illness and disability: Health statistics and health status. *Annual Review of Public Health,* 5, 83–106.

Winkleby, M. A., Jatulis, D. E., Frank, E., and Fortmann, S. P. (1992). Socioeconomic status and health: How education, income, and occupation contribute to risk factors for cardiovascular disease. *American Journal of Public Health,* 82, 816–820.

World Health Organization (WHO). (1948). Constitution of the World Health Organization. In *Basic Documents.* Geneva, Switzerland: World Health Organization.

World Health Organization (WHO). (1980). *International Classification of Impairments, Disabilities, and Handicaps.* Geneva, Switzerland: Author.

Young, A. (1985). *Long-Term Care: An Industry Composite.* New York: Arthur Young International.

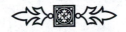

CHAPTER

3

Groundwork in Health Services Research

LEARNING OBJECTIVES

- To get acquainted with the major national-level secondary data sources currently available for health services research.
- To identify the major funding sources for health services research.
- To understand the major components of a research proposal and the general approach of proposal review.
- To become familiar with the general organizational and administrative issues related to the preparation and conduct of research.

As Chapter 1 points out, the groundwork stage of the research process requires the researcher to identify relevant data sources, explore potential funding sources, develop a research plan or proposal (to obtain funding), and get prepared organizationally and administratively to carry out the research. This chapter introduces the major national-level data and funding sources available for health services research, describes the major components of a research proposal as well as the process of reviewing research proposals, and discusses the general organizational and administrative issues related to the preparation and conduct of health services research.

DATA SOURCES

A prerequisite of any research is the availability of data. Data may be collected either through primary or secondary sources. **Primary data source** refers to the collection of data by researchers themselves. **Secondary data source** refers to the use of data collected by others. While primary data are generally more relevant, familiar, and timely than secondary data, they are also more expensive, time-consuming, and difficult to collect. Given that both funding sources and amounts available for research are declining, investigators may become increasingly dependent on secondary or existing data for research.

Data may be classified as cross-sectional, time series, or panel. **Cross-section data** are collected at one point in time. Its principal advantage is the relative inexpensiveness to obtain a large sample size. Its principal disadvantage is its transitory nature, which makes causal association difficult. **Time-series data** follow the same **unit of observation** over time. Its principal advantage is its ability to capture historical trends and changes. Its principal disadvantages are limited observations and the relative expensiveness to obtain a large sample size. **Panel data** combine cross-section and time-series data, surveying the same groups over time. Its principal advantage is its ability to capture trends and causal associations. Its principal disadvantages are attrition rates and its relative expensiveness.

This section introduces the National Center for Health Statistics, the major federal agency mandated to collect health statistics. It then summarizes the major national-level electronic databases commonly used for health services research including the Area Resource File, Behavioral Risk Factor Surveillance System, Medicare Beneficiary Health Status Registry, Mental Health Inventory, National Ambulatory Medical Care Survey, National Health Interview Survey, National Health and Nutrition Examination Survey, National Hospital Discharge Survey, National Medical Expenditure Survey, National Nursing Home Survey, and National Survey of Personal Health Practices and Consequences (AUPHA, 1992). All these data sets are available for public purchase and use. Indeed, the availability of national data has given impetus to the fast development of health services research.

The National Center for Health Statistics

The federal health statistics system is primarily located within the Department of Health and Human Services (DHHS), although other agencies such as the Department of Defense, Veterans Administration, Environmental Protection Agency, and the Bureau of Labor Statistics also collect health statistics in carrying out their functions. Within DHHS, the National Center for Health Statistics (NCHS) undertakes the majority of health statistical activities (U.S. DHHS, 1991). The NCHS was established in 1960 within DHHS as the principal federal agency to collect, analyze, and disseminate health statistics. Section 306 of the Public Health Service Act, amended to the National Health Survey Act (1956) specifies that NCHS shall collect statistics on:

- The extent and nature of illness and disability of the population of the United States (or of any groupings of the people included in the population), including life expectancy, the incidence of various acute and chronic illness, and infant and maternal morbidity and mortality;
- The impact of illness and disability of the population on the economy of the United States and on other aspects of the well-being of its population (or such groupings);
- Environmental, social, and other health hazards;
- Determinants of health;
- Health resources, including physicians, dentists, nurses, and other health professionals by specialty and type of practice, and the supply of services by hospitals, extended care facilities, home health agencies;
- Utilization of health care, including (1) ambulatory health services by specialties and types of practice of the health professionals providing such services and (2) services of hospitals, extended care facilities, home health agencies, and other institutions;
- Health care costs and financing, including the trends in health care prices and cost, the sources of payments for health care services, and federal, state, and local governmental expenditures for health care services; and
- Family formation, growth, and dissolution.

Recently, recognizing that existing national health data systems need to be more responsive to the changes occurring in the health care system, the NCHS has developed plans to revise, expand, and coordinate its data collection activities on health care utilization that currently are carried out in separate, uncoordinated surveys such as the National Hospital Discharge Survey, National Ambulatory Medical Care Survey, National Nursing Home Survey, and National Master Facility Inventory. The integrated system, called the National Health Care Survey, will collect data to monitor the nation's health, illness, and disability; the use and costs of care by incident and episode; and the outcomes and cost-effectiveness of the services provided (Panel on the National Health Care Survey, 1992; AUPHA, 1992; National Center for Health Statistics, 1964, 1965, 1966, 1975).

Area Resource File

The Area Resource File is prepared by the Bureau of Health Professions, Health Resources and Services Administration, Public Health Service, DHHS. It pools data from various sources to facilitate health analysis both cross-sectionally and longitudinally.

Each data series is available at the levels of county, state, and aggregate United States. The major unit of observation is the county, with over 6,000 counties represented. There are four major types of variables: demographics (e.g., age distribution, income, education), health professions (e.g., physicians by specialties), health facilities (e.g., hospitals, nursing homes), and health status (e.g., morbidity, natality and mortality data by cause, sex, race, and age).

The Area Resource File is an excellent data source at the aggregate county and state levels. National averages can also be easily computed from the county data. It is useful in research concerning health status and the relationship between health status and other factors, particularly for smaller geographic areas and specific population subgroups. The Area Resource File is updated annually. More frequent updates can sometimes be obtained on an ad hoc basis. The original file was created in 1986.

Behavioral Risk Factor Surveillance System

The Behavioral Risk Factor Surveillance System (BRFSS) is maintained by the Centers for Disease Control (CDC), a federal agency within the Public Health Service responsible for leadership in the prevention and control of diseases. BRFSS provides state health agencies with the funding, training, and consultation necessary to collect behavioral risk factor data. Each participating state conducts surveys of their noninstitutionalized adult population using telephone interviews. The sample size varies from 600 to 3,000 for all states. CDC also provides competitive grants to Prevention Centers around the nation for BRFSS-related activities, including development and use of research methods, data dissemination, and training.

The unit of observation is the noninstitutionalized adult population. BRFSS includes such data elements as weight control, hypertension, physical activity, obesity, mammography, alcohol consumption, seat belt use, tobacco use, HIV/AIDS, preventive health practices, and demographic information (e.g., age, sex, race, education). In addition, states may add modules of questions to meet their special needs.

This data system provides valuable information for states to monitor, develop, and evaluate health promotion and disease prevention programs aimed at reducing behavioral risk factors. BRFSS can also be used to conduct trend analysis and track progress in risk reduction over time. BRFSS was first created in the early 1980s.

Medicare Beneficiary Health Status Registry

The Medicare Beneficiary Health Status Registry (MBHSR) is developed jointly by the Agency for Health Care Policy and Research and the Health Care Financing Administration (HCFA), by linking HCFA's Medicare administrative enrollment and utilization files. The registry gathers information on 2 percent of the elderly population at the time they enter the Medicare program and at intervals of two to five years thereafter.

The unit of observation is the elderly cohort eligible for Medicare benefits. MBHSR is a longitudinal database containing information on Medicare beneficiaries regarding risk factors, functional status, sociodemographic variables, medical history, and quality of life.

By enrolling successive cohorts over time, MBHSR provides necessary information to measure the relationship between Medicare-reimbursed services and the health status of Medicare beneficiaries, analyze the use and costs of services, monitor changes in the health and utilization patterns of the elderly, project the needs of the elderly, and examine the impact of specific interventions on health status. MBHSR was implemented around 1993.

Mental Health Inventories

The Mental Health Inventories (MHIs) are maintained by the National Institute of Mental Health in the Alcohol, Drug Abuse, and Mental Health Administration. Surveys are mailed every other year to mental health organizations in the United States, including psychiatric hospitals, psychiatric services in nonfederal general hospitals, VA psychiatric services, residential treatment centers for emotionally disturbed children, freestanding outpatient psychiatric clinics, and partial-care organizations.

The unit of observation is the mental health organization. MHIs contain information on types of mental health services provided; number of inpatient beds; number of inpatient, outpatient, and partial-care additions; average daily census; patient characteristics; staffing characteristics; expenditures; and revenue by sources.

MHIs provide valuable information on the sociodemographic, clinical, and treatment characteristics of patients served by mental health facilities. MHIs were initiated in 1969.

National Ambulatory Medical Care Survey

The National Ambulatory Medical Care Survey (NAMCS) is conducted by the National Center for Health Statistics, Centers for Diseases Control, Public Health Service, DHHS. Data are obtained through a national sample of office-based physicians and a systematic random sample of physician office visits during a seven-day period. Physicians or their staff fill out an encounter form for each sampled visit. Physicians in nonoffice settings, government service, anesthesiology, pathology, and radiology are excluded.

The unit of observation is the patient visit as recorded in the patient record. Each record provides a complete description of the office visit and is weighted statistically to reflect annual utilization of private office-based practice in the United States. The number of records per survey ranges from 29,143 to 71,594. These national estimates describe the provision and utilization of ambulatory medical care services in the United States and provide information on demographic characteristics of the patient, clinical aspects of the visit, and physician specialty and practice type. The survey offers an indirect measure of health status via diagnostic information. It was initially conducted in 1973.

National Health Interview Survey

The National Health Interview Survey is conducted by the National Center for Health Statistics, Centers for Disease Control, Public Health Service, DHHS. Each week a probability sample of households are interviewed for information on all living members of the sampled households in the previous two weeks. The annual sample size is 36,000 to 47,000 households including 92,000 to 125,000 persons. The 31 major metropolitan areas have self-representing samples, allowing derivation of local measures of health status and use of health services by individuals with varying sociodemographic characteristics. The survey is a continuing nationwide household survey of the U.S. noninstitutionalized population.

The units of observation are the household and the individual members of the household. The major categories of information include region of residence, files on health conditions, doctor visits, hospital stays (in the prior 12 months), household characteristics, and personal characteristics. Specific health conditions include acute and chronic conditions, restricted activity days, bed days, work- and school-loss days, physician visits, hospital stays and long-term limitation of activity. These core questions are supplemented by additional questions on varying health topics each year. The supplemental questions are used to produce separate tapes on current health topics.

The survey is the principal source of information on the general health status of the civilian, noninstitutionalized population of the United States. It provides the most sophisticated measure of national health, illness, and disability. The "Current Health Topics" databases are valuable for policy studies on specific topics. The survey has been conducted annually since 1969, with approximately a two-year lag between survey year and availability of tapes.

National Health and Nutrition Examination Surveys

The National Health and Nutrition Examination Survey (NHANES) is conducted by the National Center for Health Statistics, Centers for Disease Control, Public Health Service, DHHS. Since 1959, the National Health Examination Survey (NHES) has been conducted in three cycles. In 1970, nutritional status was added as an additional assessment category and the survey was renamed NHANES. This expanded survey has been conducted twice to facilitate comparison. An NHANES I Epidemiologic Follow-up Study (NHEFS) was conducted in two waves to obtain longitudinal information on participants in NHANES I. NHES and NHANES were conducted through physical examinations at mobile exam sites throughout the United States. The sample sizes ranged from 6,672 persons in NHES I to over 20,000 persons in each of the NHANES surveys. NHEFS was conducted via personal interviews, interviews with proxy respondents, and review of hospital and nursing home records and death certificates.

The unit of observation is the individual person. The surveys provide measures of prevalence of a variety of physical, physiological, and psychological diseases in the U.S. general population and (since 1970) nutritional status. The objective is to collect data that can be best obtained through direct physical examination, clinical and laboratory tests, and related measurement procedures. Examples include blood pressure, visual acuity, and serum cholesterol level.

The surveys are an excellent data source on health and nutrition status. NHANES I, II, and III allow assessment of changes in the health status of the general population over time on a number of detailed health indicators. NHES Cycle I was conducted in 1959 to 1962; NHES Cycle II in 1963 to 1965; NHES III in 1966 to 1970; NHANES I in 1971 to 1975; and NHANES II in 1976 to 1980; NHEFS in 1982 to 1984 and 1986.

National Hospital Discharge Survey

The National Hospital Discharge Survey (NHDS) is conducted by the National Center for Health Statistics, Centers for Disease Control, Public Health Service, DHHS. Data are abstracted from a multistage cluster random sample of medical records of inpatients discharged from nonfederal short-stay hospitals (approximately 200,000 records per year). The survey is a continuous nationwide survey of inpatient utilization of short-stay hospitals and allows sampling at the census division level.

The unit of observation is the patient's medical records. Data elements include patient characteristics (i.e., date of birth, sex, race, ethnicity, and marital status), expected payment sources, admission and discharge dates, discharge status and disposition, length of stay, hospital characteristics (i.e., region, bed size, and ownership type), patient diagnoses, surgical and nonsurgical procedures and dates of procedures, and residence zip code. Hospital may also be used as a unit of analysis.

The survey provides measures of illness status through hospital diagnosis information and enables analysis of trends over a 25-year period so far. Interregional comparisons can also be made. The survey has been conducted annually since 1970. There is approximately a two-year lag between survey year and database availability.

National Medical Expenditure Survey

The National Medical Expenditure Survey (NMES) is conducted by the Agency for Health Care Policy and Research (AHCPR), Public Health Service, DHHS. AHCPR was established in 1989 as the successor to the National Center for Health Services Research and Health Care Technology Assessment. So far, there have been three such surveys conducted with the latest taking place in 1987.

The unit of observation is the individual person. The 1987 NMES has three components: (1) the household component that examines the general, non-institutionalized population and specific subgroups of special policy concern (i.e., the poor, the elderly, minorities, and functionally impaired); (2) an institutional population component that includes residents in nursing homes and facilities for the mentally retarded; and (3) Survey of American Indians and Alaska Natives (SAIAN) that includes all persons eligible for care under the Indian Health Service and living on or near reservations. A sample of 15,000 households (38,000 persons) were interviewed quarterly about health insurance coverage, utilization of services, cost and payment source, health status, socioeconomic, and demographic factors.

The survey provides information on expenditures for health care, use of health services, payment sources or insurance coverage, and individual health status. Results of the survey may be used to provide fairly detailed estimates of health status and access to care for different population groups, and national estimates of long-term care services and expenditures. The survey was initially started in 1977 by the National Center for Health Services Research and Health Care Technology Assessment. The second survey was conducted in 1980.

National Nursing Home Survey

The National Nursing Home Survey (NNHS) is conducted by the National Center for Health Statistics, Centers for Disease Control, Public Health Service, DHHS. The data were collected using a two-stage, stratified probability design. In the first stage, nursing home facilities are selected. In the second stage, the residents, discharges, or staff of the sampled facilities are selected. Data were collected using a combination of personal interviews and self-administered questionnaires.

The major units of observation are nursing home residents and staff of nursing home facilities. Data are collected on four major areas: (1) nursing homes (i.e., size, ownership, license and Medicare and Medicaid certification status, number of beds, services offered, staffing patterns and characteristics, and costs); (2) residents (i.e., demographics, activities of daily living, status and living arrangements prior to admission, conditions at admission and at interview, receipt of services, cognitive and emotional services, charges, sources of payment, history of nursing home utilization, and hospitalization during stay); (3) discharged residents (i.e., demographics, history of nursing home utilization, hospitalization during stay, status at discharge, conditions at admission and discharge, and sources of payment); (4) follow-up with a next of kin of the current or discharged residents (i.e., living arrangements, health, and functional status prior to admission; history of previous nursing home use; activities of daily living; and Medicaid spend-downs).

The survey provides a series of national samples of nursing homes, their residents, and their staff. It facilitates research on the general health status of the nursing home population, and the characteristics of nursing home facilities. The first NNHS was conducted in 1973, the second in 1977, the third in 1985, and the fourth in 1995.

National Survey of Personal Health Practices and Consequences

The National Survey of Personal Health Practices and Consequences (NSPHPC) was conducted by the National Center for Health Statistics, Centers for Disease Control, Public Health Service, DHHS. A national probability panel of noninstitutionalized population, 20–64 years of age, was selected using random-digit dialing. Two waves of the survey were conducted. Wave I comprises data for 3,025 respondents, and wave II (one year later) included interviews of 81 percent of the wave I respondents (2,453 interviews).

The unit of observation is the individual person. The survey provides information on a variety of personal health practices and health status. Health practice indicators include information about diet, exercise, sleeping, smoking, drinking, weight status, changes in preventive behavior due to illness, and use of preventive and acute care services. Health status measures are perceived health status and energy level, health concerns, disability, health-related limitations on activity, and various health complaints or symptoms.

The survey provides valuable information to study the relationship between personal health practices ("lifestyle") and health status. The survey was conducted in the springs of 1979 and 1980.

National Vital Statistics System

The National Vital Statistics System (NVSS) is developed by the National Center for Health Statistics, Centers for Disease Control, Public Health Service, DHHS. Data are obtained from birth and death certificates provided by States. A number of "follow-back" surveys have also been performed to obtain more detailed information from informants identified on the vital records.

The unit of observation is the individual person. NVSS is a national registration system for vital statistics including natality, fetal death, mortality, and their contributing causes. The most relevant health status databases are: Mortality—Detail, Mortality—Local Area Summary, and Mortality—Cause of Death Summary. All databases include data on age, race, sex, and residence.

The system provides the most detailed picture of vital statistics information. Vital statistics databases are annual, starting in 1968. There is approximately a two-year lag from date of vital statistics registration to public availability of vital statistics databases.

In addition to the national databases described above and summarized in Table 3–1, there are numerous other important data sources potentially useful for health services research. These include the Medicare Current Beneficiary Survey (conducted by HCFA), Nursing Home Quality Assessment (conducted by HCFA), Part B Medicare Annual Data System (prepared by HCFA), Hispanic Health and Nutrition Examination Survey, National Survey of Family Growth, U.S. Immunization Survey, National Notifiable Diseases Surveillance System, Surveillance, Epidemiology and End Results Program (prepared by National Cancer Institute); AIDS Surveillance System (prepared by Centers for Diseases Control), Occupational Injuries and Illnesses Incidence Rate Data, National Household Surveys on Drug Abuse, Drug Abuse Warning Network, and Organization for Economic Cooperation and Development's Health Data (contain various health data for 24 Western industrialized countries). Some of these sources are available as public-use databases while others disseminate data only through published reports. While these sources are less appropriate for a broad overview of U.S. health status and services, their data should be considered for more specialized policy work as needed.

FUNDING SOURCES

There are essentially four types of funding for a research project: self-funding, consultation, contracts, and grants. Self-funding involves carrying out a study using existing resources provided by the individual researcher or the researcher's institution, which will usually include data processing services, library services, and other support services as well as time and budgets for research and development work. Consulting services, while usually addressing clients' specific needs, may be integrated with research and contribute to scientific knowledge. Research combined with consulting work is common in private, nonprofit research institutions, such as Rand.

Grants and contracts are explicit research funding and may be provided by both public and private sources. The major distinction between research contracts and grants has to do with who has the final responsibility for the project and control of funding. In the case of research grants, the researcher has sole responsibility for the design of the study, any modification to it, and the implementation of the project. In research contracts, there is a joint responsibility for the conduct of the project, and the funder may have

TABLE 3–1   Major national level data sources for health services research

Source	Owner	Major Contents	Unit of Observation	First Year
Area Resource File	Bureau of Health Professions, HRSA	demographics, health professions, health facilities, health status	county, state	1986
Behavioral Risk Factor Surveillance System	Centers for Disease Control	behavioral or lifestyle risk factors, demographics	noninstitutionalized adult	early 1980s
Medicare Beneficiary Health Status Registry	Agency for Health Care Policy and Research, Health Care Financing Administration	risk factors, health status, medical history, demographics, costs of services	cohort of Medicare beneficiaries	1993
Mental Health Inventory	National Institute of Mental Health	characteristics of mental health organizations, patients, and services	mental health organization	1969
National Ambulatory Medical Care Survey	National Center for Health Statistics, CDC	provision and utilization of office-based ambulatory services	patient visit	1973
National Health Interview Survey	National Center for Health Statistics, CDC	health conditions, doctor visits, hospital stays, household characteristics, personal characteristics	household, individual members of the household	1969
National Health and Nutrition Examination Survey	National Center for Health Statistics, CDC	physical, physiological, psychological diseases; nutritional status	individual	1959
National Hospital Discharge Survey	National Center for Health Statistics, CDC	patient, treatment, hospital characteristics	patient record, hospital	1970

TABLE 3–1 *Continued*

Source	Owner	Major Contents	Unit of Observation	First Year
National Medical Expenditure Survey	Agency for Health Care Policy and Research	health expenditures, use of health services, insurance coverage	individual	1977
National Nursing Home Survey	National Center for Health Statistics, CDC	types of nursing homes, residents, discharged residents, follow-up	resident, staff	1973
National Survey of Personal Health Practices/ Consequence	National Center for Health Statistics, CDC	personal health practices, health status	individual	1979
National Vital Statistics System	National Center for Health Statistics, CDC	mortality, cause of death, fetal death	individual	1968

final control in that the contract can be stopped if the contractor fails or refuses to proceed with the research protocol as jointly agreed or amended. The key distinction, then, is whether the organization providing the money also has an active role in the study.

There are many public and private funding sources for health services research (COSSA, 1986; Annual Register of Grant Support, 1994; Durek, Burke and Kraut, 1988). Public sources include the various institutes under the National Institute of Health (NIH) of the U.S. Department of Health and Human Services (Parklawn Bldg., 5600 Fisher's Ln., Rockville, MD 20857; or NIH Bldg. 9000 Rockville Pike, Bethesda, MD 20892) such as NIH-NCI (cancer), NHL (heart and lung), NIA (aging), NIMH (mental health), NIDA (drug, alcohol), NIAAA (alcohol abuse), National Science Foundation (2101 Constitution Ave. Washington, DC 20418), Agency for Health Care Policy and Research (AHCPR), Health Care Financing Administration (HCFA), Office of Research and Demonstration (ORD), Department of Veterans Affairs (VA), National Center for Health Research (NCHR), National Center for Nursing Research (NCNR), and Office of Rural Health Policy. The Federal Information Exchange (FEDIX) has designed an electronic service to notify researchers by e-mail of grant opportunities. The participating federal agencies include DOE, NIH, NSF, ONR, NASA, FAA, AFOSR, HUD, AID, and USDA. Researchers can register their e-mail addresses and select key words from a thesaurus to develop a profile of research interests. Announcements of research opportunities will be sent via e-mail based on the correct matching of research interest and funding opportunity. The Web address for FEDIX is http://www.fie.com.

Private sources include major foundations such as the Ford Foundation, the Pew Charitable Trusts, the Robert Wood Johnson Foundation, the Lilly Endowment, the Carnegie Corporation of New York, the W. K. Kellogg Foundation, the Henry J. Kaiser Family Foundation, the Baxter Foundation, the Commonwealth Fund, the John A. Hartford Foundation, the Rockefeller Foundation, the Sloan Foundation, the Russell Sage Foundation, and the Social Science Research Council (230 Park Ave., New York, NY 10017). Additional funding sources are listed in Appendix 3.

THE RESEARCH PROPOSAL

A **research proposal** describes what specific study a researcher intends to accomplish and how. The primary purpose is to obtain the funding necessary to carry out the study. The researcher tries to convince a prospective sponsor that he or she is well acquainted with the state of the art and the accomplishments in the field, has demonstrated competency in study design and analysis, is qualified to perform the described activities, and has the necessary personnel and facilities to carry out the activities related to the project. Moreover, the proposed activities either aim at solving an immediate problem or at advancing existing knowledge in the field and eventually aiding in the solution of an identified problem. The research purpose should be within the scope of the established program objectives of the funding agency and the importance of the anticipated results sufficiently justify the expenditure of the proposed time and money.

Preliminary Work

The prelude to writing a good proposal is adequate preliminary work. The researcher reviews the funding literature and examines information regarding the funder's areas of interest and funding priorities, guidelines for proposal submission, any restrictions, size of the grants, cost-share requirements, and review procedures. The researcher should be aware of the dates and terms of proposal submission, any required forms, the contact person or office, and the correct name and address of the potential funding source. Once this information is obtained, the researcher then decides whether the proposed idea is consistent with the funding priorities, whether the proposed costs are within the given range; whether funding is short- or long-term and whether renewal is possible; whether it funds solely or requires matching and, if so, what kind; and whether there is a funding cycle and, if so, the deadlines to be met for proposal submission.

After a funding source has been identified, the investigator should contact the source prior to writing or submitting a formal proposal. Some funding agencies have specific guidelines on preapplication contact. Make sure to find out about theses guidelines prior to the contact. The preliminary contact may be made through telephone, written communication, and/or personal visit. A phone call can be made to determine the compatibility of the proposed project to the priorities of the funder, and the appropriate contact person. Phone calls can also be made for follow-up on any written communication and appointments for personal visits.

Written communication includes letters of intent, abstracts, or a preliminary proposals. A letter of intent, required by some funders, generally contains a brief description of the proposed project in terms of its objective(s) and design, an estimated budget, and some information about the researcher(s). An abstract of the proposed research project is usually accompanied by a letter of transmittal containing information about the applicant, her or his institution, and the budgetary requirements. A preliminary proposal, also referred to as a concept paper, may be required by some funders. It is an outline of the proposed project or activity and consists of such elements as the project title, the name of the submitting organization, a need statement or a statement of the problem, a statement of the objectives of the proposed project; a description of the anticipated methodology; available resources and personnel, including their roles; the benefits of the proposed project; the qualifications of the researcher(s) and site; expected support to be obtained; the estimated duration of the project; and a budget with an outline of estimated costs.

Personal visits should be preceded by adequate preparation of what to accomplish. In addition to finding out what the potential match between the proposed project and the funding agency's target, the investigator may want to obtain the following additional pieces of information during the visit: (1) the amount of funding available for new projects (as opposed to those committed to continuing ones), (2) some suggestions about what other agencies might be interested if the proposed project proves to be inappropriate for this agency, and (3) other topics of interest to the funding agency.

Format

Most funding sources require the same basic information for a research proposal although the details and required forms may vary. For examples, see Reif-Lehrer (1989), Gordon (1989), Trumbo (1989), Coley and Scheinberg (1990), and Public Health Service (1995). Appendix 4 provides a copy of the application forms for Public Health Service Grant PHS 398. Whether an application form is provided or only sketchy instructions are given, the components of a well-written research proposal generally include the following elements: a title page, a table of contents, an abstract, a detailed project description, references, a detailed budget, a human subjects review, and appendices (see Table 3–2). If a grant research officer is available in the researcher's organization, that person's help and counsel should be sought before putting together a research proposal.

Title Page

The title page identifies the proposal and provides the endorsement of appropriate organizational (e.g., university) officials. Some funding agencies, for example, the National Science Foundation and the National Institute of Health, have designed their own title pages. Whether an application form is provided or not, generally very similar

TABLE 3–2   Components of a research proposal

A.   Title Page
B.   Table of Contents
C.   Abstract
D.   Project Description
   1.   Introduction
   2.   Problem statement and significance
   3.   Goals and objectives
   4.   Methods and procedures
   5.   Evaluation
   6.   Dissemination
E.   References
F.   Budget and Justification
G.   Human Subjects
H.   Appendices

information is required, including: (1) the title of the project, (2) the name of the designated agency (i.e., funding source) to which the proposal is to be submitted, (3) the name, address, telephone number(s), and signature of the project director of the institution submitting the proposal, (4) date of proposal submission, (5) beginning and ending dates of the proposed funding period, (6) total amount of funds requested (specify first-year request for multiyear project), (7) total indirect cost, and (8) the name, address, and signature of the individual accepting responsibility for managing the funds and the designated endorsement of the institution.

Table of Contents

A table of contents may be available in the proposal application package. A brief proposal does not necessarily need a table of contents. A longer or more complex proposal generally requires a table of contents to assist reviewers in finding their way through the proposal. When included, the table of contents generally lists all major parts and divisions of the proposal.

Abstract

An abstract is a concise summary of the material presented in the proposal. Though it appears at the front of the proposal, it is written last. It should be clearly written, emphasizing the significance and need for the project, its specific objectives, study design, evaluation methods, and significance. These materials are condensed to a page or less (such as 200 to 300 words in length), although specific lengths are sometimes given in proposal guidelines.

The abstract is very important because it serves several purposes: (1) the reviewer usually reads it first to gain a perspective of the study and its expected significance; (2) the reviewer uses it as a reference to the nature of the study when the project comes up for discussion; (3) it will sometimes be the only part of the proposal that is read by those reviewing a panel's recommendation or the field readers' consensus (Miller, 1991). With these many uses, it is important that the abstract be prepared with the great care and that objectives and procedures are paraphrased using general but precise statements. Key concepts presented in the body of the proposal are highlighted in the abstract to alert the reviewer to look for them in the body of the proposal. Many funding decision makers may read only the review comments and the abstract.

Project Description

The project description, or the "narrative" section, is the main body of the proposal, the section on which the decision to accept or reject is typically based. In this section, the purpose is stated and defined, the conceptual framework and underlying premise is explained, the methods for conducting the research are described, the procedures of evaluation are explained, and the schedule of dissemination is summarized. In writing the project description, the researcher should let the language of the proposal reflect his or her knowledge of the field, and make it understandable to the least knowledgeable of the anticipated reviewers. The major components of a project description will be discussed in greater detail later.

Reference

The reference section should include the literature cited in the proposal narrative. The number of references should not exceed the page limit, if any. Unless specified by funding agency, generally any acceptable bibliographic methods may be used.

Research Budget

The research budget reflects in financial terms those activities developed in the proposal, specifying how the money will be spent. It documents the actual costs of achieving the objectives stated in the proposal. The total amount requested in the budget is determined by the needs of the project and the limitations set by the granting organization. Many major funding agencies have budget formats on computer templates. The funding agency should be contacted before developing the budget. A more detailed discussion of the budget section will follow later in this chapter. Even for a more modest project, it is a good idea to spend some time anticipating any expenses involved: office supplies, photocopying, computer disks, telephone calls, transportation, and so on.

Human Subjects

In the preparation of a proposal, investigators must follow both the sponsor's and their organizational requirements regarding human research subjects. The human subject review and approval procedures are mandated by federal statute/regulations and university policy. Violations can lead to loss of federal and perhaps nonfederal support.

Specifically, all research involving human subjects must be approved by the organization's institutional human subjects review committee. The committee is established in accordance with federal law. Most funding agencies require evidence of institutional human subjects approval prior to making a grant award for a project involving human subjects. Appropriate forms and procedures for obtaining review/approval may be obtained from the committee.

The following is adapted from the author's own agency human subjects application form.

1. Who are your subjects?
   (Briefly outline your criteria for subject selection, including information regarding the number of subjects and their anticipated ages. If your study involves the use of abnormal subjects, explain any psychological or physical characteristics they will possess.)
2. How will your subjects be recruited?
   (Describe your procedures for finding subjects and obtaining informed consent.)
3. Is there a cost involved?
   (Does consenting to be a subject lead to additional costs in tests, medical care, etc., for the subject? If so, who is responsible for the costs?)
4. What are your procedures?
   (Outline what you will do to, or require of, your subjects. Who will be your data collectors, and what training will they have or require?)
5. What are the potential risks for the subject?
   [In your estimation, do the explained procedures involve any potential risk for the subjects—physically, psychologically, socially, or legally? Could the type of data you are collecting from each subject possibly be construed as an invasion of privacy? If any of your procedures create potential risks for any of the subjects, describe: (1) other methods, if any, that were considered and why they will not be used and (2) what precautions you plan to take to reduce the possibility of such risks.]
6. What deception may be used in your study?
   (If your research involves deceiving your subjects, explain how it will be handled.)
7. Who will benefit from this study?
   [What is the significance of potential benefits to be gained by: (1) the subjects used in this investigation, (2) persons similarly situated, (3) the scientific community, and (4) humankind in general.]
8. How will subjects' privacy be protected?
   [What are your procedures for safeguarding each subject's rights with respect to the following: (1) safety and security of the individual (as described in question 5); (2) privacy and confidentially (including protection and anonymity of data); (3) embarrassment, discomfort, and harassment (i.e., would there be any stigma or repercussions from having participated in this study?)]

The following provides the instructions for writing an informed consent form for the human subjects application form.

1. A heading on top of the form indicates that it is an *Informed Consent Form.*
2. Explain the duration of the project, procedures to be followed and their purposes, including identification of any procedures that are experimental.
3. Provide evidence that the subject will be able to exercise free power of choice and no element of coercion or constraint is permitted in the obtaining of consent to participate, and an instruction that the subject is free to withdraw her or his consent and to discontinue participation in the project at any time without prejudice to the subject.
4. Describe any attendant discomforts and risks reasonably to be expected for each aspect of the study.
5. Describe the benefits that may be reasonably expected from participation in this study.
6. Include a statement of security of data (maintaining confidentiality), especially as it relates to specific individuals.
7. Include a statement on availability of compensation in the event of physical injury and how to obtain more information about this.
8. Offer to answer any inquiries concerning the procedures and include a telephone number and address for the contact person.
9. Provide a place for the subject to sign and date the form.
10. Disclose any appropriate alternative procedures that might be advantageous for the subject.
11. Prominently located on the consent form must be a statement to the effect that the subject must be provided a copy of the consent form.
12. The informed consent form must be worded at a level of understanding of the subject.
13. No statements may be made to waive or appear to waive any of a subjects' legal rights including any release of the institution or its agents from liability for negligence.

Although not common in health services research, projects involving vertebrate animals or hazardous materials must also obtain special approval before the proposal is funded. An animal use questionnaire should be completed concerning the use, procurement, and care of animals. Research involving potential hazards associated with the use of toxic materials, infectious organisms, and genetic recombination must be reviewed and approved by a committee on biosafety and hazardous waste.

Appendices

Appendices contain information that will strengthen the basic concept developed in the narrative section of the proposal. They may be items that could have been put in the main body of the proposal but in the interest of conciseness are appended. Examples include expanded vitae, letters of support, list of supportive data, publications, and so on.

Project Description

The project description, or the narrative portion of the proposal, is the most essential component of a research proposal. It consists of the following major elements: introduction, problem statement and significance, goals and objectives, procedures and methods, evaluation, and dissemination.

Introduction

An introduction section includes a brief summary of the problem of interest and the related subject. It should be clear to the lay person and give enough background to enable the reader to place the proposal in a context of common knowledge. What have other researchers concluded about this topic? What theories can be used to shed light on it and what are their major components? What relevant empirical research has been done previously? Are there consistent findings, or do past studies disagree? Are there limitations and gaps in the body of existing research that the proposed study can resolve? The introduction generally contains information showing what has been accomplished in the field, that the investigator is well acquainted with the past and current work and with the literature in the field, and that the proposed project will advance or add to the present store of knowledge in this field or be important to the solution of the problem.

Problem Statement and Significance

The problem statement and significance section describes the overall purpose of the project and its significance in meeting the funder's goals and objectives. Why is the topic worth studying? What is the practical significance of the proposed research? Does it contribute to improved understanding of health services delivery, problem solving, or the refinement of existing theories?

Goals and Objectives

In the goals and objectives section, the proposal presents a detailed description of the work to be undertaken. What exactly will be studied? Goals are general statements specifying the desired outcomes of the proposed project. Objectives are specific statements summarizing the proposed activities and including a detailed description of the outcomes and their assessment in measurable terms.

Methods and Procedures

The methods and procedures section is perhaps the most important part of the narrative portion of the proposal. In this section, the proposal describes in detail the general research plan, including research design, relevant theory and hypothesis justification, data sources, instruments to generate data and its validity, and the analysis techniques or methods to be used.

If subjects are to be selected for study, the researcher needs to address who will be studied in order to collect data. The subjects should be identified in general, theoretical terms, and in specific, more concrete terms, indicating who are available for study and how they will be reached. Will it be appropriate to select a sample? If so, how will the researcher select the sample? If there is any possibility that the research will have an impact on those under study, how will the researcher ensure that they will not be harmed by the research?

In terms of measurement, what are the key variables in the study? How are they defined and measured? Are these definitions and measurement methods consistent with or different from those of previous research on this topic? It is usually appropriate to include a copy of the questionnaire (either self-developed or available in the literature) as an appendix to the proposal.

In terms of data collection methods, procedures used to collect the data for the study need to be described. Will an experiment or a survey be conducted? Will field research be undertaken, or available data already collected by others be reanalyzed?

In terms of data analysis, the kind of analysis to be conducted should be described (e.g., multiple regression, factor analysis, etc.), and the variables to be included in each model should be specified. The purpose and logic of the analysis should be spelled out. The analysis should address research hypotheses or questions.

The researcher is often required to provide a schedule for the various stages of research, which includes time estimates for major activities to be conducted. For grant reviewers, a schedule or timeline of activities serves as a measure of the completeness and timeliness of research activities. For the investigator, it is a chronological checklist of the progress of research. Without a timeline, the researcher might not be aware when project runs behind schedule.

Evaluation

The evaluation section describes the plan of assessing the ongoing progress toward achieving the research objectives. The plan specifies how each project activity is to be measured in terms of completion, the timeline for its completion, and the conditions and mechanisms for revising program activities. A good evaluation plan enables both investigators and the funder to monitor project progress and provide timely feedback for project modification or adjustments.

Dissemination

Some funding sources require a dissemination plan to be included in a proposal. The dissemination section indicates how to make research findings available to others particularly those interested in the study outcomes. Dissemination provides research results to a regional, national, or international audience.

Researchers must recognize that grants and contracts have two different sets of rules with respect to publication. The grant usually carries the right of publication by investigators. Grantees generally encourage publication and distribution of the results of research. Under contract research, investigators may be restricted in terms of publishing their contracted research. The funding agency may be only interested in receiving reports that fit the specifications of its internal needs. Investigators should negotiate with the funding agency on publication rights prior to submitting papers for professional publication.

Budget

Typically, a proposal budget reflects direct and indirect costs. Direct costs incurred by grant activities fall within the following categories: personnel, supplies, equipment, travel, communications, publications, subcontracts, consultants, and other costs (those not included in previous categories such as computer time, service contracts, etc.). Figure 3–1 shows a budget example for a research proposal.

Personnel

Personnel costs include salaries and wages of all investigators, research assistants, and staff who will be spending full or part time on the project. All key personnel (e.g., investigators) who will participate in the proposed project should be identified by name, title, and the expected amount of time to be devoted to the project. The names of supporting personnel (e.g., graduate assistants) generally are not necessary. Unfilled positions may be marked "vacant" or "to be selected." If the individuals involved have exceptional qualifications that would merit consideration in the evaluation of the proposal, this information should be included in budget justification. Federal grants and contracts will not allow salaried personnel to be paid for overtime (i.e., extra compensation beyond the monthly rate) unless this is specifically stated in the proposal and awarded in the grant. The fringe benefit rate associated with various types of employment can be found out from the benefits office or sponsored program office of the employing agency. These percentages may change frequently.

Expendable Supplies

Expendable supplies or consumable supplies include office supplies, computer supplies, chemicals, and educational materials. Supplies and their costs may be listed under one general heading or by category. In the budget justification section, the investigator may explain why these supplies are needed for the project.

Equipment

Both the unit and total costs of equipment should be specified. Equipment is usually defined as a property with an acquisition cost of $500 or more and an expected service

DETAILED BUDGET FOR INITIAL BUDGET PERIOD DIRECT COSTS ONLY					FROM 95/10/01	THROUGH 96/09/30	
PERSONNEL (Applicant Organization Only)					DOLLAR AMOUNT REQUESTED (omit cents)		
NAME	ROLE ON PROJECT	TYPE APPT (months)	% EFFORT ON PROJ.	INST. BASE SALARY	SALARY REQUESTED	FRINGE BENEFITS	TOTALS
Scientist 1	Principal Investigator	12	20	$60,955	$12,191	$2,213	$14,404
Scientist 2	Co-investigator	12	25	$38,000	$9,500	$2,174	$11,674
Scientist 3	Co-investigator	12	25	$40,000	$10,000	$2,265	$12,265
Scientist 4	Investigator	12	15	$32,000	$4,800	$871	$5,671
GA 1		12	100	$15,000	$15,000	$90	$15,090
GA 2		12	100	$15,000	$15,000	$4,500	$19,500
					$0	$0	$0
					$0	$0	$0
SUBTOTALS					$66,491	$12,113	$78,604

CONSULTANT COSTS				
Scientist 5	$5,000			$5,000

EQUIPMENT (Itemize)		
Computer 1	$2,000	
Computer 2	$3,500	$5,500

SUPPLIES (Itemize by category)		
Postage	$500	
		$500

TRAVEL		
	$2,000	$2,000

PATIENT CARE COSTS	INPATIENT	$0
	OUTPATIENT	$0

ALTERATIONS AND RENOVATIONS (Itemize by category)	
	$0

OTHER EXPENSES (Itemize by category)		
Photocopying	$1,000	
Subcontracting	$21,000 (3 x 7000)	$22,000

SUBTOTAL DIRECT COSTS FOR INITIAL BUDGET PERIOD		$113,604

CONSORTIUM/CONTRACTUAL COSTS			
DIRECT COSTS	$0	TOTAL——>	$0
INDIRECT COSTS	$0		

TOTAL DIRECT COSTS FOR INITIAL BUDGET PERIOD	(Item 7a, Face Page) ——	$113,604

PHS 398 (Rev 9/91)   (Form Page 4) Page ____   DD
Number pages consecutively at the bottom throughout the application Do not use suffixes such as 3a, 3b

FIGURE 3–1 Example of a research proposal budget.

life of two or more years. Some funding agencies have restrictions for equipment purchases. Check proposal guidelines for specific guidelines and definitions for equipment. When developing the budget for the acquisition of expensive equipment, investigators should remember to add their state's sales tax to the vendor's quoted purchase price.

Travel

The total cost of project-related travel is summarized in the budget. The detailed breakdown of travel and its justification is provided in the budget justification section. A travel description includes mode, frequency and cost of travel. Justification includes the travel purpose and its relation to project objectives. Many funding sources do not allow foreign travel. The investigator should contact the potential funding source to determine the travel regulations.

Communications

This category usually includes postage, telephone, telegram, messenger, and fax charges associated with a project. If funding sources do not have a category for communications, such charges could be properly placed in the "other direct costs" category.

Publications

The costs incurred of preparing and publishing the results of the research are specified. Examples include technical reports, reprints, manuscripts, illustrations such as art work, graphics, photography, slides, and overheads.

Subcontract Costs

The guidelines of the potential funding agency should be checked carefully for information related to subcontracting. Usually, a subcontract proposal endorsed by the submitting agency along with a complete budget should be included in the prime proposal.

Consultant Services

The budget identifies each consultant, his or her primary organizational affiliation, compensation rate, and number of days or percent of time expected to serve. The justification section emphasizes each consultant's expertise and expected role in the project.

Other Direct Costs

Other direct costs consist of all items that do not fit into any other direct cost category, including payment to human subjects, copying fees, service charges, repair and maintenance contracts on major equipment, computer time, and postage. These categories may be itemized by unit and total costs.

Indirect costs, or overhead, are those costs incurred in the support and management of the proposed activities that cannot be readily determined by direct measurement. Examples include: (1) general administrative cost such as accounting, personnel, and administrative functions at both central and unit levels, (2) operation and maintenance including utilities and janitorial services, and (3) depreciation and use allowance. Many research institutions (such as universities) have negotiated indirect cost rates with the federal government or private foundations. These rates apply unless an agency or program specifically stipulates another. Indirect cost rates change from time to time. It is advisable to check with the grants management office before calculating indirect costs.

In addition to direct and indirect costs, some funding agencies require that grantee institutions commit to share the overall costs of a sponsored program and display the institution's share of the project in the proposal budget. Check the announcement for cost-share requirement and method.

Justification

The budget is followed by a justification section in which any unusual costs associated with the proposed project are justified. If the proposal narrative is well developed, explaining in detail the activities and anticipated objectives, the justification can be easily related to these activities. In addition, items such as annual salary increases, equipment costs, unusually high supply or travel costs, and stipend costs should be included. The researcher needs to secure the going wage rate for many budget items such as interviewers, cost of transportation, rates for using mainframe computer, and so on. A checklist for common budget items is as follows:

Personnel
- Salaries and wages for academic personnel during academic year and during summer
- Research associates
- Research assistants
- Technicians
- Secretarial staff
- Hourly help
- Fringe benefits
- Consultants
- Fees
- Domestic travel
- Foreign travel
Equipment
- Installation and freight
- Equipment rental

Communications
- Telephone and telegraph
- Photocopying
- Postage

Supplies
- Chemicals and glassware
- Animals and animal supplies
- Office supplies
- Alterations and renovation

Other costs
- Subcontracts
- Training
- Publication of reports
- Data processing

A common practical mistake in research proposals is to grossly underestimate the budget, both in time and money, required for a project. Most underestimates can be attributed to inexperience. However, the less promising funding climate for research also contributes to inadequate budget request. Unfortunately, a project with an inadequate budget is unlikely to be completed successfully.

Appendices

The appendices section includes important documentation that enhances the competitiveness of the research proposal. Examples include letters of support or endorsement, vitae, description of relevant institutional resources, and a list of references.

Letters of support or endorsement are solicited from elected officials and other organizations and individuals either required by a funding source or on the basis that their support would be essential or helpful to a funding decision. In general, letters should be addressed to the investigator's organization and sent to the investigator for submission along with the proposal. Letters should not be sent under separate cover to the funding source because they may not get there in time or may not be filed appropriately with the investigator's proposal. Some funding sources may not accept documents submitted separately. To speed up the process of securing a letter of support, the investigator may prepare a draft letter and fax it to the potential signee. Telephone discussions that summarize project ideas often do not get heard exactly as investigators think they have transmitted them.

Most sponsoring agencies require a curriculum vita and list of publications for each member and senior professional staff member in the project. Curriculum vitae may also be placed in the appendices. Vitae should be updated and current. If possible, the same format should be used. A two-page summary should be prepared highlighting important experience and publication information in the vitae.

Relevant institutional resources may be included in the appendices. Available facilities and major items of equipment especially adapted to the proposed project should be described. These facilities could include libraries, computer centers, other recognized centers, and any special but relevant equipment.

A list of references is desirable when the proposal contains 10 or more references. Otherwise, unless specifically required, references may be inserted in the text as footnotes.

Proposal Review Process

Understanding the review process helps the researcher write a more fundable grant application. Researchers need to be aware of the review process and time lapses of funding agencies. This information may be obtained in the visit if not already included in the application package. Since much of health services research is funded by the National Institute of Health (NIH), we summarize the major components of the NIH review process here (Reif-Lehrer, 1989, pp. 3–25; Public Health Service, 1991). Researchers should be aware the information provided below may not be entirely relevant in their situations.

A grant proposal to NIH is prepared by a principal investigator (PI) and submitted by his or her sponsoring institution to NIH. The proposal is received at NIH by the Division of Research Grants (DRG), which is the advisory to NIH and sets up study sections (both standing and, when necessary, ad hoc) to review research grant proposals (RO1), Research Career Development Awards (RCDA), first awards, and fellowship applications (NRSA). Knowledgeable investigators may suggest an initial review group that would be appropriate for their applications. The final decision is made by the DRG.

At the institute, the application is assigned to a health scientist–administrator (HSA), who acts as the primary institute contact for the applicant before, during, and after the review process. That person is also responsible for grant administration if the application is funded. NIH has a dual peer review system. The first level of review is by an initial review group (IRG), often referred to as a study section. The second level of review is by an advisory council. The decision to award a proposal is based on both scientific merit (judged by the study section) and program considerations (judged by the advisory council).

In the first level of review, the study section is composed of scientists who represent different geographical areas and a wide range of expertise. The study section provides initial scientific review of grant applications, assigns a priority score based on scientific merit, and makes budget recommendations. The role of the study section is only advisory. It does not make funding decisions, which are the prerogative of each institute under NIH.

The primary and secondary reviewers come to the study section review meeting with written critiques of the assigned grant proposals. The critiques focus on the proposal's scientific and technical merit, originality, methodology or research design, the qualifications and experience (or potential, in the case of a new applicant) of the investigator(s), the availability of resources, the appropriateness of the budget and timeline, and ethical issues (e.g., human subjects). The following lists some commonly used proposal review questions.

- Are research aims logical?
- Is the background or literature review adequate?
- Is there preliminary work or prior relevant experience?
- Are hypotheses appropriate, relevant to aims and procedures, and testable?
- Are data adequate?
- Is the instrument reliable and valid (having been previously tested)?
- Is the sample size sufficient and representative to draw inference to entire population?
- Are analysis methods adequate to data elements?
- Are potential contribution feasible, creative, and significant?
- Are budget and time adequate and justified?
- Are the limitations pointed out and their improvement discussed?

At the study section meeting, the primary and secondary reviewers present the critiques of their assigned proposals. A general discussion among all study section members follows, including asking further questions about the proposals or reanalyzing certain portions of the proposals. After the discussion, a recommendation is made by majority vote for (1) approval, (2) disapproval, or (3) deferral for additional information. The budget is then discussed in terms of appropriateness. For each approved proposal, all study section members then vote through secret ballot a numerical score based on a scale of 0.1 increments from 1.0 (the best score) to 5.0 (the worst score). A recommendation for a site visit may be made by the primary reviewer or the executive secretary of the study section who recognizes the need for additional information that cannot be obtained by mail or telephone.

After the study section meeting, the scores assigned by individual members for each approved proposal are averaged and multiplied by 100 to provide a three-digit rating known as a priority score. The executive secretary prepares a summary statement (often called "the pink sheets") based on the primary and secondary reviewers' reports and the discussion at the study section meeting. The summary statement is later sent to the principal investigator. The grant application is then forwarded to the advisory council for further review.

The second level of review is conducted by a national advisory council within each individual institute. The council reviews the summary statements of all approved applications from each study section together with the proposals and adds its own review based on judgments of both scientific merit and relevance to the program goals of the assigned institute. The executive secretary of a study section attends the council meeting when an application reviewed in his or her study section is discussed. The council then makes recommendations on funding to the institute staff. It may concur with or modify study section action on grant applications or defer for further review.

ORGANIZATIONAL AND ADMINISTRATIVE ISSUES

Another important preparation for research has to do with organizational and administrative issues related to the conduct of research. Before research can be started, researchers need to determine the organization and management of research work. In general, larger projects will have more formal arrangements than smaller studies. There are three main options for the organization of a research team. The hierarchically organized research team will have the status of lead researcher(s) clearly stated and usually well-defined (and sometimes narrow) roles for research assistants and other members of the team. The second option is the research team of formal equals, which is often used for multidisciplinary studies, where there is a need to draw on the different and complementary expertise of a number of people. The third option is the collaborative research team, drawing together members from different institutions who will often have somewhat different interests in the project and different contributions to make.

Regardless of how a research team is formed, it should include people with substantive, methodological, and analytical knowledge and experience related to the research topic. Substantive knowledge insures study validity, for example, whether the most relevant measures of outcome are being collected. Methodological knowledge insures that the study design is adequate for the topic and the results can be used to generalize to the population of interest. The wording and ordering of questions may also be better arranged to improve data quality. Analytical knowledge insures appropriate use of statistical methods to address research questions or hypotheses. The response format and coding scheme should be designed to allow maximum and flexible data analysis. A collaborative research team that combines the knowledge and experience of all those involved can turn out a better research product.

However, members of a research team can bring both problem-solving and problem-generating capacities (Grady and Wallston, 1988). Problems can arise because people have different research styles and work habits, in addition to differences in thinking. To reduce possible confusion, conflicts, and disputes during project implementation, the roles of members of the research team should be clearly specified. Team members should know what their roles are and how they fit into the overall research project. In funded research, one person is designated as the principal investigator (PI), who is responsible for both the scientific and financial aspects of the research. Coinvestigators or investigators are those who participate in specific aspects of the project. Research associates or assistants are assigned to investigators to assist in carrying out research activities. Prior to the conduct of research, investigators should reach an agreement, in writing, on individual responsibilities, time frame to complete specific tasks, publication credit and authorship, ways to deal with unexpected events or resolve disputes, and other mutually interested issues. The important aspect to note is to work out all foreseeable sources of conflicts in advance. A research team that carries out its activities based on individual assumptions rather than specified and agreed-upon roles will likely run into problems, adversely affecting both the research project and the interrelations among investigators.

Researchers must also think through any problems that might arise concerning access to key informants, organizations, or information. If funding needs to be sought, questions of access need to be resolved before a proposal is presented to a funding body. If the research design depends crucially on having access to key informants, organizations, sources of information, sampling frames, official statistics, and the like, it is premature to develop a research proposal for funding, without obtaining the consent or active support of potential collaborators or checking the feasibility in relation to such access issues.

Obtaining access often depends on the presentation of a study design that is meaningful and interesting to those concerned. It is usually necessary to provide a separate, shorter outline of the study for this purpose, quite different from the main proposal, focusing on the issues and questions addressed and their relevancy to the collaborators rather than on the methods and data collection techniques to be used. Researchers should actively seek inputs from potential collaborators who may be able to make suggestions on the study design, its conduct, and practical difficulties that could not have been foreseen.

Other practical details to be attended to prior to carrying out research include: negotiate with the funding agency to work out a protocol; get familiar with the research site(s); determine the level of staff support and services needed; reallocate the budget to fit with the actual situation of project implementation, including preparing a research budget that may contain subcontracts for needed services such as sampling, interviewing, or data processing; finalize the research plan with collaborators; recruit personnel; identify supplies and logistics; revise or update the timetable or schedule of research activities; train staff for data collection, processing, and analysis; conduct a human subjects review; revise the data collection instrument; and pilot-test the instrument. Careful preparation of these activities will facilitate the smooth progress of the research process.

SUMMARY

During the groundwork stage of health services research, researchers identify relevant data and funding sources, develop research proposals, and prepare organizationally and administratively to carry out the research. A rich body of data collected periodically by federal agencies, principally the National Center for Health Statistics, are available for secondary health services research. Notable examples are the National Ambulatory Medical Care Survey, National Hospital Discharge Survey, and National Medical Expenditure Survey. The various institutes under the National Institute of Health and major private foundations are the principal funders of health services research. An important step toward seeking funding for research is a well-written proposal that matches the funding purpose and level of the funder. Knowledge about how grant proposals are reviewed and preliminary research and preparation will help the researcher compose the right proposal and improve the chance of getting funded.

Key Terms

primary data source	secondary data source
cross-section data	time-series data
unit of observation	panel data
research proposal	

Review Questions

1. What are the major national-level data sources suitable for health services research? Describe the major features of these data sources.

2. Become familiar with the funding sources most likely to support the research topics of your interest. What are their requirements and restrictions?

3. Identify the major steps in a research proposal. As an exercise, write a research proposal on a topic of interest to you.

4. What is the research review process of the National Institute of Health?

5. What are the organizational and administrative issues related to research?

REFERENCES

Annual Register of Grant Support. (1994). Wilmette, IL: National Register Publishing Co.

Association of University Programs in Health Administration (AUPHA). (1992). A Report on National Electronic Databases. Washington, DC: AUPHA.

Coley, S. M., and Scheinberg, C. A. (1990). *Proposal Writing.* Newbury Park, CA: Sage.

Consortium of Social Science Associations (COSSA). (1986). *Guide to Federal Funding for Social Scientists.* Washington, DC: Russell Sage Foundation.

Durek, E., Holt, R. V., Burke, M. E., and Kraut, A. G. (1988). *Guide to Research Support.* 2nd ed. Hayattsville. MD: American Psychological Association.

Gordon, S. L. (1989). Ingredients of a successful grant application to the National Institutes of Health. *Journal of Orthopaedic Research, 7,* 138–141.

Grady, K. E., and Wallston, B. S. (1988). *Research in Health Care Settings.* Newbury Park, CA: Sage.

Miller, D. C. (1991). *Handbook of Research Design and Social Measurement.* 5th ed. Newbury Park, CA: Sage.

National Center for Health Statistics. (1964). Health survey procedure: Concepts, questionnaire development, and definitions in the Health Interview Survey. *Vital and Health Statistics,* series 1, number 2. Washington, DC: U.S. Department of Health, Education, and Welfare, Public Health Service.

National Center for Health Statistics. (1965). Origin, program, and operation of the U.S. National Health Survey. *Vital and Health Statistics,* series 1, number 1. Washington, DC: U.S. Department of Health, Education, and Welfare, Public Health Service.

National Center for Health Statistics. (1966). History of the United States National Committee on vital and health statistics, 1949–1964. *Vital and Health Statistics,* series 4, number 5. Washington, DC: U.S. Department of Health, Education, and Welfare, Public Health Service.

National Center for Health Statistics. (1975). The analytical potential of NCHS data for health care systems: A report of the United States National Committee on vital and health statistics *Vital and Health Statistics,* series 4, number 17. Washington, DC: U.S. Department of Health, Education, and Welfare, Public Health Service.

National Health Survey Act. (1956). U.S. Public Law 652. 84th Congress, chapter 510, 2d session-S, 3076.

Panel on the National Health Care Survey. (1992) *A National Health Care Survey.* Washington, DC: National Academy Press.

Public Health Service. (1995). *Application for Public Health Service Grant—Including Research Career Development Awards and Institutional National Research Service Awards.* Bethesda, MD: Office of Grants Inquiry, Division of Research Grants, National Institute of Health.

Reif-Lehrer, L. (1989). *Writing a Successful Grant Application.* 2nd ed. Boston, MA: Jones and Bartlett Publishers.

Trumbo, B. E. (1989). How to get your first research grant. *Statistical Science,* 4(2, May), 121–150.

U.S. Department of Health and Human Services (U.S. DHHS). (1991). *Current Legislative Authorities of the National Center for Health Statistics.* Hyattsville, MD: Public Health Service.

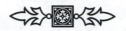

CHAPTER

4

Research Review

LEARNING OBJECTIVES

- To understand the types of research review and their purposes.
- To describe the process of research review.
- To identify the general categories of information likely to be focused on in research review.
- To become familiar with commonly used computer-based abstracting and indexing services.
- To comprehend the purpose of meta-analysis and its commonly used procedures.

As described in Chapter 1, scientific inquiry is cumulative research, with each study built on previous, related investigations. By reviewing what previous studies have accomplished and what mistakes have been made, researchers gain a comprehensive, integrated picture of the topic under investigation. Such accomplishment is particularly important today because of the huge amount of health services research conducted. Indeed, systematic and objective research reviews may become an independent research project yielding substantial information in its own right. This is especially the case because health services research is becoming more specialized, and time constraints make it nearly impossible for most researchers to keep abreast of the state of the art of all health services research topics.

This chapter introduces the method of research review with particular emphasis on its process. In addition, its strengths and weaknesses will be summarized.

DEFINITION

Research review provides a synthesis of existing knowledge on a specific question, based on an assessment of all relevant empirical research that can be found. Good research reviews are multidisciplinary, in that relevant studies from all related social science disciplines are covered, although research focuses differ across disciplines.

There are at least three uses of research review. Literature review is commonly part of the ground-clearing and preparatory work undertaken in the initial stages of empirical research. It guides the formulation of research questions or hypotheses, the design of the study, and the analysis used.

Literature review is also the initial part of the research product, appearing as the introduction in a report on empirical research (Harper, Weins, and Matarazzo, 1978). When used in this capacity, literature review has a narrow scope, typically restricted to those studies pertinent to the specific issue addressed by the primary research.

Literature review may also appear as independent research product serving different purposes (Cooper, 1989a, b). For example, reviews can focus on research methods, theories, outcomes, or what others have accomplished; criticize previous works; build bridges across related work; and identify central issues in a field.

Four independent research reviews may be identified: the **integrative research review, theoretical review, methodological review,** and **policy-oriented review.** Integrative review, by far the most frequently used, summarizes past research by drawing conclusions from many separate studies addressing similar or related hypotheses or research questions (Cooper, 1982). The reviewer aims to accomplish such objectives as presenting the state of the knowledge concerning the topic under review, highlighting issues previous researchers have left unresolved or unstudied, and directing future research so that it is built on cumulative inquiry.

Theoretical review summarizes all the existing relevant theories used to explain a particular topic and examines them in terms of major content areas, similarities, differences, and accuracy in prediction. Theoretical review provides a detailed summary of the theories and findings based on which theories were developed or tested, assesses which theories are more powerful and consistent with known findings, and refines theories by reformulating or integrating concepts from existing theories.

Methodological review summarizes different research designs used to study a particular topic and compares studies using different designs with regard to their findings. The purpose is to identify the strengths and weaknesses of different designs for a particular topic and explain to which extent differences in findings are the results of differences in designs.

Policy-oriented review summarizes current knowledge of a topic so as to draw out policy implications of study findings. Such review requires knowledge of the major policy issues and debates, as well as common research expertise.

It is possible that a comprehensive review will address several issues. For example, integrative review may cover policy impact, designs, and relevant theories, in addition to major findings. Theoretical review may also contain some integrative review components.

PROCESS

Research review is a familiar research process to most health services researchers. The common practice of literature review has been idiosyncratic, relying on the intuitive, subjective, and narrative style of the researcher. Such an approach leaves room for partial or selective coverage of the literature. Different researchers studying the same topic may select entirely different sets of studies to review without describing the selection procedures or identifying the studies that are missed. The subjectivity in selecting, analyzing, and interpreting studies has led to skepticism about the conclusions of many reviews. Due to the vast amount and diverse location of health services research, the comprehensiveness and validity of literature reviews cannot be taken for granted. Indeed, differences in review approaches create variations in review conclusions and present a threat to the review's validity.

This section presents an alternative research review process that is more systematic and objective. Specifically, there are five integrated steps in research reviews: identifying the topic, preparing a coding sheet, searching for research publications, synthesizing research publications, and reporting previous research on the selected topic. Adopting these procedures will make research review systematic and thus replicable, satisfying an important principle of scientific inquiry.

Identifying the Topic

Similar to empirical research, research review starts with topic identification. The choice of a topic for review is influenced by the interests of the researcher and the research community. In addition, the topic should have appeared in the literature for some time. A topic is probably not suitable for independent review unless there is sufficient research activity surrounding it. Similar to empirical research, the identification of a topic is also influenced by the literature review process. Researchers may encounter additional elements of a topic that were not initially identified but were considered relevant.

To assist topic identification, researchers may conduct a preliminary review of a dozen or so representative works on the topic. Such a process enables reviewers to ascertain the scope of research related to the topic, identify all needed information for the review, and further refine the topic. Generally, reviewers should adopt a broader rather than narrower definition of their topic so that worthy studies are not overlooked. If a topic has a long history within a discipline, it is likely that relevant reviews of the topic have already been conducted. These past reviews should be previewed early in the review process. A number of purposes are served in examining past reviews. Past reviews enable researchers to identify relevant bibliographies. Studying previous reviews is also consistent with the cumulative nature of scientific inquiry. Researchers will have a better sense of the scope of research based on past reviews than on individual studies. Past reviews also establish the necessity of a new review. If the topic has been recently reviewed and the approach of review was appropriate, there may be little value for another review. On the other hand, if previous reviews were conducted many years ago and many recent studies were not included, or the methodology employed in the review was problematic, reviewers will have added incentive to conduct a more current and improved review. Past reviews, thus, become the stepping stones for the new review.

Preparing a Coding Sheet

Once the topic is identified and refined, the next step is to construct a coding sheet for research review. The coding sheet will be used to collect relevant information from articles to be reviewed. The preparation of a coding sheet is all the more necessary if there are vast number of studies to be reviewed. A coding sheet enables reviewers to collect all needed information during the first reading so that the time-consuming practice of rereading research reports is avoided. The preparation of a coding sheet is also useful even for relatively small number of studies because the information collected will assist the investigator in analyzing and reporting those studies.

The information to be collected in the coding sheet should be determined based on the preliminary review and the strategy to be adopted in analyzing and synthesizing studies (refer to the "Synthesizing Research Publications" section in this chapter for details). Generally, any information to be analyzed and used in the review should be collected. It is better to collect too much than too little information, because the time spent in collecting additional information during the first reading is significantly less than if the researcher would have to go back and re-retrieve new information.

Figure 4–1 shows the general categories of information related to empirical research in which a reviewer is likely to be interested. The categories include a study's back-

1. Background Information

Source _____

Author(s) _____

Title _____

Journal _____

Year _____ Volume _____ Pages _____

2. Design Information

Primary/Secondary study _____

Random/Nonrandom _____

Control/No control _____

Matching/Statistical control _____

Pretest/No pretest _____

Type(s) of intervention _____

Population _____

Sample size _____

Response rate _____

Sample characteristics _____

Sample representativeness _____

Sampling biases _____

Other _____

3. Measurement Information

Research question or hypothesis _____

Dependent variable(s) _____

Independent variable(s) _____

Validity of measures _____

Reliability of measures _____

Statistical measures _____

Model specifications _____

4. Outcome Information

Hypothesis supported or refuted _____

Significant independent variable(s) _____

Insignificant independent variable(s) _____

FIGURE 4–1 Research review coding sheet for items of general interest.

ground, design, measurement, and outcome characteristics. In the background category, source indicates the media or information channel from which a study is retrieved. In the design category, it is possible that the general categorization as presented will not be sufficient. Reviewers may then include additional interesting design characteristics (for example, whether there were any restrictions on the types of individuals sampled in the original study, when and where the study was conducted, and whether time-series or longitudinal designs were used). In the measurement category, reviewers may document the use of particular scales, available instruments, and specific features of the analytic models (e.g., number of variables used, types of measures used for the same construct, tests of interaction terms and nonlinearity). In the outcome category, if more quantitative analysis is envisioned, more precise statistical information related to study results may be recorded. Examples are means, standard deviations, sample sizes for each comparison group (to be used for effect size calculation), association between variables (e.g., correlation coefficient), values of inferential test statistics (e.g., χ^2, t ratio, F ratio), and the strength of a model (e.g., regression R^2).

It bears reemphasis that the construction of a coding sheet is the result of, rather than a prelude to, preliminary review. The development of a coding sheet forces researchers to think ahead about the review and analysis strategy and to be precise in their thinking. The first draft of the coding sheet can then be used to *pilot-test* some additional reports. If coders other than the researcher are involved, they need to be trained in terms of how to comprehend and retrieve the relevant information. In the pilot test, different coders may be asked to code the same reports. Their differences in coding may identify ambiguities in the wording. The revised coding sheet may also be sent to "experts" or colleagues knowledgeable about the topic for further comment. The returned coding sheet may be refined based on the feedback. Researchers need not be alarmed that the completed coding sheets contain many blank spaces, an indication that studies may not report everything researchers intend to find out.

Upon completion of the coding sheet, reviewers then select the key terms associated with the topic. Table 4–1 summarizes examples of some commonly used terms used in health services research as published by the National Library of Medicine (1994) in *Index Medicus*. Note the example in Table 4–1 is not a comprehensive list of all the important areas of health care. Key terms assist reviewers in identifying relevant publications related to the topic of interest.

Searching for Research Publications

Similar to empirical research, research reviews need to specify the target population from which samples are selected. The typical target population for research reviews is all previous research conducted on the topic. However, not all previous research may be accessible to reviewers either because some research reports are hard to locate or it would be too costly and time-consuming to retrieve them. Reviewers may respecify the target once the search is complete. At a minimum, sources from which studies are retrieved and the scope of the search should be specified.

In general, there are four major sources of literature for reviewers to retrieve: (1) books; (2) journals, including professional journals, published newsletters, magazines and newspapers; (3) theses, including doctoral, master's, and bachelor's theses; and (4) unpublished work, including monographs, technical reports, grant proposals, conference papers, personal manuscripts, and other unpublished materials (Rosenthal, 1991).

The ability to gain access to health services research studies has improved in the past decade. In particular, retrieval of past research work has been facilitated by prominent national databases and the computerized literature search. Among the many ways to

TABLE 4–1   Selected key terms used in health services research, *Index Medicus*

Health	Health behavior	Health benefits plan, employee
Health care costs	Health care rationing	Health care reform
Health education	Health expenditures	Health facilities
Health facilities, proprietary	Health facility administrators	Health facility closure
Health facility environment	Health facility merger	Health facility moving
Health facility planning	Health facility size	Health fairs
Health maintenance organizations	Health manpower	Health occupations
Health personnel	Health plan implementation	Health planning
Health planning guidelines	Health planning organizations	Health planning support
Health planning technical assistance	Health policy	Health priorities
Health promotion	Health resorts	Health resources
Health services	Health services accessibility	Health services for the aged
Health services, indigenous	Health services misuse	Health services needs and demands
Health services research	Health status	Health status indicators
Health surveys	Health systems agencies	Health systems plans
Hospital administration	Hospital administrators	Hospital auxiliaries
Hospital bed capacity	Hospital charges	Hospital communication systems
Hospital costs	Hospital departments	Hospital design and construction
Hospital distribution systems	Hospital information systems	Hospital mortality
Hospital patient relations	Hospital-physician joint ventures	Hospital planning
Hospital records	Hospital restructuring	Hospital shared services
Hospital shops	Hospital units	Hospital volunteers
Hospitalization	Hospitals	Hospitals, chronic disease
Hospitals, community	Hospitals, convalescent	Hospitals, county
Hospitals, district	Hospitals, Federal	Hospitals, general
Hospitals, group practice	Hospitals, maternity	Hospitals, military
Hospitals, municipal	Hospitals, osteopathic	Hospitals, packaged
Hospitals, pediatric	Hospitals, private	Hospitals, proprietary
Hospitals, psychiatric	Hospitals, public	Hospitals, religious
Hospitals, rural	Hospitals, satellite	Hospitals, special
Hospitals, state	Hospitals, teaching	Hospitals, university
Hospitals, urban	Hospitals, veterans	Hospitals, voluntary

search for reports of previously conducted studies, the most efficient method is perhaps the use of computer-based abstracting and indexing services. A brief description of some of the most frequently used abstracting and indexing services in health services research follows.

The most common on-line abstracting service is called MEDLARS (Medical Literature Analysis and Retrieval System) compiled by the National Library of Medicine for over 100 years (National Institute of Health, 1989, 1995). MEDLARS became computerized in the early 1960s and has since served as a major source of bibliographic searches for health professionals. Its written companion, *Index Medicus,* is also a very popular source for literature search. Within MEDLARS, users have access to a host of specialized databases in the field of biomedicine, health administration, cancer, population studies, medical ethics, and more. Over the years, MEDLARS has come to represent a family of databases of which **MEDLINE** became the most well known. MEDLINE is the world's leading bibliographic database of medical information, covering over 3,500 journals since 1966 and containing information found in the publications *Index Medicus, International Nursing Index,* and *Index to Dental Literature.* MEDLINE contains abstracts of articles published by the most common U.S. and international journals on medicine and health services. *HEALTH* contains bibliographic citations covering nonclinical aspects of health care delivery. The subject areas emphasized include the administration and planning of all types of health facilities, services and personnel, health insurance, health policy, and the aspects of financial management, regulation, personnel administration, quality assurance, and licensure and accreditation that apply to health care delivery.

The *Hospital Literature Index,* published by the American Hospital Association, is another popular source. It provides the primary guide to literature on hospital and other health care facility administration, including multi-institutional systems, nursing homes and skilled nursing facilities, health maintenance organizations and other group practice facilities, freestanding facilities (e.g., surgicenters and emergicenters), health care centers of all types (e.g., academic, community, and mental health), rehabilitation centers, hospices, mobile health units, homes for the aged, and university student inpatient facilities (American Hospital Association Resource Center, 1994). The *Index* covers the organization and administration, economics, laws and regulations, policy, and planning aspects of health care delivery. The *Index* has been published quarterly since 1945.

The *Abstract of Health Care Management Studies,* an international journal with abstracts of studies of management, planning, and public policy related to the delivery of health care, aims at finding significant new studies in health care management, published or unpublished, assembling current information from journals and other pertinent literature, and publishing abstracts of studies to keep researchers and practitioners up to date on the work in the field, along with sources from which documents may be ordered (Foundation of the American College of Healthcare Executives, annual). The

Abstract is developed by the Program and Bureau of Hospital Administration, School of Public Health, the University of Michigan.

Public Health, Social Medicine and Epidemiology contains such topics as biostatistics and biometrics, health care (health education and promotion, professional education, and medical practice), epidemiology, screening and prevention, populations at risk (maternal and child health, aging and old age, and occupational health), food and nutrition, lifestyles (alcohol, smoking, drugs, health behavior, sexual and social behavior, and life events), and evaluation of intervention. The *Abstract* is prepared by the International Medical Abstracting Service (address: Excerpta Medica, P.O. Box 548, 1000 AM Amsterdam, the Netherlands).

NTIS Alert: Health Care covers such areas as community and population characteristics, data and information systems, economics and sociology, environmental and occupational factors, health care delivery organization and administration, health care measurement methodology, health care needs and demands, health care technology, health delivery plans, projects and studies, health education and personnel training, health-related costs, health resources, and health services. This publication is prepared by the National Technical Information Service, U.S. Department of Commerce, Technology Administration (address: Springfield, VA 22161; telephone: 703-467-4650).

The federal government, through its many agencies, also publishes many research reports and bibliographies. Most government documents are printed by the U.S. Government Printing Office, which issues a monthly catalogue that indexes recently published documents. The publication *Guide to U.S. Government Publications* provides an excellent introduction to potential reviewers. State governments have likewise published many research works that may be obtained from libraries or state agencies.

There are also many abstracting services that focus on general social science disciplines rather than exclusively on health. Many relevant health services research publications may be retrieved from these popular sources. For example, the *Social Sciences Citation Index* covers 50 different social science disciplines and carries over 1,500 journals. It categorizes studies based on the work cited in them as well as their topical focus. Thus, reviewers can retrieve studies that cite principal researchers in an area and screen them for topic relevance. *Psychological Abstracts* is frequently used in the behavioral sciences. Published monthly, the abstracts are generally written by authors of the articles themselves, although indexing terms are applied by the staff. All psychology-related journals are covered. *Dissertation Abstracts International* focuses exclusively on abstracts of dissertations regardless of discipline.

Although abstracting and indexing services are the major source for literature search, they are by no means the only ones used. Browsing through library shelves, obtaining topical bibliographies compiled by others, and formal requests of scholars active in the field are some of the examples. Many researchers have the habit of keeping personal "libraries" where they keep track of publications related to the topics of interest to them. Most scholars follow particular journals and keep abreast with current publications.

Professional conferences also provide excellent opportunities for scholars to exchange research experience and keep informed of what others are doing. Another popular retrieval method is to track the bibliographies in already-obtained studies. These methods, while convenient, share a potential bias: the lack of representativeness. The number of journals individuals can follow is limited. Locating bibliographies from available studies is likely to overrepresent publications that appear in particular journals. Another bias, one that affects those relying on abstracting services as well as other methods, is that published studies may be significantly different from nonpublished studies. Studies get published not solely because of scientific merit but also due to significance of findings. The tendency of many journals to favor significant findings is harmful to the truthful representation of scientific facts. Practitioners may be disheartened to find their efforts fail even though they have followed the steps of reported research without knowing that many similar attempts have been unsuccessful and unpublished. Researchers have the duty to caution readers about this flaw in the publication media, if they are not capable of overcoming it.

While it is good to be comprehensive, reviewers should also be prepared to complete the search process. The number of studies reviewed can vary significantly, depending partly on the topic and partly on reviewers' assiduity in tracking down relevant literature. The adequacy of literature search is not so much determined by the sheer number of studies retrieved as by the representativeness of those studies. Since abstracting services contain most journals in the field, they are believed to generate more representative studies than other methods. A proper protection against inadequate collection would be to include at least one major computer-based retrieval system (e.g., MEDLINE) and a couple of informal methods such as reviewing personal collections and bibliographies from available studies. Regardless of the search methods employed, reviewers should be explicit about how their search was conducted, including a discussion about the sources used, years covered, and key terms applied. Such information would enable others to retrieve similar studies, thus assuring replicability. The validity of the review can also be judged against the source materials covered in the search.

Upon completing the literature search, the reviewer has a list of titles and abstracts of studies related to the topic of interest. The next step is to obtain copies of the full-length articles and reports. Generally, the investigator's institutional library is the first place to start. However, it is possible that some articles and reports cannot be located there. A number of approaches may then be used to retrieve these studies. The reviewer can use an interlibrary loan service, available in most libraries. Contacting original authors directly to request reprints of studies and reports is another option. Dissertations may also be purchased from University Microfilms International in Ann Arbor, Michigan. Time and cost will be important factors affecting the extent of the retrieval effort. If some studies are deemed unretrievable either because they are too expensive or time-consuming to obtain, the reviewer needs to document the search effort and the percentage of studies unable to be retrieved due to various factors.

After copies of the original studies are obtained, the reviewer will have an opportunity to judge whether these studies are truly relevant to the review being conducted. Both inclusion and exclusion criteria must be explicitly stated. Commonly used exclusion criteria include wrong subject matter (i.e., title and abstract may not fully reflect the contents of the paper), flawed design (e.g., questions untestable by the methods adopted; study instrument, target population, or data sets cannot provide answers to the questions posed; poorly chosen samples; inappropriate comparison groups; too small sample size), and flawed analysis (e.g., no description about statistical procedures used, statistical tests unsuitable for the data, results not presented, or presented results are inconsistent). Such information will be valuable in reporting reviews. If researchers work as a team, all should be involved to set up the inclusion and exclusion criteria but apply the criteria to the articles independently before comparing the outcome and reconciling the differences.

Synthesizing Research Publications

There is a close relation between synthesizing and coding studies. Before studies can be synthesized, they need to be properly coded. The proper coding of studies relies on knowledge about how the studies will eventually be analyzed and synthesized. Thus, even though analysis and synthesis are performed much later, the strategy needs to be delineated before the coding sheet is designed.

Coding accuracy is important, especially when a large number of studies are involved and the coders have limited research background. A code book that provides definitions of the codes may be necessary to accompany the coding sheet. Coders need to be trained and monitored. Intercoder reliability may be checked by having different coders code the same studies. Coding may not start until a high level of coding reliability is established.

Synthesizing research publications entails categorizing a series of related studies, analyzing and interpreting their findings, and summarizing those findings into unified statements about the topic being reviewed. The traditional approach that focuses on a few selected studies places little or imprecise weight on the volume of available studies and fails to portray accurately the accumulated state of knowledge. Lack of standardization in how reviewers arrive at specific conclusions calls into question the validity of the review. Properly conducted, synthesizing research publications is a systematic process that integrates both quantitative and qualitative strategies.

Quantitative Procedures

The application of quantitative procedures in research review serves a number of purposes. Quantitative approaches tend to be more standardized, less subjective, and hence less subject to bias. The application of the quantitative review is also a response to the ever expanding literature base. Researchers' understanding of a topic can be improved by analyzing and synthesizing the results of many studies. Appropriately used, quantitative research review provides an integrated summary of research results on a specific topic and enables the reviewer to capture the findings of all relevant studies in an objective fashion.

The term that describes quantitative approaches to reviewing related studies is called **meta-analysis** (Glass, 1977; Glass, McGaw and Smith, 1981; Fitz-Gibbon and Morris, 1987; Preiss and Allen, 1995; Bangert-Drowns, 1995; Soeken, Bausell, and Li, 1995). Meta-analysis refers to statistical analyses that combine and interpret the results of independent studies of a given scientific issue for the purpose of integrating the findings. The approach in essence treats each study in the review as a case within a sample of relevant studies and applies statistical analysis to all the cases—for example to assess whether the fact that two-thirds of all the studies reviewed found a particular (statistically significant) association is itself a statistically significant finding. It allows the reviewer to synthesize the results of numerous tests so that an overall conclusion can be drawn. Generally, meta-analytic procedures are appropriate for research syntheses of studies based on experimental and quasi-experimental designs. At a minimum, for meta-analysis to be feasible, study results should be quantitative so that they can be subject to statistical analysis. Meta-analysis is an important tool to learn not only because it facilitates quantitative review but also due to its increasing popularity (Bausell, Li, Gau, and Soeken, 1995). Investigators are likely to find that meta-analyses have been conducted in almost all areas of social inquiry. Therefore, an investigator needs to be familiar with the meta-analytic technique to interpret the review literature.

There are some fundamental assumptions related to meta-analysis (Rosenthal, 1991). First, the same conceptual hypothesis or research question is assumed for all studies combined in the analysis. Second, the separate studies included in the analysis should be independent of each other. Third, the assumptions used by primary researchers in computing the results are believed to be correct. If any of these assumptions may be challenged, then the use of meta-analysis can be problematic. The techniques described below are chosen because of their simplicity and broad applicability. Readers who want more in-depth coverage of these and many more techniques should consult a meta-analysis textbook from the suggested references at the end of this chapter. For example, see Slavin (1984), Hedges and Olkin (1985), Hedges (1985), Wolf, (1986), Fleiss and Gross (1991), Hunter (1990), Eddy (1992), and Petitti (1994).

The first thing reviewers can do is to summarize the information abstracted from the studies reviewed based on the coding sheets (see Figure 4–2). The summary permits the reviewer as well as readers to quickly compare the studies in terms of their design, measurement, and results. It is a starting point for further in-depth analysis and discussion by the reviewer.

Next, the reviewer may conduct a more refined subgroup analysis, that is, group the studies into comparable categories based on a number of criteria. Examples include: (1)

Studies	1	2	3	4	5	...	N
1. Background Information							
First author	——	——	——	——	——		
Journal	——	——	——	——	——		
Year	——	——	——	——	——		
2. Design Information							
Primary/Secondary study	——	——	——	——	——		
Random/Nonrandom	——	——	——	——	——		
Control/No control	——	——	——	——	——		
Matching/Statistical control	——	——	——	——	——		
Pretest/No pretest	——	——	——	——	——		
Intervention(s)	——	——	——	——	——		
Population	——	——	——	——	——		
Sample size	——	——	——	——	——		
Response rate	——	——	——	——	——		
Sample characteristics	——	——	——	——	——		
Sample representativeness	——	——	——	——	——		
Sampling biases	——	——	——	——	——		
3. Measurement Information							
Research question or hypothesis	——	——	——	——	——		
Dependent variable(s)	——	——	——	——	——		
Independent variable(s)	——	——	——	——	——		
Statistical measures	——	——	——	——	——		
Model specifications	——	——	——	——	——		
4. Outcome Information							
Hypothesis supported or refuted	——	——	——	——	——		
Significant variable(s)	——	——	——	——	——		
Insignificant variable(s)	——	——	——	——	——		
R^2	——	——	——	——	——		
5. Other	——	——	——	——	——		

FIGURE 4–2   Summary presentation of studies reviewed.

same or similar hypotheses being tested, (2) comparable study design, (3) comparable population even though actual samples are different, and (4) similar statistics presented in the reports or available to the reviewers. Studies that share similar characteristics can then be summarized and analyzed together. The results of the subgroup analysis can be compared with the analysis done on the total studies. Such a comparison enables reviewers to evaluate whether sources and quality of research are significantly related to differences in results. If they are, reviewers can present the meta-analytic results separately for different sources of information and different levels of quality of research.

If the findings with respect to particular variables are mixed, that is, some studies indicate a positive impact whereas others show a negative impact, the reviewer may conduct a simple vote counting using a sign test to assess whether observed differences are significant (Cooper, 1989). In Formula 4.1, z_{sign} is a z score for the sign test, N_p refers to the number of studies with positive findings, and N_t refers to the total number of studies, including both positive and negative findings. The z score can be referred to a standard z table to find the associated probability.

$$z_{sign} = \frac{(N_p) - (\frac{1}{2}N_t)}{\frac{1}{2}\sqrt{N_t}} \qquad (4.1)$$

For example, if 20 among 25 studies find results in the positive direction, the z score will be 3 $\{[20 - (\frac{1}{2} \times 25)] \div \frac{1}{2}\sqrt{25})\}$ and the associated probability is less than .01, indicating the probability that the positive and negative directions have an equal chance to occur in the population is highly unlikely. Thus we are more confident about the positive impact of the variable of interest. The reviewer needs to be aware that the assumption in the sign test is that the studies are comparable. Otherwise, weighting is necessary to take into account of different sample sizes and/or qualities of study.

The most popular as well as important meta-analysis procedure is called **effect size** analysis (Fitz-Gibbon and Morris, 1987). Effect size may be defined as the size or strength of the impact of one factor on another. There are many ways to calculate effect size. The examples cited here may be used to summarize the results of studies in which there was some kind of control or comparison group so that an effect size can be calculated for each study. The concept of an effect size implies that there is a "true" population value for the effect of something and each time we run an experiment we obtain one sample of this effect. A researcher can expect the obtained effect size to fluctuate around the population value just as sample means fluctuate around the "true" population mean.

The first step to compute an effect size is to identify the effect size to be investigated. An example is weight loss due to exercise in the experiment group but not in the control group. The second step is the actual computation of an effect size for each study reviewed. The following formulas (4.2–4.4) may be used depending on which information is available in the published reports.

$$\text{Effect Size} = \frac{(\text{mean } y \text{ for } E\text{-group}) - (\text{mean } y \text{ for } C\text{-group})}{SD \text{ of } y} \qquad (4.2)$$

$$\text{Effect Size} = t\sqrt{(1/n_E) + (1/n_C)} \qquad (4.3)$$

$$\text{Effect Size} = \frac{2r}{\sqrt{1 - r^2}} \qquad (4.4)$$

In Formula 4.2, y stands for the outcome measure (weight) that is affected by the program or the "treatment" received (exercise) by the experimental group (E-group) but not by the control group (C-group). SD of y stands for the pooled standard deviation of y (or the average standard deviation of the two groups), which may be retrieved directly from the reports.

In situations where data have already been processed, the effect size can be computed based on the given information. Formula 4.3 assumes that t values are calculated and presented. In the formula, n_E is the sample size for the experiment group, and n_C for the control group. Formula 4.4 uses correlation between y (weight change) and group membership (experiment versus control).

The substantive interpretation of the size of the effect may be made by reference to other information. For example, have there been previous meta-analyses with which findings of this study can be compared? At the time of the study, what is in the literature about this intervention? The most informative interpretation occurs when an effect size is compared with other effect sizes using similar variables. Cohen (1988) has suggested that effect sizes of about 0.20 are small, 0.50 are medium, and 0.80 are large. The practical significance of effect size needs to be taken into account in interpreting effect size. The same effect size of life saved is certainly more significant than number of pounds lost. Effect size may also be converted into dollar figures to highlight the significance. For example, 0.3 hospitalization days averted may translate into hundreds of dollars saved per person.

The standard error measures how accurately the effect size has been measured. Formula 4.5 may be used to calculate the standard error. The smaller the standard error, the more accurate is the measurement. The 95 percent confidence interval of an effect size may be calculated using Formula 4.6. The reviewer may graphically display effect sizes calculated for different studies with effect sizes displayed at the vertical axis and studies on the horizontal axis. The graphical display presents an informative summary of the distribution of effect sizes.

$$ES \text{ for Effect Size} = e = \sqrt{ES^2/2(n_E + n_C) + [(1/n_E) + (1/n_C)]} \qquad (4.5)$$

$$\text{Effect Size} + 1.96e \text{ and Effect Size} - 1.96e \qquad (4.6)$$

Once the reviewer has calculated effect sizes for all studies, she or he then averages these effects to obtain the mean. A mean effect size based on all studies calculated may also be computed using Formula 4.7 where ES refers to the effect size, and w is a weight. Since effect sizes likely come from studies with very different sample sizes, it is a common practice to weigh individual effect sizes based on the number of subjects in their respective samples.

$$\text{Mean of } ES = \frac{\Sigma w \times ES}{\Sigma w} \qquad\qquad \text{where} \quad w = \frac{1}{e^2} \qquad\qquad (4.7)$$

To test for homogeneity of effect sizes (H), that is, whether obtained effect sizes were random samples estimating a single effect size (appearing homogeneous) or coming from different populations (appearing heterogeneous), researchers use Formula 4.8. The result of the homogeneity test will be compared with a chi-square for $df = k - 1$, where k is the number of studies. If the value is larger than the critical value in the chi-square table, the result becomes significant and suggests the effect sizes did not appear to come from a single population value (i.e., heterogeneous). The homogeneity statistic indicates whether an intervention has a consistent impact on an outcome variable.

$$H = \Sigma(ES - \text{Mean of } ES)^2 \times w \qquad\qquad \text{where} \quad w = \frac{1}{e^2} \qquad\qquad (4.8)$$

Table 4–2 applies the above formulas with a research review example about the impact of a health promotion exercise intervention on weight loss among overweight adults. The example uses five studies and assumes only sample size and t statistic information are available from the reports.

Meta-analysis is proposed as a more rigorous approach to research reviews, but it does not entirely resolve the question of partial or selective coverage. Further, different quantitative procedures employed by reviewers may create variations in the conclusions of reviews. Meta-analysis is merely a useful tool. Its successful application hinges on an extensive and systematic literature search and the presence of sufficient quantitative information in published reports. To make computations possible, authors should routinely report the exact test statistics (e.g., r, t, F, z) along with their degrees of freedom and sample sizes. Editors and reviewers should also require the reporting of these statistics.

A common criticism of meta-analysis is that poor studies are summarized together with good ones. To adjust for study quality, a system of weighting can be used. A weight of zero can be assigned to a study of extremely poor quality. A study twice as good as the average can be weighed twice as heavily. However, weighting itself may introduce bias if researchers assign heavier weight only to studies whose results they favor and lower weights to those they oppose. A more objective way would be to have each study weighed by "outside" experts who do not have a vested interest. Or, if reviewers were to weigh themselves, they could weigh each study twice, once after reading only the design section of the study, the other after reading both the design and results. The reason for the first weighting is to insure that one weighting is made uninfluenced by the results of the study. If both weightings are comparable, there is less likelihood for bias to be introduced associated with weighting.

TABLE 4–2 Example of effect size analysis

Studies	1	2	3	4	5	Total
n (Experiment)	100	150	200	250	300	
n (Control)	100	150	200	250	300	
$(1/n_E) + (1/n_C)$	0.02	0.01	0.01	0.01	0.01	
t	4.86	2.32	5.14	3.50	10.20	
ES	**0.69**	**0.27**	**0.51**	**0.31**	**0.83**	
$ES\backslash 2$	0.47	0.07	0.26	0.10	0.69	
$2(n_E + n_C)$	400	600	800	1000	1200	
$(1/n_E) + (1/n_C)$	0.02	0.01	0.01	0.01	0.01	
SE for ES = e	**0.15**	**0.12**	**0.10**	**0.09**	**0.09**	
$ES + 1.96e$	0.97	0.50	0.71	0.49	1.00	
$ES - 1.96e$	0.40	0.04	0.32	0.14	0.67	
95% CI of ES	**(0.97,**	**(0.50,**	**(0.71,**	**(0.49,**	**(1.0,**	
	0.40)	**0.04)**	**0.32)**	**0.14)**	**0.67)**	
w	47.21	74.33	96.80	123.49	138.03	479.87
$w \times ES$	32.45	19.91	49.76	38.66	114.96	255.73
Mean of ES						**0.53**
$(ES - \text{Mean of } ES)$	0.15	-0.27	-0.02	-0.22	0.30	
$(ES - \text{Mean of } ES)^2$	0.02	0.07	0.00	0.05	0.09	
$(ES - \text{Mean of } ES)^2 \times w$	1.13	5.22	0.04	5.97	12.42	
Homogeneity						**24.77**

Qualitative Procedures

Even though quantitative approaches are preferred in research reviews, there are circumstances in which the use of quantitative procedures is inappropriate. A basic premise of quantitative approaches is that the studies reviewed address an identical conceptual hypothesis. If studies address different hypotheses, although related to the same topic, quantitative methods may not be appropriate.

Quantitative approaches are likely to gloss over details, ignoring idiosyncrasies related to differences among studies. The reviewer should be aware that not all studies are of the same quality. Studies can be incomplete in their description of design, measurement, and results. Incomplete description of statistical values will affect the performance of quantitative synthesis. Reporting errors may be found in statistical analyses. Inconsistency may be noted between results reported in the tables and in the text. When studies present insufficient statistical information or when there are obvious errors in the choice of statistical procedures as well as calculations, the reviewer cannot use quantitative approaches.

The qualitative approach to research review aims at overcoming the deficiencies associated with the quantitative approach. Specifically, qualitative narratives provide an opportunity for the reviewer to address the nonquantifiable features of the study, such as settings and background, interesting anecdotes and cases, as well as the historic evolution of the topic. The qualitative approach is frequently used in theoretical reviews where relevant theories are compared and summarized. The implications of the results and their policy relevancy may be analyzed using qualitative approach. In sum, a complete research review should integrate both quantitative and qualitative approaches.

Reporting Previous Research

In reporting the findings of a research review, the reviewer may follow a similar format used in reporting empirical research, including such sections as introduction, methods, results, and discussion. The introduction section presents an overview of the theoretical and conceptual issues related to the topic and summarizes previous reviews on the topic and issues left unresolved. The methods section describes specific steps in literature search and specific approaches adopted in analyzing and integrating study results. The results section provides a sense of the representativeness of the sampled reviews and presents cumulative findings on the literature reviewed. The discussion section serves to summarize the major findings, draw implications of the findings, and suggest direction for future research.

Specifically, in the introduction section, the reviewer reports: (1) the research topic or problem and its significance, (2) a historical overview of the theoretical issues related to the topic, (3) a historical overview of the methodological issues related to the topic, (4) historical debate surrounding the topic, (5) summary of previous reviews on the topic and highlights of the findings, and (6) the need for the current review as a result of unresolved controversies surrounding the topic, new development of issues related to the topic, and/or significant increases in recent studies on the topic.

In the methods section, the reviewer reports: (1) sources from which studies were retrieved, including which abstract and indexing services were used, which bibliographies were consulted, which years were covered during the search, which key terms were used to assist the search, which other informal sources were consulted, and the percentage distribution of materials selected from each of the sources; (2) inclusion and exclusion criteria for selecting studies to be reviewed, an assessment of the impact of these criteria (e.g., how many studies were excluded by each criterion), and how these criteria were actually applied (e.g., how many studies were included and excluded from reading the titles, abstracts, and the full texts, respectively); (3) a summary of the different hypotheses or research questions related to the topic; (4) a systematic review of the different prototypes of studies reviewed, including descriptions of designs, population and sample characteristics, variables, models, and statistics applied; and (5) a discussion of specific approaches (e.g., meta-analytic techniques) used in analyzing, integrating, and synthesizing study findings, the statistics needed for applying these techniques, whether weights were assigned and if so, how, and how missing information was handled.

In the results section, the reviewer records: (1) descriptive results of the studies reviewed, including types of studies, sources of studies, publication dates, hypotheses or research questions, population and samples, measurement characteristics, and the like; (2) the results of each hypothesis and/or research question tested, along with a breakdown of the relationship between results and different types of studies (e.g., published versus nonpublished, experiment versus nonexperiment, random versus nonrandom, etc.); (3) results of other tests conducted (e.g., vote counts, effect size analysis, etc.); and (4) a qualitative summary of findings not captured in the quantitative analysis.

In the discussion section, the reviewer records: (1) a summary of major findings of the research review; (2) a comparison of current findings with previous reviews, if available; (3) a discussion of the theoretical and practical implications of the findings; (4) a summary of the limitations of the current review; and (5) a discussion of the direction for future research surrounding the topic reviewed.

STRENGTHS AND WEAKNESSES

The principal strength of research review is its contribution to the advance of scientific knowledge. Scientific knowledge is cumulative knowledge and research review provides a critical assessment of the state of research related to a given topic, thus suggesting fruitful direction for future research. Research review based on a systematic rather than an idiosyncratic approach is important to maintaining the credibility of conclusions, particularly at a time when research review plays an increasing role in the definition of knowledge.

Research review also has the advantage of being efficient. Money spent in retrieving studies is usually far less than in collecting primary data. The staff necessary to carry out the review is far less than in most primary studies. The time requirement for research review is also significantly less demanding than for primary research. In addition, the schedule is more predictable and less subject to outside factors.

The principal disadvantage of research review is that it is constrained by the materials available for review. Inconsistencies, missing information, and many other quality variations among published reports invariably create problems for the reviewer. Assumptions have to be made and compromises sought to make use of current studies. Research review on some topics may not be feasible if a limited number of studies have been conducted on these topics.

Some of the limitations of research review represent pervasive concerns in primary research as well. For example, when the reviewer encounters access problems, particularly to unpublished studies, that could have a significant bearing on the outcome of the review, the representativeness of the research review is threatened. The cost of data collection, even though significantly less than most primary studies, would be much higher based on the approaches specified in this chapter than based on traditional approach. Should a researcher with limited funding be discouraged from undertaking research review? Certainly not. Just as primary research can never be perfect, the perfect review is merely an ideal. The steps are presented as guidelines, not prerequisites, for conducting research review. They may also assist us in assessing reviews conducted by others.

SUMMARY

Research review is an efficient method of synthesizing existing knowledge on a topic. It can be used both as part of an empirical investigation or independently, focusing on theories, methodology, or policies. The integrative research review, the most commonly used review, consists of five integrated steps including identifying the topic, preparing a coding sheet, searching for research publications, synthesizing research publications, and reporting previous research on the selected topic. Properly used, these steps will make research review systematic and replicable, contributing to the advancement of scientific knowledge.

Key Terms

research review
theoretical review
policy-oriented review
meta-analysis

integrative research review
methodological review
MEDLINE
effect size

Review Questions

1. What are the types of research reviews and their respective purposes?

2. Identify commonly used computerized abstracting and indexing services used in health services research.

3. What are the strengths and weaknesses of research review as a scientific inquiry?

4. Do the following exercise as a way to learn the process of research review. The purpose of this exercise is to conduct an integrative research review on a health services research topic of interest to you. Your review should follow the five-step process delineated in this chapter. It is possible that the class may be divided into groups with each member of a group responsible for one step of the process.

   First, conduct a preliminary review to identify the topic to be reviewed.

   Second, prepare a coding sheet based on the preliminary review, pilot-test the coding sheet using additional studies, and then revise the coding sheet.

   Third, ascertain the key terms used in your search. You may want to consult *Index Medicus* or other index publications for verification. Identify a computer-based abstracting service available in your library (e.g., MEDLINE) and conduct the search using your key terms. You may want to limit your initial search to a few years. Perform a parallel manual search and compare the differences between the two approaches.

Fourth, record relevant study information on the coding sheets. If feasible, have different coders code the same studies and compare the results. If there are too many differences between the coders, you may want to revise the coding sheet or design a code book that accompanies the coding sheet. Then recode the articles.

Fifth, based on the information abstracted on the coding sheets, prepare a summary table of the major variables of interest. If applicable, conduct an effect size analysis using the formulas and the example from Table 4.2 as a reference. Make qualitative assessments of the studies being reviewed, in particular, focusing on the uniqueness of study settings, interventions, and sample characteristics.

Finally, prepare a formal report of your review using the following sections: introduction, methods, results, and discussion. Consult the relevant sections for contents to be included in the review.

REFERENCES

American Hospital Association Resource Center. (1994). *Hospital Literature Index.* Chicago, IL: American Hospital Association, quarterly.

Bangert-Drowns, R. L. (1995). Misunderstanding meta-analysis. *Evaluation and the Health Professions,* 18, 304–314.

Bausell, R. B., Li, Y. F., Gau, M. L., and Soeken, K. L. (1995). The growth of meta-analytic literature from 1980 to 1993. *Evaluation and the Health Professions,* 18, 238–251.

Cohen, J. (1988). *Statistical Power Analysis for the Behavioral Sciences.* 2nd ed. New York: Academic Press.

Cooper, H. M. (1982). Scientific guidelines for conducting integrative research reviews. *Review of Educational Research,* 52, 291–302.

Cooper, H. M. (1989a). *Integrating Research: A Guide for Literature Reviews.* 2nd ed. Newbury Park, CA: Sage.

Cooper, H.M. (1989b). The structure of knowledge synthesis: A taxonomy of literature reviews. *Knowledge in Society,* 1, 104–126.

Eddy, D. M. (1992). *Meta-analysis by the Confidence Profile Method: The Statistical Synthesis of Evidence.* Boston: Academic Press.

Fitz-Gibbon, C. T., and Morris, L. L. (1987) *How to Analyze Data.* Newbury Park, CA: Sage.

Fleiss J. L., and Gross A. J. (1991). Meta-analysis in epidemiology, with special reference to studies of the association between exposure to environmental tobacco smoke and lung cancer: A critique. *Journal of Clinical Epidemiology,* 44, 127–139.

Foundation of the American College of Healthcare Executives. (annual). *Abstracts of Health Care Management Studies*. Ann Arbor, MI: Health Administration Press.

Glass, G. (1977). Integrating findings: The meta-analysis of research. In *Review of Research in Education*, Vol. 5. Itasca, IL: F. E. Peacock.

Glass, G., McGaw, B., and Smith, M. (1981). *Meta-analysis in Social Research*. Beverly Hills, CA: Sage.

Harper, R., Weins, A., and Matarazzo, J. (1978). *Nonverbal Communication: The State of the Art*. New York: John Wiley.

Hedges, L. V. (1985). *Statistical Methods for Meta-analysis*. Orlando, FL: Academic Press.

Hedges, L. V., and Olkin, I. (1985). Statistical Methods for Meta-analysis. New York: Academic Press.

Hunter, J. F. (1990). *Methods of Meta-analysis: Correcting Error and Bias in Research Findings*. Newbury Park: Sage.

National Institute of Health. (1989). *National Library of Medicine: MEDLARS*. (Publication no. 89-1286). Bethesda, MD: U.S. DHHS, Public Health Service, August.

National Institute of Health. (1995). *National Library of Medicine: Fact Sheet*. Bethesda, MD: U.S. DHHS, Public Health Service, February.

National Library of Medicine. (1994). *Index Medicus: Subject Section*. (Publication no. 94-252, vol. 35, no. 6). Bethesda, MD: U.S. DHHS, Public Health Service, June.

Petitti, D. B. (1994). *Meta-analysis, Decision Analysis, and Cost-Effectiveness Analysis: Methods for Quantitative Synthesis in Medicine*. New York: Oxford University Press.

Preiss, R. W., and Allen, M. (1995). Understanding and using meta-analysis. *Evaluation and the Health Professions*, 18, 315–335.

Rosenthal, R. (1991). *Meta-analytic Procedures for Social Research*. Newbury Park, CA: Sage.

Slavin, R. E. (1984). Meta-analysis in education: How has it been used? *Educational Researcher*, 13, 6–15, 24–27.

Soeken, K. L., Bausell, R. B., and Li, Y. F. (1995). Realizing the meta-analytic potential: A survey of experts. *Evaluation and the Health Professions*, 18, 336–344.

Wolf, F. M. (1986). *Meta-analysis: Quantitative Methods for Research Synthesis*. (QASS series 07-059). Beverly Hills, CA: Sage.

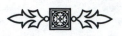

CHAPTER

5

Secondary Analysis

LEARNING OBJECTIVES

- To become familiar with the types of secondary analysis.
- To identify the general categories of secondary data sources.
- To describe administrative records research analysis, content analysis, published statistics analysis, and historical analysis.
- To understand the strengths and weaknesses of secondary analysis.

DEFINITION

Secondary analysis is any reanalysis of data collected by another researcher or organization, including the analysis of data sets collated from a variety of sources to create time-series or area-based data sets (Singleton, Straits, and Straits, 1993; Stewart and Kamins, 1993). Secondary analysis is commonly applied to quantitative data from previous studies.

Secondary analysis differs from **primary research** in that primary research involves firsthand collection of data by the researcher or research team. The data are gathered through the research and did not exist prior to the research. By contrast, secondary analysis uses available data collected by other researcher(s) for completely different research purposes or not for any research purpose at all. Since secondary analysis does not require researchers to have contact with subjects, it is sometimes referred to as nonreactive or unobstrusive research.

TYPES

There are several ways to classify the types of secondary analysis. The classification may be based on the number of databases used both cross-sectionally and longitudinally, the sources of data, and the methods adopted to analyze secondary data.

Number of Databases Used

The simplest approach is to use a single data set, either to replicate the original researcher's results or to address entirely different research questions. A second approach is to use a single data set that is extended by the addition of data from other sources, thus providing a richer and more comprehensive basis for the secondary analysis study. The more complex secondary analysis involves the use of multiple data sets, to provide an overall assessment of findings on a topic.

Secondary data sets may be cross-sectional, capturing one moment in time, or longitudinal, recording data elements over a series of time periods. Most secondary data sets are designed to study some phenomenon by taking a cross section of it at one time and analyzing that cross section carefully. Exploratory and descriptive studies are often cross-sectional. Many explanatory studies are also cross-sectional. Explanatory cross-sectional studies have an inherent problem. Typically, their aim is to understand causal processes that occur over time, yet their conclusions are based on observations made at only one point in time.

Longitudinal studies are designed to permit observations over an extended period. Three special types of longitudinal studies are **trend,** cohort, and **panel studies.** Trend studies are those that study changes within some general population over time. Examples would be a comparison of U.S. health care expenditure, utilization, and outcomes over time, showing the extent of compatibility. Cohort studies examine more specific sub-populations (cohorts) as they change over time. Typically, a **cohort** is an age group, such as those people born during the same year, but it can also be based on some other time grouping, such as people discharged from the same hospital, having the same insurance coverage, and so forth. Panel studies are similar to trend and cohort studies except that the same set of people is studied each time.

In general, it is more difficult to find multiple data sets over a series of time periods than to find one such data set. Longitudinal studies have an obvious advantage over cross-sectional ones in providing information describing processes over time. But often this advantage comes at a heavy cost in both time and money, especially in a large-scale survey. Panel studies, which offer the most comprehensive data on changes over time, face a special problem: panel attrition. Some of the respondents studied in the first wave of the survey may not participate in later waves. The danger is that those who drop out of the study may not be typical, thereby distorting the results of the study. Another potential problem occurs when questions have been altered from one study to the next so that the questions for different waves may not be entirely comparable. The problem does not always disappear even when questions remain constant, because the meaning of concepts may have changed over time, so that the same question may not be measuring the same concept. A good example is the reduced buying power of the U.S. dollars. Comparisons of total national health expenditures across different years would be less meaningful if the dollars were not adjusted for inflation. In using published time series data, researchers need to be aware that the earliest points in their series may be composed of corrected data while more recent points in their series may be uncorrected or partially corrected. Greater errors may be contained in the latter than in the former.

Sources of Data

The variety of secondary data is tremendous. A secondary data source may be classified as produced either specifically for a research purpose or not for a research purpose.

Research-Oriented Secondary Data

Research-oriented secondary data include all data sets collected by others for research rather than other purposes. There are numerous examples of such secondary data sets. Chapter 3, where available data sources were introduced, enumerated some regularly collected data sets by government agencies (in particular, the National Center for Health Services Research), including the Area Resource File, National Ambulatory Medical Care Survey, National Health Interview Survey, National Hospital Discharge Survey, National Medical Care Expenditure Survey, to name just a few. These data sets are stored on computer tapes that are available for public use, often for a fee. Additional data sources can be found in the *Social Science Data Archives*.

The fundamental difference between research- and nonresearch-oriented secondary data has to do with quality both in terms of data collection and documentation. Research-oriented data sets were generally collected according to strict scientific procedures of sampling and measurement. To the extent errors occur, they were more likely to be properly documented. Nonresearch-oriented data sets are comparatively less strict on both accounts. The sampling procedures may be inaccurate and measurement may be idiosyncratic rather than tested. Incomplete or missing data are also more common. Documentation of data collection procedures and measurement are less refined. Thus, extra caution needs to be taken when researchers use secondary data that were not collected for research purposes.

Nonresearch-Oriented Secondary Data

Nonresearch-oriented secondary data include public documents, official records, private documents and records, mass media, and physical, nonverbal materials. **Records** are systematic accounts of regular occurrences. Examples of public documents and official records include proceedings of government bodies, court records, state laws, city ordinances, directories, almanacs, and publication indexes such as the *New York Times Index* and *The Reader's Guide to Periodic Literature* (Stewart and Kamins, 1993; Singleton, Straits, and Straits, 1993). Private documents and records refer to information produced by individuals or organizations about their own activities, including diaries, letters, notes, personnel and sales records, inventories, tax records, and patient records. Examples of mass media include television, newspaper, radio, periodicals, movies, and so on. Examples of physical, nonverbal materials consist of works of art (paintings and pictures), artifacts, and household collections.

Of particular interest to health services researches with regard to government documents are the numerous volumes of official statistics such as vital statistics from birth, death, marriage, and divorce certificates and population demographics from census data. State laws require that all births and deaths be recorded. The variables in birth records include demographic information about the newborn child, as well as information about the parents (e.g., names of mother and father, address, age, and occupation). Death records contain biographic information of the deceased; cause of death; length of illness; whether injuries were accidental, homicidal, or self-inflicted; and the time and place of death. These data make possible research ranging from a study of fertility patterns in an area to epidemiological investigation about the incidence and prevalence of disease.

The census data, collected and maintained by the U.S. Bureau of the Census, provide detailed information about the demographic characteristics of the populations of the states, counties, metropolitan areas, cities and towns, neighborhood tracts and blocks. In addition, the Bureau of Census conducts regular censuses of business, manufacturers, and agriculture and other institutions, as well as the *Current Population Survey,* a monthly survey of a representative sample of households throughout the fifty states. These data, when used with other health-related data sets such as health services utilization, enable researchers to examine many topics central to health services research (e.g., the relationship between population characteristics and health services use).

Of particular interest to health services researches with regard to private records are administrative records kept by hospitals and other health institutions. Health-related administrative records are collections of documents containing mainly factual information compiled in a variety of ways (e.g., directly from those concerned, or indirectly from employers, doctors, and agencies acting as informants) and used by health organizations to record the development and implementation of decisions and activities that are central to their functions. Examples are health service records, insurance membership and payment records, organizational accounts and personnel records, and hospital revenues and expenditures.

The potential for research analysis of health administrative records is expanding as more organizations are transferring such records from manual systems of files, forms, and cards to computerized systems, including CD-ROM (Stewart and Kamins, 1993), in the process redesigning them as health information systems that can be analyzed quickly and routinely to produce summaries of particular aspects of the data. This also makes it easier to provide suitably anonymous extract tapes for health services research purposes. The computerization of many record systems facilitates linkages of different databases such as hospital patient records, population censuses, and sample surveys. In linking different databases or extracting the required information from records or computer files, it is essential that sufficient time and resources be allocated to the tasks of familiarization with the contents, preparation of basic or additional documentation with reference to the specific questions addressed by the study and pertinent data items, and, in some cases, sorting out whether missing values can reliably be imputed or estimated. Perhaps the most common mistake is to think of data from records as ready-to-use research data, whereas they usually require more preparation, care, and effort than an equivalent secondary analysis of a research-oriented data set.

Methods of Secondary Analysis

Methods used to analyze available data take many forms. The type of analysis chosen is usually a function of the research purpose, the design, and the nature of the data available. For example, descriptive accounts of a topic differ from tests of general hypotheses. Longitudinal designs entails different analytic methods than cross-sectional surveys. The quality of available data also dictates the proper analytic procedures to be used. When data were collected by some nonrandom means, no statistical estimates of sampling errors are possible, and the use of analytical statistics is limited. For the most part, health services researchers use quantitative methods to analyze available data. For a glimpse of some of these methods, refer to Chapter 14. In addition to those commonly used quantitative methods, there are some methods that are less frequently used by health services researchers but commonly used by other social scientists in secondary analysis.

Content analysis is a research method appropriate for studying human communication and aspects of social behavior (Carney, 1972; Krippendorff, 1980; Holsti, 1969). The basic goal is to take a verbal, nonquantitative document and transform it into quantitative data. The usual units of analysis in content analysis are words, paragraphs, books, pictures, advertisements, and television episodes. Contents can be manifest or latent. Manifest content refers to characteristics of communication that are directly visible or objectively identifiable, such as the specific words spoken or particular pictures shown. Latent content refers to the meanings contained within communications that have to be determined by the researcher. For example, what constitutes sexual harassment in the workplace? What is the process of implementing informed consent in health services organizations? Coding may be used to transform raw data into more quantitative forms that can then be counted and analyzed. The results of content analysis can generally be presented in tables containing frequencies or percentages, in the same way as survey data. Content analysis has the advantages of economy in terms of both time and money, being unobtrusive and safe, and the opportunity to study a topic over a long period of time. Its disadvantage includes the study of *recorded* communications only. Content analysis is frequently used to analyze the symbolic content of communication, especially verbal materials from the media. Content analysis may also be used in health services research. For example, the study of health legislation may illuminate everyone's understanding about why U.S. health care delivery has evolved into its current form.

Analyzing *published statistics* is another way researchers use available data (Jacob, 1984). Analyzing published statistics is different from using secondary data, because published statistics are aggregate information and cannot be traced to the individual level from which the aggregation is made. For confidentiality and privacy reasons, aggregate data may be the only available information to study a particular topic. At the least, published statistics should always be used as a supplemental evidence to the research. Examples of published statistics include *The U.S. Fact Book: The American Almanac, Demographic Yearbook* available through the United Nations, the countless data series published by various federal agencies, chamber of commerce reports on business, and public opinion surveys published by George Gallop. The unit of analysis involved in the analysis of published statistics is often not the individual but rather some aggregate elements such as countries, regions, states, counties, and cities. In using aggregate statistics, researchers should guard against committing **ecological fallacy,** which refers to the possibility that patterns found at a group level differ from those that would be found on an individual level. Thus, it is usually not appropriate to draw conclusions at the individual level based on analyzing aggregate data.

Researchers need to be assiduous in tracking down important information that may not be available in the published reports. For example, the data found in published sources are often extracted from other studies that include more information about sampling error. Consequently, the investigator needs to go to the original source cited in the report to track down more information.

The principal advantage of using published statistics is economy in terms of time and money. The principal disadvantage is the limitation of what exists. The analysis of existing statistics depends heavily on the quality of the statistics themselves. Often existing data do not cover everything the researcher is interested in, and the measurements may not be exactly valid representations of the concepts the researcher wants to draw conclusions about.

Examples of research based on published statistics include study of rates of crimes, accidents, diseases, and mortalities. Health services researchers may find data of great interest and relevance from such publications as the annual *Statistical Abstract of the United States,* published by the U.S. Department of Commerce, and *Health United States,* published by the U.S. Department of Health and Human Services. These sources facilitate comparative studies of health indicators across countries. Examples include physician–population ratio, hospital beds–population ratio, days of hospitalization per capita, death rates (number of deaths per 1,000 population) and, more specifically, infant mortality rate (the number of infants who die during their first year of life among every 1,000 births).

Historical analysis involves attempts to reconstruct past events (descriptive history) and the use of historical evidence to generate and test theories (analytical history) (Babbie, 1992). The basic evidence primarily consists of authentic documents, such as testimony, and organizational records, such as charters, policy statements, and speeches. Since historical research is largely a qualitative method, there are no easily listed steps to follow in the analysis of historical data. Generally, *verstehen* (translated loosely as "understanding") is necessary. In other words, in interpreting historical data, researchers need to mentally take on the circumstances, views, and feelings of the participants and compare and critically evaluate the relative plausibility of alternative explanations. Examples of historical analysis include the study of health-seeking patterns by different cultures, and Marmor's account of the evolution of Medicare program for the elderly (Marmor, 1970).

STRENGTHS AND WEAKNESSES

The principal advantage of secondary analysis is economy, achieved through money, time, and personnel saved in data collection and management. For example, administrative records can be used for research and evaluation without additional demand for data collection. The savings vary depending on the quality of the data set, including proper documentation, format compatibility, and ease of access.

With the development of computer-based analyses in health services research, it has become relatively easy for researchers to share their data with one another. The multiple sources of secondary data enable researchers to conduct inquiry into many areas of interest. Vast quantities of information are collated and recorded by organizations and individuals for their own purposes, well beyond the data collected by researchers purely for research purposes. They are typically large in number and are often available for a considerable span of time.

Because of the economy and availability of secondary data, secondary analysis is fast becoming one of the most popular methods of health services research. For example, research in health economics is largely based on the secondary analysis of macrolevel, time-series data consisting of a large number of national statistical indicators and measures collated from a variety of official surveys and statistical series.

In addition to savings on time, cost, and personnel, the use of available data may afford the opportunity to generate significantly larger samples than primary research, such as surveys and experiments. Large sample size is important to researchers because it allows more sophisticated multivariate analysis and enhances confidence in research results because studies performed on large data sets generally provide more reliable estimates of population parameters.

Secondary data particularly administrative records may be viewed as more objective and therefore credible because the purpose of data collection is not research oriented and personal biases are less likely to be introduced. A particular problem with research is the **reactive effect:** changes in behavior that occur because subjects are aware they are being studied or observed. Research using available data may still encounter this problem if the sources of data are surveys. But many available data sources such as administrative records are nonreactive.

Secondary analysis affords the opportunity to study trends and change over a long period of time. Available data often are the best and only opportunities to study the past and trends. To study the evolution of health care delivery and financing, for example, necessitates the use of data collected in the past. Because of the commitment and cost involved, researchers rarely conduct longitudinal surveys over a long span of time. Longitudinal studies for the most part rely on available data.

Secondary analysis is also the general approach used to carry out area-based research, especially cross-national comparative studies. Secondary analysis of existing data is likely to remain by far the most common approach to carrying out international comparative studies, especially for studies that seek to cover large numbers of countries and/or trends over time. Aggregate national statistics from each country derived from official statistics and censuses, for example, enable the performance of international, macrolevel comparative studies. Secondary analysis of multisource data sets is also used to study geographical patterns and variations within countries, sometimes using existing compilations of area-based statistics, sometimes using data sets specially collated for counties, cities, or other areas. Thus, when the units of analysis are countries or social units rather than individuals and groups, secondary analysis may be the only viable research option.

The principal weakness of secondary analysis is the extent of compatibility between the available data and the research question. Secondary data such as surveys, records, and documents must be found rather than created to the researcher's specification. Searching for relevant data sources is by no means easy. While the material to study a given topic may exist, how does the researcher know where to look for it? To a large extent, identification of relevant data hinges on the general knowledge of the investigators.

Once identified, the value of available data will depend on the degree of match between the research questions to be addressed and the data that happen to be available. Often, available data will not be ideally suited to the purposes the researcher has in mind. Creativity is needed to reconstruct original measures that approximate the variables of interest.

Because of potential compatibility problems, the design of secondary studies may have to be started from back to front. Instead of designing the study and then collecting the necessary data, the researcher obtains details of the contents and characteristics of a set of secondary data and then identifies the corresponding research model. One key disadvantage is that the scope and content of studies are constrained by the nature of the data available from secondary data. Even when relevant data exist, they may not provide the particular items of information required to address the question at issue. In other words, information may be present but the definitions and classifications applied may be incompatible with those the researcher wishes to use.

Accessibility to available data may pose a challenge to investigators. Some data sets extracted from government records are routinely released for public use. Data compiled by government agencies are mandated for public use without restrictions. In other cases, access may need to be specially negotiated, and there may be constraints on access due to confidentiality and ethical concerns. In yet others, laws specifically prohibit the release of such data for confidentiality reasons.

Another limitation of secondary data, particularly administrative records that were not collected for research purposes, is that records are frequently incomplete or inaccurate. There may be large blocks of missing data as a result of nonrigorous data recording, which may not matter for administrative purposes but present serious problems for a research analysis. In the pressures of the day, recorders may forget to keep track of all the relevant information.

The decision to accept or reject a data set based on quality concerns hinges on several factors. First, is there an alternative data set that might have superior quality and that is available or accessible to the researcher at a reasonable cost? If such alternative exists, it should be used. A second factor is the magnitude of errors and their significance to the research outcome. If the errors are large and significant, the data set may not be tolerated. If the errors are minor or inconsequential toward study findings, the data set may still be used with the limitations duly stated. A third factor has to do with the purpose of the study. Is it an exploratory study that may tolerate larger measurement errors, or is it a causal modeling that seeks to confirm or disconfirm a set of hypotheses? A study on which important theoretical or policy implications are to be drawn requires a data set of acceptable quality. It may be wise to abandon such a study rather than conduct it with flawed data.

Another disadvantage or caution is that the process of examining secondary data can be time-consuming. Some researchers may think that because the data are already collected and stored on computer, they can begin analysis immediately. This may not always be the case. When an investigator gathers the data firsthand, he or she is aware of their limitations and errors and can adjust the analyses accordingly. In contrast, if the investigator has not participated in data collection, he or she may have to spend hours getting familiar with the documentation and data structures.

SUMMARY

Secondary analysis is any reanalysis of data collected by another researcher or organization. Secondary analysis may be based on the number of databases used both cross-sectionally and longitudinally, the sources of data, and the methods adopted to analyze secondary data. The principal advantage of secondary analysis is economy, achieved through money, time, and personnel saved in data collection and management. Its principal weakness is the extent of compatibility between available data and the research question.

Key Terms

secondary analysis	primary research
trend study	cohort
panel study	records
content analysis	ecological fallacy
historical analysis	reactive effect

Review Questions

1. What is the difference between secondary analysis and primary research?

2. What are the major types of secondary analysis?

3. What secondary data sources can you identify?

4. What are the strengths and weaknesses of secondary analysis as a scientific inquiry?

5. Do the following exercise as a way to learn the process of conducting secondary analysis.

Choose an available data set, either from published sources or other researchers, and study the measurement carefully. Based on the measurement available, try to conceptualize a research topic of interest to you. Describe, in detail, what measures will be used by you to study your topic. Describe any limitations you might encounter (e.g., missing variables, inaccurate approximates, etc.).

REFERENCES

Babbie, E. (1992). Chapter 12: Unobtrusive research. In E. Babbie, *The Practice of Social Research*. Belmont, CA: Wadsworth Publishing Co.

Carney, T. F. (1972). *Content Analysis: A Technique for Systematic Inferences from Communications*. London: Batsford.

Holsti, O. R. (1969). *Content Analysis for the Social Sciences and Humanities.* Reading, MA: Addison-Wesley Publishing Co.

Jacob, H. (1984). *Using Published Data.* Beverly Hills, CA: Sage Publications.

Krippendorff, K. (1980). *Content Analysis: An Introduction to Its Methodology.* Beverly Hills: Sage.

Marmor, T. R. (1970). *The Politics of Medicare.* London: Routledge and K. Paul.

Singleton, R. A., Straits, B. C., and Straits, M. M. (1993). Chapter 12: Research using available data. In R. A. Singleton, *Approaches to Social Research.* 2nd ed. New York: Oxford University Press.

Stewart, D. W., and Kamins, M. A. (1993). *Secondary Research: Information Sources and Methods.* Newbury Park, CA: Sage.

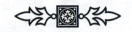

CHAPTER

6

Qualitative Research

LEARNING OBJECTIVES

- To understand the major purposes of conducting qualitative research.
- To differentiate various terms related to qualitative research.
- To explain the major types of qualitative research including participant observation, focused interview, and case study.
- To describe the process of qualitative research.
- To identify the strengths and weaknesses of qualitative research.

PURPOSE

Qualitative research serves four major purposes; as an exploratory study method; as a complement to large-scale, systematic research; as a method for certain research purposes; and as an alternative when other methods cannot be properly used. Qualitative research is particularly oriented toward exploratory discovery and inductive logic. Inductive analysis begins with specific observations and builds toward general patterns. The objective is to let important analytic dimensions emerge from patterns found in the cases under study without presupposing what these dimensions are.

Qualitative research is often used to complement quantitative approaches such as survey and experiment. Qualitative research may be used when investigators know little about the subject, because the less they know, the more they can be open to other possibilities. It is often conducted first, providing leads and feedbacks for more structured or large-scale quantitative explanatory research. Quantitative research, such as surveys and experiments, on the other hand, generally requires a certain amount of prior knowledge about the topic to provide guidance for instrument design or intervention manipulation and control. In areas where measurements have not been developed and tested, it is appropriate to first gather descriptive information about the subject areas and then develop measures based on the gathered information. Qualitative research also plays confirmatory and elucidating roles. It adds depth, substance, and meaning to survey and experimental results.

The qualitative research method is more appropriate for certain objectives, topics, problems, and situations than other methods. These include the study of: (1) complete events, phenomena, or programs; (2) developmental or transitional programs and events; (3) attitudes, feelings, motivations, behaviors, and factors associated with the changing process; (4) complex events with interrelated phenomena; (5) dynamic or rapidly changing situations; (6) relationships between research subjects and settings; and (7) processes or how things happen rather than outcomes or what things happen.

Qualitative research may be used as an alternative when methodological problems and ethical concerns preclude the use of other methods. For example, qualitative research is more appropriate and less intrusive in situations where experimental designs and the administration of standardized instruments would affect normal operations. When subjects are unable (e.g., illiterates, mentally ill, young children) or unwilling (e.g., social deviants) to participate in a formal survey or experiment, qualitative research may be used as a viable alternative. From an ethical standpoint, the control and manipulation necessary for experiments (e.g., creating certain medical conditions such as disabilities) are not always feasible, and qualitative research is often a preferred alternative.

DEFINITION

The term *qualitative research* is used to serve as a contrast to *quantitative research* because qualitative research embodies observations and analyses that are generally less numerically measurable than methods typically considered as quantitative research (e.g., survey and experiment). This classification does not mean there are no quantitative elements in qualitative research. Qualitative research may also involve counting and assigning numbers to observations. The term is used simply because qualitative statements and concepts, rather than quantitative numbers, represent the bulk of qualitative analysis.

Although we have used the term *qualitative research,* several other terms are often applied to the methodological approach examined here (Patton, 1990). The term **field research** is often used because qualitative researchers observe, describe, and analyze events happening in the natural social setting (i.e., field). Indeed, fieldwork is the central activity of qualitative inquiry. Going into the field means having direct and personal contact with people under study in their own environments (Babbie, 1992). Qualitative approaches emphasize the necessity and importance of going to the field and becoming close to the people and situations under study so that researchers become personally aware of the realities and details of daily life. The term *field* is not used in this book because quantitative research may take place in the field (e.g., interview survey).

Another often used term is **observational research,** or **participant observation.** The term is used because observation is a primary method of qualitative research. Qualitative researchers observe for the purpose of seeing the world from the subject's own perspective. "Observation" is not selected because this term is basic to all scientific inquiry rather than limited to qualitative research. However, qualitative observation differs from other forms of scientific observation in two important ways. First, qualitative observation emphasizes direct observation, usually with the naked eye, rather than indirect observation, which characterizes respondents' answers in questionnaires or interviews. Second, qualitative observation takes place in the natural setting rather than a contrived situation or laboratory.

Case study is another term often associated with qualitative research because qualitative research typically examines a single social setting (i.e., case), such as an organization, a community, or an association. However, while case studies may use qualitative approaches, they may also use quantitative methods such as surveys and quasi experiments. In addition, not all qualitative studies are concerned with detailed description and analysis of study settings.

Qualitative studies may also be termed **ethnographic,** which refers to the description of a culture after an extensive field research. The primary method of ethnographers is participant observation. However, qualitative research is not limited to the study of culture. There are large numbers of additional topics pertinent to qualitative research including physician–patient relationship, the experience of dying, living through HIV/AIDS, building regional health delivery network, and so on.

Qualitative research is also related to **phenomenological inquiry** focusing on the experience of a phenomenon for particular people. The phenomenon being experienced may be an emotion (e.g., loneliness, jealously, anger), a relationship, a marriage, a job, a program, an organization, or a culture. In terms of subject matter, phenomenological inquiry holds that what is important to know is what people experience and how they interpret the world. In terms of research methodology, phenomenological inquiry believes the best way for researchers to really know what another person experiences is to experience it through participant observation.

Heuristics, a form of phenomenological inquiry, focuses on intense human experience from the point of view of researchers. It is through the intense personal experience that a sense of connectedness develops between researchers and subjects in their mutual efforts to elucidate the nature, meaning, and essence of a significant experience. Qualitative research encompasses both the research subject and the method of phenomenological inquiry but is much broader in both areas. In addition to individuals, qualitative research may focus on a group, organization, community, or any social phenomenon or entity. In addition to participant observation, qualitative research may include focused interviews, case studies or other methods suitable for qualitative fieldwork.

The field of **symbolic interactionism** contributes to qualitative observation and analysis. The symbolic interactionist focuses on a common set of symbols and understanding that have emerged to give meaning to people's interactions. The importance of symbolic interactionism to qualitative research is its special emphasis on symbols and their interpretations by those who use them in explaining human interactions and behaviors.

Qualitative research may be defined as research methods used to provide detailed descriptions and analyses of issues of interest in terms of how and why things happen the way they do. It aims at gaining individuals' own account of their actions, knowledge, thoughts, and feelings. Qualitative analysis provides rich descriptions of individuals' own account of their perspectives focusing on meanings, interpretations, attitudes, and motivations. By capturing insiders' view of reality, qualitative researchers can understand the substance and logic of views that may seem to be implausible to outsiders. Qualitative research is an excellent way of gaining an overview of the process of a complicated event or problem.

TYPES

There are many types of qualitative research methods. Three of the major ones are participant observation, **focused interview,** and case study (Rubin, 1983; Yin, 1989; Patton, 1990; Bailey, 1991; Babbie, 1992; Singleton, Straits, and Straits, 1993).

Participant Observation

To fully understand the complexities of certain phenomena, merely relying on surveying what people say is limited because people may be unwilling to share important details especially if they are sensitive. Direct participation in and observation of the phe-

nomena are critical. Observations enable researchers to go beyond the selective perceptions of others and experience the setting firsthand.

In participant observation, researchers study a group or organization by becoming
part of that group or organization (e.g., hospital, managed care organization). Participation may be open or disguised. In open participation, investigators make known their
role as researchers to group members. However, the group leader or head of the organization always needs to be informed and his or her collaboration sought. The choice of
open versus disguised participation depends on whether knowledge of the study by
members will significantly affect their normal behavior.

As participants, researchers pay close attention to the physical, social, and human
environment surrounding the topic under study, the formal and informal interactions,
and unplanned activities. Informal interactions in the research setting include activities,
hierarchy of command, span of control, channels of communication, and languages
used and their meanings from the perspective of those being observed. Qualitative analysis must be faithful to facts and enable readers to understand the situation described. The
goal is to describe the problem under study to outsiders based on an understanding of
the insiders' perspectives.

Participant observation has many advantages. It sensitizes researchers to the research
setting and the members within. By becoming part of the group, researchers are more
likely to see events from the perspective of insiders. By directly observing operations and
activities within the setting, researchers gain a better understanding of the context and
process of activities. The firsthand experience acquired through participant observation
helps address the whys and hows of research questions.

Focused Interview

There are three types of qualitative interviews: the informal conversational interview,
the standardized open-ended interview, and the general interview guide approach
(Patton, 1990). In an informal conversational interview, neither specific questions nor
general topics are predetermined. Rather, they emerge naturally. Questions are spontaneously asked based on the natural flow of conversation. Informal conversational interview takes place most often in participant observation.

The standardized open-ended interview consists of a questionnaire instrument with
a set of questions carefully worded and sequenced. Each respondent is asked the same
set of questions in the same sequence. Instructions on probing accompany the questionnaire so that probing is consistently used by different interviewers toward different
respondents. The standardized open-ended interview is used when it is important to
minimize variation in the questions posed to interviewees, particularly when studies
involve many interviewers. The downside of this approach is that it is less flexible or
spontaneous.

The general interview guide approach has an outline of issues to be explored during the interview. The issues are unstructured and open-ended (i.e., there is no formal questionnaire) and of variable length (e.g., questions may take up to several hours). The issues in the outline were prepared before the interview but need not be taken in any particular sequence. The wording of the issues can be changed during the interview so long as the essence is maintained. Their sequence can also be altered to fit in with the actual flow of the interview. The outline of issues or interview guide simply serves as a basic checklist during the interview to make sure that no relevant issues are left out. Often, new findings during the interview may determine subsequent questions. Respondents are free to answer the questions in their own words, either briefly or at length. Respondents' answers are recorded by hand or, with their permission, a tape-recording device. This approach is most frequently used during focused interviews.

Focused interviews may be conducted with one individual or a group of individuals. The latter is often referred to as **focus group study,** or focus group. Focus group study involves interviewing a small group of people on a particular topic. A focus group typically consists of 6 to 12 people who are brought together in a room to engage in a guided discussion of some topic for up to two hours. Participants for the focus group are selected on the basis of relevancy to the topic under study, although they are not likely to be chosen through probability sampling methods. This means that participants are not statistically representative of any meaningful population, but the purpose of the study is to explore rather than to describe or explain in any definitive sense. At least two investigators should be present during focus group study, one serving as moderator and the other as recorder. The moderator, guided by the outline of issues, facilitates and controls the discussion to make sure that the discussion is not dominated by one or two people who tend to be highly verbal and that everyone has an opportunity to talk and share their views. Facilitating and conducting a focus group study requires considerable group process skill. Recording can be done in the same room or in an adjacent room where the focused group activities can be observed. Focus group study can also be videotaped and analyzed later.

Participants talk about their perceptions of the issues raised by the facilitator, hear one another's views, and provide additional comments. Although the depth of information about individual motivations and views may be more shallow than in individual focused interviews, group discussions can yield additional information about group interactions and dynamics as people react to views they disagree with. Participants are not required to reach any consensus on any issues. The objective is to allow people to provide their own views on the topic of interest in the context of other people's views. A given study may consist of one or more focus groups.

The focused interview has several advantages (Patton, 1990). It is flexible, has high face validity, and low cost. The focus group study is an efficient data collection method, because during one setting investigators can gather information from 6 to 12 people instead of only just one person. The process also enhances data quality as participants provide checks and balances on each other that reduce inaccurate information and extreme views. Further, it allows investigators to assess whether relatively consistent, shared views exist among participants on certain issues.

The focused interview has several weaknesses. The number of questions to be asked or issues explored is limited since it takes time for respondents to think about each open-ended question and then to say what they think. This is particularly true in focus group study where each participant responds to the same questions. Focus group study also affords the researcher less control than individual interviews. When participants share opposing views and are nonconciliatory, the interview may be difficult to conduct. The focused interview requires greater facilitating skill on the part of investigators. Another weakness of the focused interview is note-taking. It is difficult to take notes while also facilitating the interview. Usually the interview is tape-recorded and transcribed later. The transcription of notes is also time-consuming. Finally, data resulting from focused interviews are usually difficult to analyze.

Case Study

A case study may be defined as an empirical inquiry that uses multiple sources of evidence to investigate a real-life social entity or phenomenon (Yin, 1989). It is particularly valuable when the research aims at capturing individual differences or unique variations from one setting to another or from one experience to another.

The case study method is flexible and diverse. It may be a small project carried out by a single researcher or a large one carried out by a team of researchers over several years. It may focus on a single case or multiple cases. A single case often forms the basis for research on typical, deviant, or critical cases. Multiple case designs can be limited to two or three settings or extend to dozens of cases, either to achieve replication of the same study in different settings or to compare and contrast different cases.

A case can be a person, an event, a program, an organization, a time period, a critical incident, or a community. Regardless of the unit of analysis, a case study seeks to provide a richly detailed portrait of a particular unit so that an in-depth and comprehensive understanding can be achieved.

When the case study focuses on one individual, that individual is interviewed over an extended period of time to obtain detailed accounts of his or her personal history and the events he or she has experienced. The individual case study is commonly used to study ethnic or cultural groups who are difficult to locate and whose experiences are more distinctive and less well known. For example, an individual case study can be conducted on health-seeking patterns of ethnic groups. To complement and substantiate the individual's personal account, the researcher refers to a variety of other sources of evidence, such as interviews with other people (family, friends, and colleagues who have had contact with the subject), documentary sources (records), and observation of relevant social settings and events.

A case study may focus on a particular social entity, such as a single local community, to describe and analyze certain aspects of community life, such as politics, religious activities, crimes, health, and the like. For example, a community case study can be performed to study a community-based health care network, including community organizing, needs assessment, restructuring, and evaluation. The term **sociography** may be used for community-based studies, to denote the social mapping of a community's institutions, structure, and patterns of relationships. A community case study can focus on one or more communities.

A case study may be conducted for social groups, such as families, work units, or interest groups. A group case study can focus on typical as well as deviant groups. For example, a case study can be conducted on health interest groups in terms of their influences on national health policy and regulations.

A case study may be conducted for organizations or institutions such as health services organizations, schools, regulatory agencies, and the World Health Organization. For example, a case study of a health maintenance organization (HMO) can reveal its impact on cost containment and quality care.

In a case study, the type and quantity of data collected and analyzed can also vary enormously. Researchers usually use several methods of data collection, including the analysis of administrative records and other existing documents, in-depth interviews, structured surveys, and participant observation. Data obtained through multiple sources enable researchers to obtain a more complete account of the relevant issues under study. The costs and timetables for case study designs thus vary significantly. A case study may be extended into a longitudinal study with periodic follow-up data collection and analysis.

PROCESS

Qualitative research may be considered as a process consisting of a number of essential components: preparation, access, design, data collection, analysis, and presentation. It must be emphasized that qualitative research rarely proceeds smoothly in a sequence of steps. The components merely summarize the major efforts involved in qualitative research even though they may not always occur in the same order.

Preparation

As is true with other research methods, qualitative research starts with a review of all relevant literature related to the topic. Such a review enables the researcher to ascertain the current extent of the knowledge regarding the topic and the existing gaps. Since qualitative research is likely concerned with exploratory issues, there might be limited relevant literature existing prior to the study. However, researchers may still gain an understanding as to the types of problems likely to be encountered in such types of study. If the investigator will study an organization, a relevant literature source would be the organization's charts, mission statements, annual reports, as well as other pertinent statements. Researchers should avoid going in cold. Familiarity with relevant literature and background materials will prepare them well during the field study.

Access

The choice of a research setting hinges on a number of considerations, including whether the site is consistent with the researcher's interests, whether it is accessible, and whether rapport with informants is possible. It is also possible that several sites may be selected in order to obtain enough informants for the study. In other situations, the site is predetermined and is linked with the problem of investigation.

Gaining access to the group or setting a researcher wishes to study depends on the nature of the group or setting. If the setting is a public place, the researcher may not need to negotiate for access. If it is a formal organization, permission from a responsible person of the organization is critical. If researchers are to conduct a study in a hospital, they need to approach the administrator to obtain permission and cooperation. The general purpose of the study as well as its significance should be explained. Strict confidentiality should be guaranteed.

However, researchers may want to be ambiguous about the detailed research objectives for several reasons. The revelation of the detailed study objectives may distort the outcome of the research if the host agency is able to alter its normal course of action. In addition, at the beginning of a qualitative research, researchers may not know exactly what they are looking for. Researchers should not commit themselves too narrowly, because when research questions are changed along the way, the host agency may perceive them as being dishonest. Further, if the study objectives are contrary to the interests of the organization or group within, researchers may be denied access or provided barriers to access. While most often the administrator has formal control over access to patient populations, persons dealing with the patient on a day-to-day basis, such as physicians, nurses, technicians, and receptionists, can be critically important in facilitating or hindering real access (Grady and Wallston, 1988).

One approach often used to obtain entry is the known-sponsor approach (Patton, 1990). Investigators rely on the legitimacy and credibility of another person or agency to establish their own legitimacy and credibility. Before using this approach, researchers need to be certain that the known sponsor is indeed a source of legitimacy and credibility and can provide halo feelings that are beneficial.

In identifying informants, researchers should recognize informal leadership. The help of group leaders is often critical. Researchers should also try to select a representative cross section of people, representing different sociodemographic groups, organizational units, and tasks. Atypical individuals should also be sought. To select the ideal mix of informants, researchers need to be familiar with the setting. The familiarity may be gained through a background reading of the organizational literature.

Access may also be gained with a snowball strategy that locates additional contacts through informants. Once researchers have established trust and rapport with the informants, they will reveal additional names of people who can provide more information about the questions of interest.

Regardless of which methods are used to gain access, researchers should be clear about the actual reasons people allow themselves to be interviewed. Some commonly encountered reasons are:

- interest (respondents are interested in the research topic or participating in research);
- legal/agency requirement (e.g., as part of the contract, as agency's policy);
- public information (e.g., public officials, politicians, agencies that spend tax dollars);
- coercion or disincentive (e.g., superior–inferior relation, to avert penalties and other problems);
- reward or incentive (e.g., financial and nonfinancial benefits associated with participation);
- clarification (e.g., to tell your side of the story, to change an opinion or perception);
- seeking support (e.g., to look for assistance);
- pique or pleasure (e.g., whistle-blower, an opportunity to praise something);
- catharsis (e.g., to let out the impact of a traumatic experience);
- sociability (e.g., fond of conversation);
- courtesy (e.g., being polite and cooperative).

Design

In qualitative research, investigators do not attempt to manipulate the research setting. This naturalistic characteristic makes qualitative research design rather flexible. In general, the features of qualitative research design (e.g., operational measurement, hypotheses, and sampling methods) cannot be completely specified prior to fieldwork. Qualitative design needs to remain open to permit adjustment as warranted by the fieldwork. The design unfolds after investigators have become familiar with the major issues to be studied and the opportunities and obstacles afforded by the research setting. Once specified, qualitative design may also change during the course of the study as a result of new or unforeseen events.

The flexibility of research design does not mean qualitative researchers should not think about design. To the contrary, researchers will be better prepared if they know what they are looking for and how to look for it ahead of data collection. One important way to strengthen the validity and reliability of qualitative research is through **triangulation,** or the combination of several methods in the study of the same topic, including both quantitative and qualitative methods. Examples of triangulation types include data (i.e., the use of a variety of data sources in a study), investigator (i.e., the use of several different researchers or evaluators), theory (i.e., the use of multiple perspectives to interpret a single set of data), and methodology (i.e., the use of multiple methods to study a single problem or program) (Denzin, 1994).

Specifically, design considerations include the unit of analysis, the preliminary sampling procedures, the researchers' roles in the study, and the ethical implications of the fieldwork. Methods of data collection (through observations and interviews), primary questions to be explored, and analysis strategy, to be covered in detail in later chapters, are also addressed in the design phase.

Unit of Analysis

In qualitative research, the unit of analysis varies significantly depending on research purposes or what researchers intend to accomplish at the end of the study. The same study may also use several units of analysis. Examples include individuals, groups, cultures, brief actions such as incidents, longer actions such as events and activities, meanings, relationships, and the research setting itself. The choice of the unit of analysis determines the ensuring strategies on data collection, analysis, and reporting.

Sampling

In qualitative research, typically both the research sites and subjects are predetermined based on their availability and accessibility. Random sampling is usually not possible. Rather, small nonrandom sampling characterizes the selection of research sites and subjects. In situations where a choice can be made in selecting research sites or subjects, attempts should be made to be as representative in the selection of sites and subjects as possible. For example, if a qualitative research is conducted to investigate statewide hospital conditions, one may not be able to study more than one or two sites given the time constraint. Therefore, the representativeness of the choice of hospitals becomes significant. A purposive or quota sampling technique may be relied on so that the hospital(s) chosen should share certain important characteristics as the average hospitals in the state, such as urban and rural location, the socioeconomic status of the patients in the community, and the size of the hospital(s). Even when probability sampling methods are impossible or inappropriate, the logical link between representativeness and generalizability still holds for qualitative research.

Other commonly used qualitative sampling methods include **time sampling, typical case sampling, extreme** (deviant) **case sampling, intensity sampling,** and **stratified purposeful sampling** (Patton, 1990). Time sampling is based on sampling periods (e.g., months of the year) or units (e.g., hours of the day) of time. It is used when activities are believed to vary significantly at different time periods or units. Typical case sampling provides a detailed profile of one or more "typical" or usual cases to demonstrate the major features of the topic under study. Extreme or deviant case sampling focuses on cases that are different from typical cases to provide examples of unusual or special situations. Intensity sampling focuses on information-rich cases that strongly demonstrate the topic under investigation. Intensity cases are not unusual because they are not extreme cases. Stratified purposeful sampling is a combination of typical case sampling and extreme case sampling. Cases are first stratified into different categories of interest (e.g., above average, average, and below average) and then samples are selected from each.

Roles

Researchers need to be clear about their roles during research and how much they will reveal themselves as researchers. At one extreme, researchers may play the role of complete observers who only watch events and activities but do not participate. At the other extreme, they may assume the role of complete participants who take part in events and activities just like members of the group. In between, researchers can combine observation and participation by playing the role of participant observers that emphasizes participation or assuming the role of observer participants that stresses observation.

Researchers should also determine whether to make known their role as researchers. If they choose to reveal their true identities, they need to build up rapport with and seek trust and cooperation from the subjects. They must also consider whether the subjects' behavior will be affected by their presence. If researchers hide their true identities, they must consider the ethical consequences of such deception.

Ethical Implications

In designing and implementing qualitative research, researchers should consider several ethical issues that might be relevant to their studies. The first concern is the potential risk into which research subjects might be put. Examples of risk include bodily harm, side effects, undue stress, legal liabilities, loss of benefits, and ostracism by colleagues. When researchers are unsure about potential ethical or legal implications, they should consult with the institutional review board (IRB) for clarification. A large project usually has an ethical counselor on staff to deal with anticipated and unanticipated ethical issues.

Before data are gathered, researchers should obtain informed consent from subjects. During the study, subjects should be given opportunities to ask questions or refuse to be studied. After the study, confidentiality should be maintained in data storage, processing, analysis, and reporting. If researchers have made any promises to study subjects including both financial (e.g., cash) and nonfinancial (e.g., study report) reward, they should live up to their promises in a timely fashion so that continued cooperation from subjects can be maintained.

Data Collection

In general, qualitative researchers use multiple sources of evidence to address a broad range of issues related to a topic, and to validate study findings. The most common methods of data collection are observations, interviews, and case studies. Observations consist of detailed descriptions of subjects' activities, behaviors, actions, interactions, and organizational processes and dynamics. Interviews provide subjects' views about their experiences, ideas, perceptions, feelings, and knowledge. Case studies include a variety of relevant information about the setting under study.

Qualitative researchers also rely heavily on existing data sources, including media publication (e.g., newspaper clippings, articles), administrative documents (e.g., proposals, project reports), formal studies (e.g., consulting reports, evaluations performed previously), figures (e.g., organizational charts, diagrams, maps), service records (e.g., clients' for major services), personnel records (e.g., directories, telephone listings), financial records (e.g., budgets), personal records (e.g., diaries, calendars, appointment books), communication (e.g., letters, memoranda), survey data (e.g., census records), and administrative records (e.g., data previously collected about the site).

There are three major ways to record data during field study, relying on memory, manual or electronic note-taking, and tape recording. Relying on memory is used in informal interviews. It permits an informal conversation without interruptions so that the interview will appear more natural. However, an individual's memory is usually faulty. Typically, only an approximation of the actual interview can be reproduced.

Note-taking is used in more formal interviews. It enables researchers to record subjects' responses verbatim. It is also flexible in that researchers may ignore repetitions and digressions by subjects. Typewriters or portable (laptop) computers can be used to facilitate note-taking. In recording field notes, researchers should assign a code and date to each interview so that notes can be easily sorted. In addition to recording subjects' perceptions on the issues under study, researchers can also jot down their own feelings, reactions, insights, interpretations, and reflections to facilitate later analysis. However, they should clearly indicate which are subjects' responses and which are theirs. The downside of note-taking is that it can be distracting, tends to slow down the interview, and reduces the spontaneity of the conversation.

Tape recording provides complete coverage of interview without interrupting the interview. However, respondents may be uneasy to provide forthright answers because their responses are now "on record." In addition, transcription of tape recording is a time-consuming process. It may take five hours to transcribe one hour of tape recording. However, nonverbal behavior cannot be tape-recorded. A camera or videotape recorder may be used to make a visual record of an interview.

Recording is not limited to interviews. Qualitative researchers also take notes of things they observe and their thoughts related to the observation. Some researchers use a Stenomask to facilitate note-taking. A Stenomask is a sound-shielded microphone attached to a portable tape recorder. Researchers can dictate to the recorder during observation without attracting the attention of subjects.

To collect data properly, researchers need to improve their interviewing skills. They should have an inquiring mind and not be trapped by their personal perceptions and preconceived ideologies. Before the interview, they should have a general ideal of the topic and issues being studied and the type of information to be collected. Such an understanding allows the research to be conducted with focus.

During the interview, researchers should be good listeners. They must maintain neutrality and not ask leading questions or offer personal opinions. Probing when necessary should be kept neutral. They should be sensitive and responsive to subjects. Researchers should understand the interview setting may affect responses. For example, interviews conducted in an office setting are more formal than those conducted in a public place such as a cafeteria or in the subjects' own homes. The methods of recording interviews can also affect responses. Subjects are most self conscious when they are being tape-recorded and most relaxed during information conversation.

Analysis

Because qualitative research is relatively unstructured, there are few guidelines and procedures that govern qualitative data analysis. In general, researchers should be watchful for biases and seek multiple sources of evidence to corroborate research findings.

One major objective of qualitative analysis is description. Researchers provide detailed descriptions of insiders' views of the issues of interest. Qualitative descriptions use anecdotes, examples, and quotes from subjects. Descriptions may be organized chronologically, covering various periods and processes of the program and the events within those periods; in terms of importance, focusing on critical events and major activities relevant to primary research questions; or around major unit of analysis, such as research sites, individuals, or groups. Qualitative descriptions aim at answering the "how" questions.

Based on detailed descriptions, a qualitative analysis then integrates concepts and ideas to help explain and interpret the actions, activities, and beliefs described. The underlying meanings are explored, guided by existing theoretical frameworks. Results are attached significance and generated into patterns. Themes and concepts are identified and become the components of grounded theories. This level of qualitative analysis answers the "why" questions.

To assist qualitative analysis, researchers think about analysis early on during data collection. As soon as data are collected, they are coded and organized along different categories to facilitate later analysis. Examples of these categories are background, bibliographies, settings, biographies, issues, relationships, concepts, examples, supporting data, and quotes. The frequent review and editing of field notes is the beginning of qualitative analysis. Computers can be used to facilitate the filing and analysis process. Word processing allows the investigator to set up a filing system with relative ease. Software programs designed for qualitative data analysis can be used to help analyze filed notes.

Presentation

There are many ways to present the results of qualitative research. Results of qualitative research may be published as a book or journal article or as a report submitted to the funding agencies. A summary of the findings may be presented at conferences or published by the media. The styles of writing also vary significantly, from a narrative style to a format with tables, graphics, and pictures. A more structured format is suggested below and is composed of six major sections: introduction, setting, design, findings, discussion, and bibliography.

In the introduction section, the author describes the issue or problem being studied, its significance, as well as a review of the relevant theoretical and practical literature. In the section about research setting, the author provides a brief account of the historical development, current characteristics (both qualitative and quantitative), and major problems or issues related to the setting that the author studied, as well as a discussion about why this setting was selected. In the design section, the author summarizes the methods adopted in entering into the site, sampling subjects, establishing rapport, and collecting and analyzing data. In the findings section, the author summarizes major results of the study, with many pertinent examples as supporting evidence. The raw data drawn from field notes and other sources are organized into meaningful subsections reflecting the major themes and research questions. Illustrative examples and quotes are provided throughout the presentation of results. The qualitative findings are presented in combination with quantitative data. In the discussion section, the author analyzes the findings in terms of the underlying meanings, patterns, alternative perspectives, and policy or theoretical implications. The bibliography section can be drafted from the beginning of the study and augmented later with new citations when necessary.

The presentation of study results is tied to the specific audiences. For example, if the major audience involves professional colleagues in the same field, the contribution to theory development is likely to be important. If the audience consists of policymakers or practitioners, the policy and practical implications become more important. If the audience is the funding agency, the fulfillment of the research objectives and the rigor of the research become important concerns. Because of potential differences among audiences, a successful presentation may need more than one version of the study report.

STRENGTHS AND WEAKNESSES

The main strength of qualitative research is the validity of the data obtained: individuals are interviewed in sufficient detail for the results to be taken as true, correct, complete, and believable reports of their views and experiences. The question why can usually be answered through qualitative research. However, validity in qualitative research largely hinges on the skill, competence, and rigor of the researchers conducting the investigation.

Qualitative research is more effective for studying certain topics that are difficult to be analyzed quantitatively. Qualitative methods are better suited for the study of attitudes, meanings, perceptions, feelings, behaviors, motivations, interrelations among factors, changes, complexities, idiosyncrasies, and contextual background.

Qualitative research is also a less expensive approach both in terms of money and personnel required to conduct the research. Other research methods may require expensive equipment or a large research staff, but qualitative research can typically be undertaken by one or a few researchers. For example, survey research generally incurs greater expenses in sampling, data collection, and analysis. Similarly, experiments, while generally on a smaller scale than surveys, can be more complex and expensive to conduct.

Flexibility is another strength of qualitative research. The design and scope of the research may be modified at any time to account for changing situations or conditions.

The major weakness of qualitative research has to do with its lack of generalizability. The depth and detail of qualitative research typically derive from a small number of respondents or case studies that cannot be taken as representative, even if great care is taken to choose a cross section of the type of people or sites. With its qualitative rather than quantitative focus, qualitative research rarely yields descriptive statements about the characteristics of a large population. The conclusions reached as a result of qualitative research are generally regarded as less definitive.

Reliability is another potential problem with qualitative research. Even though qualitative measures are detailed and comprehensive, they are also personal and idiosyncratic. Another researcher studying the same topic may use entirely different measures, or analysis strategy, and may come to a different conclusion.

When a case study is carried out by an active participant (in a social group or an organization, for example), ethical issues may arise, and there may be practical difficulties in combining the sometimes conflicting roles of group member and researcher.

Qualitative research also places great demand for research skills. The in-depth interview requires researchers to demonstrate adequate prior knowledge of the subject and sufficient sensitivity to research subjects. Other important skills for qualitative researchers include the ability to observe details and conduct analysis and interpretation based on observations as well as the study of available data. Qualitative research benefits from good writing and presentation skills more than other research methods. Capable qualitative researchers must have observational, interviewing, interpretive, and writing skills.

SUMMARY

Qualitative research may be used as an exploratory study method; as a complement to large-scale, systematic research; as a method for certain research purposes; or as an alternative when other methods cannot be properly used. Other terms often used to denote qualitative research include field research, observational research or participant observation, case study, ethnographic study, phenomenological inquiry, and heuristics. Three of the major types of qualitative research methods are participant observation, focused interview, and case study. The process of qualitative research consists of a number of essential elements: preparation, access, design, data collection, analysis, and presentation. The strengths of qualitative research include its relatively high validity, its appropriateness for topics that are difficult to be analyzed quantitatively, its relatively low cost, and flexibility. Its major weaknesses include the lack of generalizability and reliability.

Key Terms

qualitative research

observational research

case study

phenomenological inquiry

symbolic interactionism

focus group study

triangulation

typical case sampling

intensity sampling

field research

participant observation

ethnographic

heuristics

focused interview

sociography

time sampling

extreme case sampling

stratified purposeful sampling

Review Questions

1. What purposes does qualitative research serve?

2. Draw distinctions among the various terms used to denote qualitative research.

3. How do researchers conduct a focus group study? Why do they conduct them?

4. What are the components in qualitative research? What does each component entail?

5. What are the various ways of data collection in qualitative research? Assess their pros and cons.

REFERENCES

Babbie, E. (1992). Chapter 11: Field research. In E. Babbie, *The Practice of Social Research*. Belmont, CA: Wadsworth Publishing Co.

Bailey, K. D. (1991). Chapter 10: Observation. In K. D. Bailey, *Methods of Social Research*. New York: Free Press.

Denzin, N. (1994). *Handbook of Qualitative Research*. Thousand Oaks, CA: Sage.

Grady, K. E., and Wallston, B. S. (1988). *Research in Health Care Settings*. Newbury Park, CA: Sage.

◧

Patton, M. Q. (1990). *Qualitative Evaluation and Research Methods.* 2nd ed. Newbury Park, CA: Sage.

Rubin, H. J. (1983). *Applied Social Research.* Columbus, OH: Charles E. Merrill Publishing Co.

Singleton, R. A., Straits, B. C., and Straits, M. M. (1993). Chapter 11: Field research. In R. A. Singleton, *Approaches to Social Research.* 2nd ed. New York: Oxford University Press.

Yin, R. K. (1989). *Case Study Research: Design and Methods.* Newbury Park, CA: Sage.

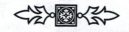

CHAPTER

7

Experimental Research

LEARNING OBJECTIVES

- To describe the major elements of experimental research.
- To understand the major types and designs of experimental research.
- To identify major threats to validity in research designs.
- To explain the strengths and weaknesses of experimental research.

PURPOSE

The major purpose of **experimental research** is to study causal relationships (Cochran, 1957; Campbell and Stanley, 1966; Kirk, 1968; Broota, 1989). A causal relationship may be established when the independent variable is associated with and influences the dependent variable, and rival explanations about this relationship have been eliminated. The simplest experimental study seeks only to ascertain whether there is a direct link between two factors, whether changes in a given factor produce changes in another factor. A more complex experimental study seeks to assess the importance or magnitude of the changes caused (i.e., the size of the effect). Still more complex experimental research examines the relative effects among a host of relevant factors on the dependent variable of interest. Experimental research is believed to be better suited than other research methods for explanatory studies whose goal is to provide more definitive answers to questions about causal relationships.

DEFINITION

Experimental research involves planned interventions carried out so that explicit comparisons can be made between or across different intervention conditions to test a research hypothesis. The term **demonstration** is sometimes used to indicate interventions carried out primarily to extend or test the applicability of already existing knowledge rather than to add to scientific knowledge. In experimental research, the unit of analysis may be individuals, families, small groups, organizations, or communities. The essential elements of experimental research in the natural as well as social sciences are experimental and control groups, randomization, pretest and posttest, and the application of the intervention factor.

Experimental and Control Groups

The word group refers to individuals defined by the service or program they receive or do not receive. The **experimental group** includes those individuals or other units of analysis that receive the intervention such as service or program. The **control group** includes those individuals or other units of analysis that do not receive the intervention, or receive an alternative form of intervention.

Ideally, the control group consists of subjects or other units who are as similar as possible to those in the experimental group except that they do not receive the experimental intervention or program. In reality, the similarity between the experimental and control groups varies for each study. A common practice is to divide control groups into two kinds: those made equivalent by random assignment, which generally assures a nonbiased distribution of the various characteristics; and those that do not employ random assignment and are termed *nonequivalent* (Fitz-Gibbon and Morris, 1987). The former are also referred to as true control groups, and the latter, **comparison groups.** Comparison groups refer to control groups selected through nonrandom methods and are so called to distinguish them from true control groups. If random assignment into experimental and control groups is not possible, then researchers should try to find a group as similar as possible on key characteristics to the experimental group.

The use of control groups allows researchers to account for the effects of the experiment itself. Participation in an experimental intervention or program can sometimes impact the outcome independent of the experiment or program itself. A classic example in medical research is that patients who participate in experimental treatment have appeared to improve. But it is not clear how much of the improvement has resulted from the treatment and how much from participation. The use of a control group that does not receive the treatment or receives a placebo would allow researchers to assess the true impact of the treatment.

In social science experiments, control groups are used not only as a guard against the effects of participation but also to account for events that occur outside the experimental setting in the course of experiments. To the extent that both experimental and control groups are subject to the effects of outside events, the biases experienced will likely cancel out, and the true effect of the experiment can still be determined.

Experimental research is not limited to using one experimental group and one control group, although they are the minimum groups required. Often an experimental design uses more than one experimental and/or control group. When using multiple experimental and control groups, researchers should specify the differences among the groups clearly. In analysis, the impact of each level of intervention should be examined separately, and the combined intervention effect should also be assessed.

Randomization

Randomization means taking a set of units and allocating them to an experimental or control group by means of some random procedure. Randomization is not equivalent to **random sampling,** which consists of selecting units in an unbiased manner to form a representative sample from a population of interest.

In a true experimental design, random sampling is used to select a representative number of units such as people or groups for study from a target population. This process is needed to ensure that study results are generalizable to the population of interest. Randomization procedures are then used to allocate each member of the sample to experimental or control groups, regardless of individual characteristics or preferences. This process aims at ensuring validity of the study by eliminating self-selection. When people voluntarily participate in the intervention, they are likely to be different from those choosing not to, so that the impact of the experimental factor will be confounded with the impact of selection effects.

The best way to accomplish randomization is through probability sampling, which ensures that each individual unit has an equal chance of being selected and allocated to either the experimental or control group. From a sampling frame composed of all the units in the population under study, researchers can select subjects by numbering all units and picking numbers based on a random number table. The odd-numbered subjects are then assigned to the experimental group and the even-numbered subjects to the control group. Tossing a coin is another way of assuring that subjects have equal chance of being selected in either group.

Randomly selected subjects are more likely to resemble the population from which they are selected. Since both experimental and control groups are randomly selected, they will also resemble each other. Randomization is the most effective way of eliminating alternative explanations. It automatically controls for factors that might have been neglected but that might influence results. Individual characteristics or experiences that might confound the results will be almost evenly distributed between the two groups. In addition, randomization allows the proper application and accurate interpretation of inferential statistics to analyze the experimental results.

In addition to randomly selecting subjects from the population and randomly assigning them to the experimental and control groups, sometimes it is necessary to administer a placebo to the control group. In testing the effects of new drugs, for example, medical researchers frequently administer a placebo (such as sugar pills) to the control group so that members of the control group believe they, like the experimental group, are receiving an experimental treatment. Often, their health might improve due to the placebo effect. However, if the new drug is effective, those receiving the drug will improve more than those receiving the placebo.

Sometimes, knowledge of the experiment can make researchers or experimenters become biased in assessing outcomes. In medical research, the experimenters, especially those who developed the experimental drug, may be more likely to "observe" improvements among patients receiving the drug than among those receiving the placebo. Similarly, in health services research, opponents of a particular cost-saving program are more likely to "note" quality deterioration among patients using new programs. This bias could be reduced if researchers responsible for administering the drug or assessing program outcomes would not be told which subjects were receiving the intervention and which were receiving the placebo. Conversely, researchers who have knowledge about which subjects are placed in experimental or control groups are not given the responsibility to administer the experiment or evaluate the outcomes. Such **double-blind experiments** reduce prejudice because neither subjects nor researchers or experimenters know which is the experimental group and which is the control group. Another way to reduce experimenter bias is to make the operational definitions of the outcome measures more precise. For example, researchers would make fewer errors in reading patients' temperature than assessing how lethargic patients are.

Although randomization is crucial for experimental results to be valid, in many practical situations, as in health services research, it is not always feasible. People might object to random "chancy" assignment to interventions that last a long time and are likely to significantly affect their lives. It might be unethical to withhold certain interventions or programs from those in the control group. Often subjects in the experimental group are predetermined. Researchers then have to use alternative methods to ensure the comparability between the experimental and control groups. Fitz-Gibbon and Morris (1987, pp. 28–29) have illustrated that the following approaches may be used instead.

One approach may be called the *two new interventions,* or *programs, approach.* Because new programs usually are more attractive, researchers may use a second new program as a control for the main intervention program. Subjects can be randomly assigned to one new program or the other. The second new program can be a version of the main intervention without the more costly components. It can also be a true competitor to the intervention program that is used by others in the community.

Another approach is the *borderline control-group strategy.* This strategy is appropriate when the people most in need must be given a particular program (e.g., Medicaid recipients or people with a special need). The measure of who is most needy is not always accurate. The borderline group refers to those who are immediately above the cut-off point. Many of them are also in need of the program. For example, if low income is used to decide who gets the program, the borderline people will be those whose income is slightly higher than the cut-off point. In such a case, the nonborderline, most needy people must be assigned to the intervention program, but the borderline group can be randomly assigned to the intervention program or the control group. This approach allows for a comparison to be made within a similar population, that is, the borderline group. Information regarding the value of the program is also valuable for policy decisions on whether or not to expand the program.

A further example is the *taking turns* (or *delayed program*) *approach.* Sometimes groups can take turns to receive the intervention or program. For example, a worksite health promotion program may be introduced to different divisions of the company employees in different time periods. Because divisions can be randomly assigned to their turn, a true control group is achieved even though all people will eventually be given the program. Starting out on a small scale is also a cautious strategy in implementing new programs.

One commonly used nonrandom assignment method is called *matching,* the attempt to make the control group as similar to the experimental group as possible. The matching process could be efficiently achieved through the creation of a quota matrix including all the relevant characteristics to be matched. For example, if demographic similarities are important between experimental and control groups, researchers may select control group subjects based on the demographics of the predetermined experimental group so that the average demographic characteristics of the experimental group are comparable to those of the control group. For example, they should have about the same average age, sex, racial composition, and so forth. If the experimental group is selected by means of a pretest, then the pretest should also be introduced to the control group so that subjects from both groups are exposed to the same outside stimuli other than the experimental intervention or program. Finally, researchers should record the similarities and differences between control and experimental groups. To the extent that subjects from both experimental and control groups can be demonstrated to be similar in all important characteristics except for the intervention, the validity of the finding will be enhanced.

Random sampling cannot always generate representative samples. When the sample size is small and the population heterogeneous, random sampling may produce a non-representative sample, and matching may be the only viable alternative. Matching and randomization can sometimes be combined to produce more comparable groups. Beginning with a pool of subjects, researchers first create strata of subjects similar in characteristics that need to be matched. Then, from each of the strata, subjects are randomly assigned to experimental and control groups. This procedure is called the *stratified random sampling procedure.* See Chapter 11 for additional random sampling procedures.

Before using the matching process to assign subjects to experimental and control groups, researchers should understand the conditions of matching. First, the variables being matched should be truly critical and are expected to affect the outcome of the intervention if not taken into account. Second, since most of the statistics used to evaluate experimental results are based on randomization, nonrandom sampling will limit the choices of statistics for data analysis.

Testing

Both experimental and control groups are tested or observed before and after the intervention and at the same points in time (Fitz-Gibbon and Morris, 1987). Tests given before an experimental intervention or program are called **pretests,** which stands for preprogram or preexperiment tests. Similarly, tests given after the experimental intervention or program are called **posttests.** Comparisons of the "before" and "after" information for experimental and control groups are used to assess the impact of the intervention or program. In the simplest experimental design, subjects are pretested on a dependent variable (e.g., weight), exposed to an intervention (e.g., weight control program), and then posttested in terms of the dependent variable (e.g., weight). Differences noted between pre- and posttests on the dependent variable are then attributed to the influence of the intervention.

Researchers may wish to make some measurement during the time the intervention or program is being implemented. These tests are termed **midtests,** or *midprogram tests,* and indicate the impact of the intervention or program over time. Likewise, a series of measurement or tests may be conducted well after a program finishes, thus allowing the assessment of the long-term impact of the intervention or program. Series of tests given at equal intervals before and after the program are called **time-series tests.** Generally at least three measures are desirable in order to draw a trend line. These three measures must be on the same instrument, for example, the same test or questionnaire. A series of tests administered systematically before a program starts may reduce the need for a control group because the results of these pretests can be used to project the outcome when there is no intervention.

Intervention

An experiment essentially examines the effect of an intervention factor (i.e., independent variable) on a dependent variable. The independent variable is the cause and the dependent variable the effect. Typically, the independent variable takes the form of an experimental stimulus, which is either present or absent, that is, a dichotomous variable having two attributes.

It is essential that both independent and dependent variables be operationally defined for the purpose of the experiment. Such operational definitions might involve a variety of observation methods. Taking a drug, subjecting to a treatment, eligibility for a service, participation in a workshop, undergoing exercises, receiving certain information, having a particular experience or an event, responses to a questionnaire, and the like, are some common health-related interventions. More complex experimental designs are also available, for example, using several levels of intensity in the intervention treatment or carrying out repeated follow-ups of the two groups in order to differentiate the immediate, short-term impact from the longer-term impact, as these may differ in strength and in character.

TYPES

Many types of experiments may be conducted including **laboratory** (or controlled) **experiment, field experiment, natural experiment,** and **simulation.**

Laboratory Experiment

Traditionally, we tend to equate the terms *experiment* and *laboratory experiment.* Laboratory experiments may be defined as experiments conducted in artificial settings where researchers have complete control over the random allocation of subjects to treatment and control groups and the degree of well-defined intervention. They represent the ideal prototype of true experiment. However, the laboratory experiment is rarely used in health services research due to the practical constraints on random assignment as well as the manipulation of intervention. Another reason for its limited use in health services research is the highly interactive health services environment where a multiplicity of social, economic as well as health-related factors interact. This environment is very difficult to be recreated in an artificial setting.

Field Experiment

Health services and many social scientific experiments often occur outside laboratories or the controlled environment, typically in real-life settings. Health policy research (e.g., Rand's insurance and utilization experiment) provides the best example of true experiments carried out in real-life settings and, in some cases, with samples sufficiently large and representative for the results to be extrapolated to the national level.

Field experiments refer to experiments conducted in a natural setting. The experimental observations are unobtrusive and take place as subjects are going about their normal activities. For example, one may observe the interaction or lack thereof between physicians and patients in clinical encounters or study the triage system at work in the emergency department of urban hospitals. Field experiment has high external validity and is particularly suitable for applied research that focuses on problem solving.

The major weakness of field experiments is the low level of control compared with laboratory experiments. Researchers may not be able to assign subjects randomly to the various treatment conditions or to control groups due to ethical considerations or subject preferences. Consequently, in the field experiment, it is usually more difficult to ensure that there are no systematic differences between experimental and control groups. In addition, because of the unobtrusive nature of field experiments, it may be inappropriate to obtain informed consent prior to the field experiment. The lack of informed consent can have both legal and ethical consequences.

Natural Experiment

Experiments in real-life settings, however, are still somewhat artificial in that they occur purely for research purposes and researchers have control over the random allocation of subjects to treatment and control groups. Many times practical and ethical considerations may rule out experiments on some topics, such as the effects of lack of access to care on health status, so that research (if done at all) must rely on truly naturally occurring events in which people have different exposures that resemble an actual experiment. This type of natural experiment may also be called a social experiment, where, in the course of normal social events, nature designs and executes experiments that researchers may observe and analyze.

Simulation

Simulation, or modeling, is a special type of experiment that does not rely on subjects or true intervention (Stokey and Zeckhauser, 1978). A **model** is a representation of a system that specifies its components (variables in health services models) and the relationships among the components. Simulation is a special kind of model—a model in motion, and one that is operating over a period of time to show not only the structure of the system (what position each variable or component occupies in the system and the way components are related or connected) but also the way change in one variable or component affects changes in the values of the other variables or components. Simulation is an imaginative "acting out" of how a program is supposed to be implemented and achieve its effects. Because of increasing access to computers and the availability of sophisticated software for the analysis of research data, a great deal of simulation and modeling can be done with the use of computer software.

The major advantages of simulation are economy, visibility, control, and safety. Operation of a simulation may not only be much cheaper than operation of the real event, but it can also provide trial runs that will help avoid costly mistakes in the real operation. Simulation can heighten the visibility of the phenomenon to be studied by making the phenomenon more accessible to the investigator. It clarifies the phenomenon by separating the essential components of the system from the irrelevant or less relevant features. Researchers often have a greater level of control over the simulation of an intervention than over the actual intervention itself. Another feature of control is the possibility that certain conditions can be manipulated in order to observe the difference in the results of the simulation. Simulations have potential use in situations that are theoretically important but will cause harm, embarrassment, or other moral and ethical problems if human subjects are used in a natural environment.

The major disadvantage of simulation is its artificiality. By its very definition a simulation is merely an imitation or copy of the real event. As a working model or substitute, there is always the possibility that the simulation is so inaccurate or incomplete that conclusions gained from it are not applicable to the phenomena being modeled, and thus the findings will be invalid. Particularly in social modeling, in which the social system may be highly complex, researchers may have little assurance that all the essential components are included in the model or that the relationships between components are specified correctly. Since simulation is only as good as the assumptions used in its construction, it is a useful approach when significant amount of empirically based knowledge is available. It is less useful or even misleading in areas about which little knowledge is available.

The requirement of highly quantitative skills may present problems for some researchers. A complex simulation, particularly a computer simulation, may not only require costly computers or other machines but also entail programming (software) costs and complex mathematical problems. Researchers unable to solve complex mathematical problems or do sophisticated computer programming, and without consultants available to solve these problems, may be unable to perform the simulation.

VALIDITY THREATS

For any experiment to be valid, researchers should guard against potential validity threats. The two types of validity researchers are most concerned with are **internal valid-**

ity and **external validity** (Campbell and Stanley, 1966). An experiment is internally valid if it shows that the study outcome is only caused by the hypothesized independent variables, rather than any extraneous variables. External validity is related to the generalizability of the experimental results. An experiment is considered externally valid if its effect can be generalized to the population, setting, treatment, and measurement variables of interest.

One threat to internal validity is **history,** which refers to events happening in the course of the experiment, other than the manipulated independent variable. They may affect the outcome of the experiment.

Another threat to internal validity is **maturation,** which refers to any changes to research subjects due to the passage of time rather than of the experimental intervention. In the course of an experiment, particularly one of long duration, subjects may change psychologically (e.g., become more knowledgeable) or physically (e.g., become stronger or weaker). These changes are not results of the experiment, but may affect experimental outcome.

Testing, a frequent rival explanation for research findings, refers to changes caused by measurement rather than the experiment. For example, individuals having repeated measurements generally improve their score because each measurement serves as a practice opportunity.

Instrumentation refers to changes in study outcome due to characteristics of the measuring instrument or procedure rather than the experiment itself. For example, if not properly trained, different interviewers may conduct interviews differently. The results of the interviews may differ due to the manner in which the interviews are conducted.

Statistical regression, or *regression toward the mean,* is another threat to internal validity. It is the tendency for extreme subjects to move (regress) closer to the mean or average with the passage of time. This phenomenon is likely to affect experimental results when subjects are selected for an experimental condition because of their extreme conditions or scores. The more deviant the score, the larger the error of measurement it probably contains. On a posttest, it is expected the high scorers will decline somewhat on the average and the low scorers will improve their relative standing, regardless of the intervention.

A further threat to internal validity, **selection** occurs when there are systematic differences in the selection and composition of subjects between the experimental and control groups.

Attrition, the withdrawal of subjects from an experiment, is another threat to internal validity. Attrition poses the greatest threat to internal validity when there is differential attrition, that is, when the experimental and control groups have different dropout rates. Invariably, those subjects who drop out differ in important ways from those who remain, so that the experimental conditions are no longer equivalent in composition. The reasons for subjects to withddraw from the experiment include dissatisfaction with the experience, being too sick to participate, declined interest, geographic relocation, and so on. Differential attrition rate usually defeats the purpose of random assignment.

The factors that might affect representativeness or external validity of the research include interaction effect of testing, the interaction between selection bias and intervention, the reactive effects of the experimental arrangements, and multiple-treatment interference. Interaction effect of testing occurs when a pretest increases or decreases the subjects' sensitivity or responsiveness to the experimental variable, thus making the results unrepresentative of the population who have not received any pretest. Interaction between selection bias and the intervention occurs when subjects selected are not representative of the population and may respond better or worse than the general population toward the intervention. When control group subjects are exposed to part of the experimental intervention as a result of inadequate experimental arrangements, the generalizability of the true experimental effect will be limited. Multiple-treatment interference occurs when multiple treatments are applied to the same subjects, largely because the effects of prior treatments are not usually erasable. It then becomes difficult to determine the true cause of the outcomes.

Researchers should not only be wary of potential threats to validity during the design phase of a study; they need to look out for potential threats in the actual implementation of the design. For example, they need to know that significant differences in time spent on the intervention or program between experimental and control groups could cause biases. A program that provides lengthy contact periods with subjects may turn out better results independent of the actual quality of that program. In analyzing program results, therefore, they need to take into account the actual time allocated to the program and the participation records of subjects.

Differential attrition rates is another cause for concern. The loss of subjects will lead to loss of data, which may affect program results. If subjects who performed less well or were less motivated dropped out of a new program, for example, the new program would obtain higher average results simply because of the loss of certain participants.

Researchers should also be concerned about potential confounding factors. A confounder is something extraneous to the program that happens to one group (either the experimental or control group) but not to the other group and that could influence the outcome measures for the program. With a one-group design, where a control group is absent, a confounder is an extraneous event that occurs at the same time as the program and might be expected to influence the program's outcome measures. Large numbers of experimental units (groups, employees, teams) provide some protection against confounders. In general, when comparing experimental groups with control groups consisting of many cases, differences in what happens to them, apart from the program itself, will tend to average out.

Contamination is another potential problem during the implementation stage. It refers to the phenomenon that the methods or components of the intervention program are used to some extent by the control group. Contamination may be less of a problem when experimental and control groups are at different sites so that control groups are less likely to be aware of the experiment.

DESIGNS AND THREATS TO VALIDITY

There are many configurations of experimental and nonexperimental (i.e., quasi-experiment) designs as summarized by numerous authors over the years (Finney, 1955; Cochran, 1957; Campbell and Stanley, 1966; Kirk, 1968; Cook and Campbell, 1979; Miller, 1984; Fitz-Gibbon and Morris, 1987; Broota, 1989; Black, 1993; Singleton, Straits, and Straits, 1993; Creswell, 1994). In implementing these designs, researchers must be guarded against potential threats to validity summarized above. In this section, based on previous researchers' work, we introduce the more commonly used designs and evaluate potential threats to validity for these designs.

Nonexperimental Designs

Nonexperimental, or nonequivalent comparison group, designs often are used when the experimental treatment is administered to intact groups, such as work units, making random assignment of individual subjects impossible. The simple notation employed in the classic work by Campbell and Stanley (1966) is used here to diagram the various designs. Specifically, the diagrams use the following symbols:

R indicates random assignment
O indicates an observation or a measurement being made
X indicates the experimental intervention or program

Design 1: The Simple Case Study Design

Figure 7–1 illustrates the simple one-group case study experimental design. X stands for the experiment or intervention (i.e., the independent variable), and O_1 for the outcome measurement of the experiment or intervention (i.e., the dependent variable). Time moves from phase 1 (preintervention) to phase 2 (postintervention).

The fatal drawback of this design is that there is no baseline measurement to provide comparison with the intervention outcome. Thus, it is impossible to tell whether there is an improvement in outcome. Other threats to internal validity of the simple case study design are attrition, maturation, and history.

Design 2: The Before-and-After Design

A second nonexperimental design, the one-group before-and-after design (see Figure 7–2), consists of measuring or making observations of one group of subjects (the

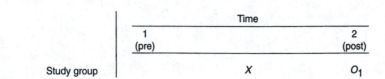

FIGURE 7–1   Design 1: The simple case study.

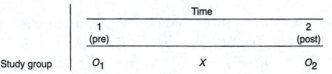

FIGURE 7–2   Design 2: The before-and-after design.

pretest), implementing an intervention or a program (the independent variable), and measuring the subjects at the end of the intervention or program (the posttest). The preintervention observations are represented by O_1, the independent variable by X, and the postintervention observations by O_2.

This is an improvement over Design 1 because it at least provides a basis for comparison. The attrition threat is controlled in the Design 2 study, because the preintervention observation makes it possible to determine whether those who dropped out before the second observation differed initially from those who remained. Only the data from those subjects observed both before and after the intervention would be used in analyzing the effects of the independent variable.

However, Design 2 is still subject to major threats to validity. Two of the threats found in Design 1, maturation and history, also affect the one-group before-and-after design. The longer the period of the experiment, the more likely that these two threats will happen and confound the results. Other potential threats to internal validity include testing, instrumentation, and, statistical regression. Unless objective reference or norm groups are available for comparison, considerable problems will occur when trying to establish any judgments about program X on the basis of this design.

Design 3: The Comparison Group Posttest-Only Design

As symbolized in Figure 7–3, the rows represent separate groups. X stands for the intervention or program and the blank space under X for the no-intervention comparison group. O measures the outcome of the dependent variable, and each group is measured just once (i.e., postintervention). This third nonexperimental design, the posttest-only design, like Design 2, is an improvement over the simple case study design in that it provides a set of data from the comparison group with which to compare the postintervention results. While Design 2 provides preintervention results on the same group, Design 3 provides the results of a comparison group.

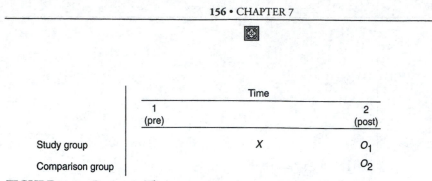

FIGURE 7–3   Design 3: The comparison group posttest-only design.

Design 3 generally is an improvement over the previous two nonexperimental designs in terms of controlling threats to internal validity. The threat of history is largely controlled, as subjects in the two groups should experience the same major external events. The absence of a pretest, avoids testing bias. Instrumentation can be controlled if the same instrument or measurement is consistently administered to both groups. Selection bias is the most serious threat to internal validity. Without the random assignment of subjects to the study and comparison groups, there is no control of possible preintervention differences. Indeed, there is no formal way to tell whether the two groups are comparable. Another threat to internal validity is attrition, which is uncontrolled because no pretest data exist by which the investigator may find out whether subjects who drop out of a study are comparable to those who remain. To the extent differences exist between those who drop out and those who remain in the study, study results may not be generalized to the population with confidence. Differential attrition rates between study and comparison groups can also bias the study results. Maturation may become a problem if the study is of long duration and if maturational factors are operating differently in the two groups.

Design 4: The Nonequivalent Comparison Group, Pretest–Posttest Design

Design 4 is a pretest–posttest design with a nonequivalent (nonrandomized) comparison group (see Figure 7–4). Prior to intervention, measurement was made in both study and comparison groups. This design is an improvement over Design 3 with the addition of pretests for both the study and comparison groups. The pretest results provide the opportunity to examine the similarity of the two groups, which is crucial to assess the impact of the intervention. Except for the lack of randomization in sample selection, this design is similar to the classic experiment true control group, pretest–posttest design (Design 7). It is frequently used in health services research when random assignment is not possible. The inclusion of a comparison group, especially one highly similar to the study group in known respects, makes it superior to previously introduced nonexperimental designs. If the groups are similar in important characteristics, then the design controls for history, maturation, testing, and regression to the mean.

Design 5: The Single Group, Time-Series Design

Design 5 uses the subjects in the experimental intervention or program as their own control group (see Figure 7–5). The same measurement is made on intervention or pro-

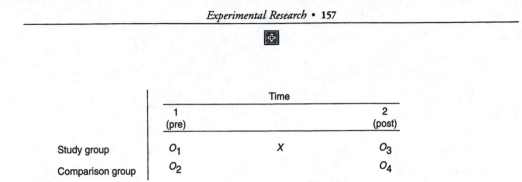

FIGURE 7–4 Design 4: The nonequivalent comparison group, pretest–posttest design.

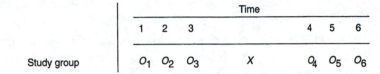

FIGURE 7–5 Design 5: The single group, time-series design.

gram subjects at regular intervals several times before and after the intervention. The impact of the intervention or program can be assessed by comparing the trend of measurement before the intervention with that after the intervention. If the intervention has any impact, the two trends will be significantly different. This design is a much better one than the before-and-after design because obtaining a series of measurements before and after the intervention provides a more accurate picture of the intervention effect. The essence of the time-series design is the presence of a periodic measurement process and the introduction of an experimental change into this time series of measurements.

However, history may represent a potential threat to internal validity. Even if you note a clear change in the observations following the implementation of program *X,* it is difficult to know for certain whether *X* caused the change or whether *X* just happened to occur at about the time that the measures would have changed anyway, because of some other outside events. Such coincidences, however, may be ruled out by obtaining additional contextual information.

Design 6: The Time Series with a Nonequivalent Control Group Design

Design 6 is like Design 5, except with the addition of a nonequivalent control group (see Figure 7–6). It also incorporates the prepost, nonequivalent control group design (Design 4). Two groups of subjects are measured regularly both before and after the intervention or program, which is available to one group but not the other. The addition of a comparison group makes it possible to control for external events that might take place during the course of the intervention or program. In other words, subjects from both groups will be subject to the same external influence. The alternative explanation for the results due to external influence or history can often be ruled out. In addition, the selection–maturation interaction is controlled to the extent that, if the study group showed in general a greater rate of gain, it would show up in the preintervention observations as well.

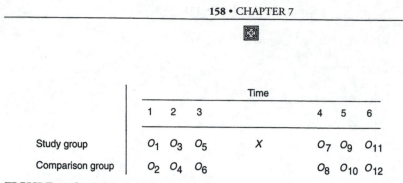

FIGURE 7–6 Design 6: The time series with a nonequivalent control group design.

Experimental Designs

The single most important difference between experimental and nonexperimental designs is randomization, or the random assignment of subjects to experimental or control groups. Randomization is present in experimental designs but absent in nonexperimental designs. Randomization is represented by the letter R. Similar to previous symbols, the study period is shown as time moves from left to right. The rows represent study or experiment and control groups. O stands for observation or measurement of the dependent variable(s). X stands for the intervention or program of the independent variable(s).

Design 7: The True Control Group, Pretest–Posttest Design

Design 7 is the classic true experimental design (see Figure 7–7). It is like Design 4 except that the control group was formed by random assignment. Research subjects are randomly assigned to either the experimental or control groups. Subjects assigned to the experimental group will receive experimental intervention or program X. Subjects assigned to the control group will not receive experimental intervention or program X. However, they may get an alternative program (X'). The pretest–posttest control group design involves measuring both the experimental and control groups at approximately the same time before and after the intervention or program. The pretest results can be used to assess the similarities or equivalency between the two groups. The posttest results are used to assess the impact of the intervention or program (X). For example, if subjects from the experimental group have performed significantly better than those from the control group as reflected in the posttest–pretest difference, we may attribute the difference to the effect of the intervention or program X.

This is a very good design and permits a powerful test to be made between program X and the alternative. Generally, threats to internal validity are dealt with successfully. For example, comparison of O_1 and O_2 provides a check on the randomization procedure with regard to initial differences on the dependent variable between the experimental and control groups. Given sufficient sample size, the randomization procedure should eliminate biases associated with selection and regression to the mean. In terms of history, any event in the external environment that would produce a difference between the pretest and posttest in the experimental group ($O_1–O_3$) would also do so in the con-

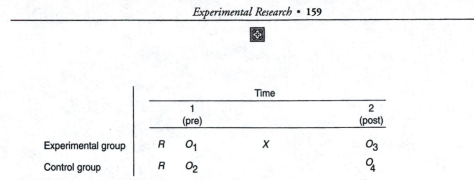

FIGURE 7–7   Design 7: The true control group, pretest–posttest design.

trol group (O_2–O_4). Likewise, this design effectively controls for other potential threats to internal validity including maturation, testing, and instrumentation, because they will affect both groups and not affect differences between the posttests, O_3 and O_4. This design permits the assessment of possible attrition effects by comparing the pretest results of those who drop out for both groups. However, even though Design 7 adequately controls the threats to internal validity, it is still susceptible to threats to external validity, which reflects the extent to which the experimental results may be generalized.

Design 8: The True Control Group, Posttest-Only Design

Design 8, the true control group, posttest-only design, is a simple true experimental design. Subjects are randomly assigned to experimental or control groups. No pretest or measurement is given. Instead, intervention or program is administered to the experimental group. The control group does not receive any intervention. Measurement is made after the intervention for both groups (see Figure 7–8). It is like Design 7 except that no pretest is used. Except for the use of subject randomization—Design 8 resembles the nonexperimental, comparison group posttest-only design (Design 3). Unlike Design 3, however, Design 8 controls for the common threats to internal validity adequately (e.g., testing, maturation, regression to the mean, instrumentation). This design effectively eliminates the possibility of an interaction between the pretest and the experimental manipulation. It is therefore useful when a pretest (such as attitude measures) might interfere with the program effects in some way. It may also be used when a pretest is not available or would take too much time. The random assignment of subjects to either the experiment or control groups, especially if numbers in the groups were large enough, is generally sufficient to ensure approximate equivalence.

Design 9: The Solomon Four-Group Design

The Solomon four-group design (Design 9), is another true experimental design. It is relatively complex and integrates both Designs 7 and 8 (see Figure 7–9). There are two experimental groups and two control groups. Randomization procedure is used in assigning subjects to each of the four groups. Pretest measurement is used for one pair of experimental control groups but not for the other. The same intervention is implemented in both groups. Posttest measurement is used for all four groups at about the same time.

	Time		
	1 (pre)		2 (post)
Experimental group	R	X	O_1
Control group	R		O_2

FIGURE 7–8   Design 8: The true control group, posttest-only design.

	Time		
	1 (pre)		2 (post)
Experimental group 1	R O_1	X	O_3
Control group 1	R O_2		O_4
Experimental group 2	R	X	O_5
Control group 2	R		O_6

FIGURE 7–9   Design 9: The Solomon four-group design.

The Solomon four-group design combines the strengths of the two previous experimental designs and enables the researcher to make additional comparisons. For example, the effectiveness of randomization may be assessed by comparing the pretests between Experimental Group 1 and Control Group 1 (O_1 and O_2). A positive result will build confidence in the random assignment of Experimental Group 2 and Control Group 2 where no pretest is conducted. A comparison between the outcome of Experimental Group 1 and Experimental Group 2 (O_3 and O_5) shows the extent of interaction between pretesting and intervention. A comparison between the outcome of Control Group 1 and Control Group 2 (O_4 and O_6) indicates the extent of testing effect. The effect of the intervention or independent variable(s) can be examined by (1) comparing O_3 and O_5, (2) comparing O_4 and O_6, and (3) comparing O_3 and O_5 and O_4 and O_6 (minus pretest effect). This design also effectively controls for threats to internal validity. However, the design may be twice as expensive due to the addition of two extra groups.

Design 10: The Time Series with an Equivalent Control Group Design

Design 10 is like Design 6, except with the addition of random assignment (see Figure 7–10). Two groups of subjects are randomly selected, measured regularly before the program and then one group gets program X, but the other does not; the other might get an alternative program or no program. This is a very powerful design effectively controlling for all threats to internal validity. However, it is also a very expensive design and is seldom used.

				Time				
		1	2	3		4	5	6
Study group	R	O_1	O_3	O_5	X	O_7	O_9	O_{11}
Comparison group	R	O_2	O_4	O_6		O_8	O_{10}	O_{12}

FIGURE 7–10 Design 10: The time series with an equivalent control group design.

STRENGTHS AND WEAKNESSES

The principal advantage of a controlled experiment lies in its validity in studying causal processes. Because the experiment reflects direction of influence and controls for extraneous variables, it is high in internal validity and provides relatively accurate inferences about cause and effect.

Experimental research is longitudinal in that observations are required for at least two points in time (before and after the intervention), so that the experiment provides the opportunity for studying change over time. In an experiment, investigators generally observe and collect data over a period of time and measure at more than one interval. The intervention itself may be of short duration, such as a few hours, or last a long duration, such as months. Even short intervention provides more opportunity to study change than does a cross-sectional study such as survey research.

For many decades, the randomized controlled experiment was presented in textbooks as the norm or ideal to strive for in the design and conduct of social research. However, because of the applied nature of health services research, the utility of experiment cannot be taken for granted. Researchers must critically evaluate whether an experimental research design is more appropriate than other designs for the particular issue or question under study.

The principal disadvantage of experiment has to do with its limit in generalizability or external validity. For example, the health behavior or social processes observed in an artificial environment (i.e., laboratory) will be drastically altered, or simply not occur at all, if examined out of its natural social setting. If the stringent requirements of experimental research designs are to be met, the design often becomes feasible only with small and untypical groups, in which case the conclusions cannot be generalized with any certainty. Experiment is designed to show the effect of a particular factor net of all other factors that may produce or moderate the same effect. But there may be little practical value in seeking a precise separation of these factors if, in the real world, they operate together. For example, in a controlled medical experiment, patients are generally not representative of all patients with a particular condition. Therefore, it cannot be known how the treatment being evaluated will work within the larger population of patients. Moreover, treatment in such an experiment is usually not at varying levels of intensity or in combination with other interventions. A narrower range of outcomes typically is considered.

Experimental designs may simply not be feasible for many of the topics and questions addressed by social scientists, including health services researchers. For example, people cannot be randomly assigned to experience poor health outcomes. Experiments are appropriate for research on unidirectional causal processes (i.e., where the influence works one way only). But when reciprocal causal processes (i.e., where a change in X produces a change in Y, and a change in Y also produces a change in X) are expected, other types of study (e.g., qualitative research) may be more appropriate and effective. Apart from practical constraints on the type of treatment that can be tested, feasibility problems arise also in relation to people's willingness to be experimental guinea pigs in research. Many people are simply not "available" for participation in experiments, and volunteers may not be representative. This tends to limit experimental research to captive populations, such as students in schools and other education institutions, recipients of a government benefit program (e.g., Medicaid, WIC), employees in a company, and so on.

Many of the controls required in experimental research may be difficult or impossible to realize in health services or other social science research especially when a natural setting is used. When a double-blind process cannot be implemented, the experimenter's expectations may affect the results of the experiment either through cues given (perhaps subconsciously) to the research subjects, who then conform to the experimenter's wishes, or through the misinterpretation of the experimental results to conform more closely with his or her hypothesis. In other instances, ethical and time considerations make it infeasible to study behavior in artificial settings. In addition, conducting true experiment with large and representative sample is typically more complex and costly than other designs. Because of these limitations, nonexperimental (or quasi-experimental) designs are more widely used in health services research.

SUMMARY

Experimental research involves planned interventions carried out so that explicit comparisons can be made between or across different intervention conditions to test research hypotheses. Its essential elements consist of experimental and control groups, randomization, pretest and posttest, and the application of the intervention factor. Experiment may be conducted in the laboratory, or natural environment with or without controls, or in the field without controls. Simulation is a special type of experiment which does not rely on subjects or true intervention. The principal strength of experiment lies in its validity in studying causal processes. Its principal weakness has to do with the limit in generalizability, or that it tends to be low in external validity.

There are also many configurations of experimental and nonexperimental designs.

Examples of nonexperimental designs are the simple case study; the before-and-after design; the comparison group, posttest-only design; the nonequivalent comparison group, pretest–posttest design; the single, group-time series design; and the time series with an equivalent control group design. Examples of experimental designs include the true control group, pretest–posttest design; the true control group, posttest-only design; the Solomon four-group design; and the time series with an equivalent control group design.

For any experiment to be valid, researchers should guard against threats to both internal and external validity. Threats to internal validity include history, maturation, testing, instrumentation, statistical regression or regression toward the mean, selection, and attrition. Threats to external validity include interaction or reactive effect of testing, the interaction between selection bias and the experimental variable, the reactive effects of the experimental arrangements, and multiple-treatment interference.

Key Terms

experimental research	demonstration
experimental group	control group
comparison group	random sampling
randomization	double-blind experiment
matching	pretests
posttests	midtests
time-series tests	laboratory experiment
natural experiment	field experiment
simulation	model
internal validity	external validity
history	maturation
testing	instrumentation
selection	statistical regression
contamination	attrition

Review Questions

1. What are the essential elements of an experiment?

2. In designing studies, if randomization is not feasible, what can researchers do to ensure comparability between the experimental and control groups?

3. Describe commonly used experimental and nonexperimental designs. What potential threats to validity must we guard against for each of these designs?

REFERENCES

Black, T. R. (1993). *Evaluating Social Science Research.* Thousand Oaks, CA: Sage.

Broota, K. D. (1989). *Experimental Design in Behavioral Research.* New York: John Wiley.

Campbell, D. T., and Stanley, J. C. (1966). *Experimental and Quasi-experimental Designs for Research.* Chicago: Rand McNally.

Cochran, W. G. (1957). *Experimental Designs.* New York: John Wiley.

Cook, T. D., and Campbell, D. T. (1979). *Quasi-experiment: Design and Analysis Issues for Field Settings.* Chicago: Rand McNally.

Creswell, J. W. (1994). *Research Design: Qualitative & Quantitative Approaches.* Thousand Oaks, CA: Sage.

Finney, D. J. (1955). *Experimental Design and Its Statistical Basis.* Chicago: University of Chicago Press.

Fitz-Gibbon, C. T., and Morris, L. L. (1987). *How to Design a Program Evaluation.* Newbury Park, CA: Sage.

Kirk, R. E. (1968). *Experimental Design: Procedures for the Behavioral Sciences.* Belmont, CA: Brooks/Cole.

Miller, S. H. (1984). *Experimental Design and Statistics.* London: Methuen.

Stokey, E., and Zeckhauser, R. (1978). *A Primer for Policy Analysis.* New York: W. W. Norton and Co., Inc.

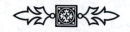

CHAPTER

8

Survey Research

LEARNING OBJECTIVES

- To describe the major elements of survey research.
- To understand the major types of survey research.
- To explain the strengths and weaknesses of survey research.

PURPOSE

Survey is the most commonly used method of data collection (Converse, 1987). It is extensively used both inside and outside the scientific community for different purposes (Bailer and Lanphier, 1978; Miller, 1991; Fowler, 1993; Singleton, Straits, and Straits, 1993). Social scientists, including health services researchers, use surveys for both descriptive and explanatory research purposes. The descriptive survey seeks to show the distribution of certain characteristics, attitudes, opinions, feelings, or experiences within a population. Explanatory survey examines the causal relationships among variables and attempts to explain how these variables are related. The survey offers an effective means of description and provides extraordinarily detailed and precise information about large heterogeneous populations. Guided by theories and using multivariate statistics, researchers are able to examine factors associated with the problems of interest.

Outside the scientific community, the survey is widely used by both the public and private sectors. The federal government conducts or sponsors many major surveys (including health-related surveys) each year for the purpose of gathering information, planning, and decision making. The news media conducts opinion polls to gauge public reactions to important events, policies, programs, and political candidates. Businesses (including health services organizations) conduct surveys to test market new products and services, assess consumer satisfaction with current products and services, and compile consumer profiles.

The survey is most popular with researchers because it enables a wide range of topics to be covered. The survey may be used to discover factual information such as age and income. It may be used to ascertain attitudes, beliefs, opinions, and values. Knowledge questions are often surveyed as well. A survey can record reports of past behavior as well as future intentions. Properly constructed, the survey can explore factors associated with a phenomenon of interest and thus test a particular hypothesis.

Indeed, the survey is such a basic method that it can be found in many other types of research. A research review of existing studies may find many of the findings are the result of surveys. Similarly, in secondary analysis, many of the secondary data sets may originate from surveys. Qualitative research, particularly case study, may integrate the survey component in its data collection. Experiments commonly use surveys to collect data measuring the impact of intervention. Evaluation research may also use survey findings to assess program impact.

DEFINITION

Survey research can be defined as the use of a systematic method to collect data directly from respondents regarding facts, knowledge, attitudes, beliefs, and behaviors of interest to researchers, and the analysis of these data using quantitative methods.

Typically, survey research consists of the following characteristics: large and randomly chosen sample, systematic instrument, and quantitative analysis (Bailer and Lanphier, 1978; Cox and Cohen, 1985; Miller, 1991; Fowler, 1993; Singleton, Straits, and Straits, 1993). A large sample of respondents randomly chosen from the population of interest will make the survey findings more representative and generalizable. Usually, probability sampling procedures are used to select the survey sample to ensure precise estimates of population characteristics. Chapter 11 examines probability and nonprobability sampling methods.

Survey research uses a systematic questionnaire or interview guide to ask questions of respondents. Regardless of whether the survey obtains information through an interview or a questionnaire, the data collection instrument and procedures tend to be standardized for all respondents. Questions are written beforehand and presented or asked in the same order for all respondents. During the interview, since changes in the wording of questions or in the behavior of interviewers (tone of voice, friendliness, appearance, etc.) may influence responses, interviewers are trained to present questions with exactly the same wording, order, and manner. They are also trained in the use of introductory and closing remarks, transitions from topic to topic, and supplementary questions or probes to gain a more complete response. Such standardization is necessary to enhance data reliability by minimizing measurement error and to facilitate hypotheses testing. If the purpose is to acquire preliminary data in an area in which little research has been done, in order to generate hypotheses, a less structured approach such as unstructured interviewing is generally used.

The results of the survey are numerically coded and analyzed quantitatively, typically with the aid of computer statistical software. Quantitative data analysis techniques depend on whether the survey's purpose is descriptive or explanatory. Surveys that are primarily descriptive make use of simpler forms of analysis. Explanatory surveys that sort out the relationships among the variables of interest require the use of more sophisticated data analysis techniques. Chapter 14 describes commonly used statistical methods for analyzing research data.

PROCESS

Survey research consists of three major components: planning, administration, and analysis. Each has a number of interrelated elements.

Planning

Select a Topic

This first step in planning a survey research is the same as in other types of research. Researchers decide on a topic of interest, select a problem to study within the identified topic, and formulate general hypotheses or research questions based on the selected problem. See Chapter 2 for conceptualizing health services research topics.

Review the Literature

Similar to other types of research, the next step is to review the relevant literature from journal articles, books, and other published and nonpublished materials to determine what is known about the topic and what work remains to be done. During the course of this review, the researcher clearly states the research objective(s), refines the problem, and specifies the research hypothesis or question in operational terms. A unique element in survey research is that researchers also search for and evaluate existing measures, scales, or instrument that may be incorporated or adapted in the prospective survey.

Select the Unit of Analysis

The survey unit of analysis may be anything that can be counted, including either individuals or groups of individuals, such as household, organization, city, and the like. The choice of the unit of analysis is determined by the research objectives, specified hypothesis, or research question. If the population of interest as specified by the research objectives are individuals, then data need to be collected at the individual level. If the population of interest are groups of individuals, then data need to be collected from samples of groups. If the research objective is to examine causal relationships at the individual level, but the data are collected at the aggregate level, then the investigator commits the error of ecological fallacy. To avoid such an error, researchers need to collect data at the appropriate level.

Assemble the Survey Instrument

The next step is to assemble the instrument to be used for data collection. The survey instrument or questionnaire may be constructed by the researchers themselves or adapted from available instruments used by others. The particular variables selected depend on which characteristics should be studied in order to meet the research objectives. The advantage of using others' instrument is that reliability and validity measures of the instrument are likely to be available. The disadvantage is the degree of match between the researcher's interest and the available measures. Chapter 12 provides a detailed discussion of the preparation of research instruments.

Select the Survey Mode

Researchers need to also determine the appropriate survey mode or type to use for the study (Aquilino and Losciuto, 1990). Three common survey modes are questionnaires, personal interviews, and telephone interviews. Questionnaires may be self-administered in person or by mail. The choice of survey mode depends on a number of factors, including the research topic, type of respondents, sample size, and resources available to the researchers. Certain research topics are more amenable to interviews than question-naires and vice versa. For example, if the purpose is to assess the knowledge level of the respondents, interview or in-person administration of a questionnaire are more proper modes than a mail questionnaire survey, because the latter cannot control for the possi-bility of respondents seeking outside help. In terms of respondents, the questionnaire is more appropriate for better-educated respondents and the interview for less-educated respondents. The geographic distribution of respondents is also an important consider-ation. A well-dispersed survey population are better reached by a mail questionnaire or a telephone interview than a face-to-face interview. Survey sample size also dictates the mode chosen. The self-administered questionnaire survey is more likely to be used for larger samples and the interview for smaller samples. Among resources important to sur-vey research are funding and personnel. The most expensive and time-consuming mode of survey research is the face-to-face interview, the major costs being incurred from direct interviewing time and travel to reach respondents. The least expensive mode is the questionnaire survey. Chapter 13 provides more detailed comparisons of the pros and cons of the data collection methods.

Design Survey Sampling

Survey sampling design depends on the characteristics and distribution of the popu-lation of interest, the availability of sampling frame, the survey mode chosen, as well as the overriding factor of cost (Kalton, 1983). For example, if population subgroups are disproportionately represented, a stratified sample may be chosen. If respondents are widely dispersed geographically, the most efficient sampling procedure for locating respondents is the use of the cluster sampling method. If mail survey or telephone inter-view is used, simple random or systematic sampling may be used, provided that an ade-quate sampling frame that contains the list of addresses or phone numbers can be obtained. Decisions about the survey mode and sampling are closely related and made concurrently. Telephone interview requires access to a telephone directory comprising the target population. Mail survey is only feasible where a mailing list is available. Finally, the sampling decision is influenced by cost and the resources available. Face-to-face interviews are the most costly, followed by telephone interviews and mail surveys. Chapter 11 examines various sampling methods.

Administration

Pretest the Survey Instrument

Whether the survey mode is an interview or questionnaire, the instrument should be pretested prior to actual use. A pretest consists of selecting a small but representative group of people and administering the survey instrument to them. Probability sampling is not required in selecting the group for pretest. The key is to choose those who share the major characteristics of the target population. A pretest is especially necessary if the instrument is newly designed for the purpose of the current study. Respondents are typically followed up and asked their views of the instrument in terms of clarity, choice of words, missing items, and length. A pretest is conducted to help determine whether further revision is needed, add new items or categories, and improve the clarity of wording.

Obtain Access to Respondents

The next step is to obtain access to respondents. If respondents are from particular organizations, permission from the appropriate organizational administrators is needed. Endorsement from those who have an appeal to the respondents is also useful. A cover letter introducing the purpose and significance of the study may also facilitate access. In interviews, the cover letter is usually read to the respondent. In mail questionnaires, the cover letter is sent with the questionnaire either as a separate sheet or attached to the questionnaire. The major contents of a general survey cover letter are:

- indicate the general purpose and significance of the research
- specify the researcher(s) and sponsor(s)
- explain how respondents are selected for the study
- summarize the benefits of the study to the respondents and others
- list the incentives, if any, for participating in the study
- assure complete confidentiality
- estimate the time needed to finish the survey
- provide a telephone number for possible questions by respondents
- give directions as to how and when to return the completed survey

Administer the Survey

Surveys may be administered by mail, in-person, or via telephone. Sometimes, a combination of these methods can be used. For example, questionnaires may first be mailed to respondents. Nonrespondents may be followed up with telephone interviews.

Follow-up on Nonrespondents

The final step of field administration involves following up on nonrespondents to encourage their participation and increase the response rate (James and Bolstein, 1990; Cox and Cohen, 1985). Response rate is one important guide to the representativeness of the sample because nonparticipants may differ in some important ways from respondents. A high response rate indicates less chance of significant response bias than a low response rate. Although no agreement exists as to what constitutes an adequate response rate, some researchers believe that in social science surveys, response rates of approximately 80 percent for face-to-face interviews, 70 percent for telephone interviews, and 50 percent for mailed questionnaires are generally considered acceptable. Response rates are generally higher for interviews than mail questionnaires. Reasons for the high response rate generally include the intrinsic attractiveness of being interviewed (having someone's attention, being asked to talk about oneself, the novelty of the experience), the difficulty of saying "no" to someone asking for something in person (respondents are more reluctant to turn down an interviewer than they are to throw away a mail questionnaire), and the fact that the importance and credibility of the research are conveyed best by a face-to-face interviewer who can show identification and credentials.

There are many ways to enhance the response rate for a given survey. Examples include a shorter questionnaire, sponsorship by a relevant authority, novel and appealing format, and paying respondents. Regardless of which alternatives have been used, a follow-up mailing is a required sequence for increasing return rates, particularly in large-scale mail surveys. In general, the longer a potential respondent delays replying, the less likely that person will do so at all. Properly timed follow-up mailing(s), then, provides additional stimuli to respond.

Follow-up methods vary by survey modes. Since response rates are typically lower for mailed questionnaires, follow-up efforts are especially important with this mode. Usually, questionnaires are coded so that researchers know who have not responded. Researchers should monitor the returns of the questionnaires intensely to look for clues for sending out the second follow-up mailing. A return rate graph can be drawn that records the number of questionnaires returned for each day after the mailing. This information will enable researchers to know how long it takes for the first batch of questionnaires to be returned, when the peak is reached, when it tails off, and what the cumulative number and percentage of returns are. The dates of subsequent follow-up mailings should be noted on the return rate graph as well to monitor the effects of follow-up mailings.

The first follow-up mailing is typically sent out to all nonrespondents about four weeks after the original mailing, to allow time for completion and for mailing in both directions. The return rate graph will indicate that the return has stopped or significantly dropped down. A new questionnaire is included with each follow-up mailing along with a cover letter that contains a thorough explanation of why each respondent's cooperation is important to the validity of the findings, and all the basic information in the original cover letter. If the questionnaire is truly anonymous, follow-up questionnaires are sent to all persons in the initial sample. The cover letter includes a statement that expresses appreciation for those who have already sent in their completed questionnaire and encourages those who have not to do so immediately. In practice, three follow-up mailings (an original and two follow-ups) seem to be the most efficient.

In telephone interviews, follow-up procedures include calling back at different times of the day and/or different days of the week. In face-to-face interviews, neighbors or those knowledgeable about the whereabouts of the respondents may be contacted and asked as to when people are usually at home or how they might be contacted. The field administration phase concludes when follow-up efforts have been completed with initially unresponsive persons in the sample.

Analysis

Process the Data

Before data can be analyzed, they have to be processed. Data processing entails correcting data-inputting errors, dealing with missing values, and recoding variables into conceptual categories to facilitate analysis. Chapter 13 details these and other procedures in data processing.

Analyze the Data

Data analysis applies appropriate statistical methods to survey data to test research hypothesis or answer research questions. Chapter 14 provides coverage of commonly used statistical methods for analyzing survey data.

TYPES

There are many ways to categorize the different types of surveys used by health services researchers. Surveys may be self-administered or administered by an interviewer either in person or through the telephone. Survey may be cross-sectional capturing one point of time, or longitudinal providing a series of observations.

Self-Administered Questionnaire

The **self-administered survey** refers to the fact that respondents are asked to complete the questionnaires themselves by reading the questions and entering their own answers. There are many ways of conducting self-administered surveys. The most common way is the use of a mail survey. The basic method is to send respondents through the mail a copy of the questionnaire, accompanied by a cover letter explaining the purpose of the study and a self-addressed, stamped envelope for returning the completed questionnaire. If feasible, researchers may consider the use of a self-mailing questionnaire that requires no return envelope, making the return of questionnaires easier. The questionnaire may be folded so that the return address appears on the outside. Such a design minimizes the chance of losing the envelope.

There are several postal options for mailing out the questionnaire and getting them returned. To mail out the questionnaire, the researcher can choose between first-class postage and bulk rate. First-class mail is faster and more certain, but bulk rate is cheaper. To get the questionnaires returned, the researcher can choose between business-reply permits and postage stamps. The advantage of using business-reply permits is that questionnaires are only paid when returned. It is particularly appropriate for surveys that have a very low response rate per mailing. Its disadvantage is that for those returned questionnaires, the researcher pays for the mailing plus an additional surcharge. The use of the business-reply permits may seem less appealing to some respondents who consider it to be less personal. Since bulk rate and business-reply permits require establishing accounts at the post office, it is more appropriate if the survey is large in scale. The advantage of using stamps is that it may be more appealing to respondents and money may be saved if the response rate per mailing is high. The disadvantage is that questionnaires will be paid whether people return them or not. Before deciding on a particular option, the researcher needs to visit the local post office to find out the actual arrangements and rates.

In addition to the mail survey, researchers may consider administering the questionnaire simultaneously to a group of respondents gathered at one place. This approach is feasible when respondents can be assembled together. Its advantages include savings on time and money (e.g., stamps), higher response rate, and the presence of researchers to provide introduction and assistance.

Furthermore, questionnaires may be delivered by mail and picked up later by the research staff at a designated time. The research staff also then have the opportunity to check for completeness. Conversely, questionnaires can be hand delivered by the research staff who explain the purpose of the study with a request that the respondents mail the completed questionnaires back to the researchers.

Interview Survey

In **interview surveys,** respondents do not complete the questionnaire by themselves. Rather, researchers or interviewers sent by researchers ask the questions and answer categories (if applicable) orally and then record the respondents' choices or answers. The interview process typically involves the following aspects: selecting the interviewers, training the interviewers, and conducting the interview (Fowler and Mangione, 1990; Suchman and Jordan, 1990).

Select the Interviewers

The field administration of the survey instrument begins with the recruitment of interviewers if the interview method is chosen and the respondents are too numerous for the researchers to interview alone. The desirable qualities of interviewers include a high sense of responsibility, a pleasant personality that enhances respondents' trust and cooperation; an interest in the research topic and in talking with people; an absence of prejudices toward the respondents; an ability to listen carefully and articulate in conversation; and legible handwriting that records responses clearly and accurately.

Train the Interviewers

In training interviewers, researchers first provide information about the study's general purpose, specific objective(s), significance, sponsor, sampling method, planned uses, general guidelines, and procedures. Even though the interviewers may be involved only in the data collection phase of the project, it will be useful to them to understand what will be done with the interviews they conduct and what purpose will be served. Motivation will be higher when interviewers know the purpose of the study and can identify with it (Billiet and Loosveldt, 1988; Babbie, 1992).

Interviewers are then acquainted with the interview schedule or questionnaire item by item. The interview schedule consists of instructions to the interviewer, the questions to be asked, and the response categories. Each question and answer category is read out aloud and explained as to the purpose. Questions or comments from the interviewers are then addressed. Interviewers must be able to read the questionnaire items fluently, without stumbling over words and phrases. They must be taught to follow question wording exactly.

The interviewers must be familiar with the instructions and specifications prepared in conjunction with the questionnaire, which are explanatory and clarifying comments about how to handle various situations that may occur with regard to specific questions in the questionnaire. They must be able to follow the instructions and determine when some questions will not fit a given respondent's situation and how the question should be asked in that situation.

Interviewers should learn how to record responses, especially when the questionnaire contains open-ended questions. Since open-ended questions aim at soliciting respondents' own answers, it is important that interviewers record the answers exactly as told without attempting to summarize or paraphrase. Interviewers should not worry about how the responses are to be coded. Researchers will decide on coding open-ended questions after the survey has been completed.

Basic interview techniques and rules are taught in terms of how to establish rapport with respondents and gain their cooperation, ask questions and probe in a manner that will not bias the response, record observations, and deal with interruptions and digressions. When respondents reply to a question with an inappropriate answer, probing is required. For example, the question may present an attitudinal statement and ask the respondent whether he or she strongly agrees, somewhat agrees, somewhat disagrees, or strongly disagrees with the statement. The respondent may reply that he or she agrees with the statement. The interviewer should follow this reply with: "Would you say you strongly agree or agree somewhat?" If necessary, interviewers can explain that they must check one or the other of the categories provided.

To decrease the number of missing answers or "don't knows," interviewers can be instructed to probe for answers. For example, interviewers may ask "If you have to choose an answer, which one do you consider as the most appropriate choice?" Interviewers can also help explain potentially confusing questionnaire items. If respondents clearly misunderstand the intent of a question or indicate that they do not understand, interviewers can clarify the question so that responses are relevant.

Probes are more frequently required in eliciting responses to open-ended questions. It is imperative that probes be completely neutral and must not affect subsequent responses. They should be written in the questionnaire whenever a given question is suspected of requiring probing for appropriate responses so that all interviewers will use the same probes whenever they are needed. This practice will reduce the effect of interviewer bias.

Demonstrations are held for interviewers on how to actually conduct the interview. Preferably, researchers should interview a representative cross section of true respondents. After the demonstrations, they should invite interviewers to address any of the questions or concerns they might have. Then, interviewers are paired off to complete mock interviews themselves. Once the practice is completed, interviewers should discuss their experiences and ask any additional questions they may have. Next, interviewers are provided opportunities for real interviews under close supervision. When researchers are truly satisfied with the performance of a given interviewer, that person may then be allowed to conduct independent interviews. Continual supervision of the work of interviewers is necessary over the course of a study. Researchers should read the completed survey and resolve any problems in a timely fashion.

Conduct the Interview

During the interview, interviewers should dress properly, remain courteous, tactful, and nonjudgmental throughout. Dress and appearance may send signals as to a person's attitudes and orientations. Generally, interviewers should dress cleanly, neatly, and in a fashion not too different from that of the people they are interviewing. In demeanor, interviewers should be pleasant, friendly, interested, and relaxed without being too casual or clinging. They should try to communicate a genuine interest in getting to know the respondents but not engage in any debate or argument about anything that is reported. The information gathered in the course of the interview should not be revealed to anyone except the supervisor. Interviewers may be required to sign an agreement not to disclose the contents of the interview.

Interviewers can observe as well as ask questions. For example, observations can be made regarding the quality of the dwelling, the presence of various possessions, respondents' general reactions to the study, and so forth. Interviewers can record these observations at the margins of the survey instrument.

Researchers should regularly check completed instruments to ensure that the survey questionnaire is properly filled out. At the initial stage of the study, they should sit in on interviews to make sure that respondents are interviewed properly. Throughout the study, researchers should remain available to interviewers to answer questions and provide assistance. Regular meetings with interviewers may be arranged to provide opportunities for interviewers to raise questions and receive solutions.

Telephone Survey

Interviews may be conducted in person or via the telephone (Lavrakas, 1987). The **telephone survey** is becoming more and more common given the wide availability of telephones. Telephone use is becoming omnipresent in the U.S. and many other countries. Most U.S. households now have telephones. However, certain groups are still underrepresented, such as rural people and the poor. On the other hand, many families have more than one telephone listing (e.g., one at home, one in the car), thus creating a problem of double counting. Another potential selection bias, caused by unlisted numbers (typically richer people request that their numbers not be published), has been reduced through the random digit dialing procedure. Known residential prefixes are sampled and the last four digits of the telephone number are selected by means of a table of random numbers.

Computers play an increasingly significant role in telephone interviews. A computer-assisted telephone interviewing, or CATI, system can greatly facilitate data collection, particularly for large scale survey (Baker and Lefes, 1988). The interviewer can sit in front of a computer terminal wearing a telephone-operator headset. The interviewer dials the number or the central computer randomly selects a telephone number and dials it. When the respondent answers the phone, the interviewer reads the instructions and interview schedule displayed on the computer screen. When the respondent answers the question, the interviewer types that answer into the computer terminal—either the code category for the appropriate answer to a closed-ended question or the verbatim response to an open-ended question. All answers are immediately stored in the computer so that researchers can begin analyzing the data before the survey is complete, gaining an advanced view of how the results will look.

Cross-Sectional Survey

Cross-sectional survey (one survey for one sample) is by far the most commonly used survey design. In a cross-sectional survey, data on a sample or cross section of respondents representing a target population are collected within a short period of time. Data collection may be through interviews or self-administered questionnaires. Although a cross-sectional survey may ask prospective (future), contemporaneous (now), or retrospective (before) questions, it is limited by the amount and accuracy of the information that individual respondents can capably report due to memory and recall capability. Because the cross-sectional survey collects data at one point in time, it does not adequately show the direction of causal relationships or rule out alternative rival explanations.

Longitudinal Survey

The **longitudinal survey** follows a single sample or another similar sample with repeated (at least two) surveys, over a period of time. Unlike cross-sectional surveys where the same questions are asked for all respondents, longitudinal surveys may be designed as multipurpose surveys. In addition to a set of core questions that are asked in each survey, noncore questions or topics may be included on an ad hoc basis to take into account the latest developments and interests.

Longitudinal surveys may be carried out at predetermined intervals: quarterly, annually, or biannually. Or they may be conducted on a continuous basis, that is, with interviews spread out evenly across the calendar year so that the data are not affected by seasonal variations.

The two major types of longitudinal surveys are trend studies and panel studies. A trend study includes conducting a series of cross-sectional surveys to collect data on the same items or variables with randomly selected samples of the same population. Even though different samples are selected, they all represent the same population of interest. A trend study can also be designed as a cohort study when the impact of a development, such as aging or health behavior is to be studied. A cohort consists of persons (or other units, such as households or organizations) who experience the same significant event within a specified period of time (e.g., a particular illness) or have some characteristic in common (e.g., same date of birth or marriage, same illness or symptom, membership in the same organization, etc.).

A panel study takes as its basis a representative sample of the group of interest, which may be individuals, households, organizations, or any other social unit, and follows the same unit over time with a series of surveys. Whereas trend studies focus on variables and their changes over time, panel studies focus on individuals and their changes over time, because the same individuals are repeatedly studied over time. In a panel study, a more personalized relationship with study members is needed to promote their active interest in the study, in order to reduce sample attrition and nonresponse rates.

A longitudinal survey is initiated when cross-sectional surveys or other sources of data reveal new trends that they cannot fully describe or explain. A longitudinal survey provides strong inferences about causal direction and more accurate studies of processes of change. Thus it is unique in its ability to answer questions about causes and consequences and hence to provide a basis for substantiated explanatory theory.

However, the longitudinal survey, especially panel study, represents a small component of survey research, mainly for economic reasons and the difficulty with follow-up respondents. The continued implementation of a longitudinal survey requires the commitment of both long-term funding and a secure organizational base. However, both are difficult to maintain. There are substantial practical problems associated with sample attrition and nonresponse. The failure to trace sample members at each subsequent wave of the study and their inclination to drop out of it are likely to increase over time, so that the subgroup that is successfully covered up to completion of the study may no longer be fully representative.

Change presents another obstacle to longitudinal survey. In a prolonged longitudinal survey, the methods of data collection and the instrument itself may change over time, to take account of maturation and aging. For example, children may be interviewed directly as they reach maturity, whereas personal interviews pose greater problems as people reach old age. The questions addressed at the start of the study may be overtaken by events, or simply cease to attract the same degree of interest. But changing questions from one study to the next may affect the comparability of information obtained over time. Even when questions remain constant, particular concepts may have changed meaning over time, so that the same variable may not be measuring the same construct. Changes in research staff are also more likely and may produce discontinuities in the approach or methods adopted for the study.

Finally, the inadequate development of a theoretical framework and methodologies to be used for analyzing longitudinal data presents another obstacle. The analysis of data from a longitudinal survey is usually substantially more difficult and costly than equivalent analysis of a cross-sectional survey. Longitudinal analysis of linked data from a series of surveys frequently involves extremely large data files.

STRENGTHS AND WEAKNESSES

Survey research is probably the best method to describe the characteristics of a population too large to observe directly. Probability sampling yields a group of respondents whose characteristics may be taken to reflect those of the larger population. Carefully constructed standardized measurements provide data consistent across all respondents so that the responses of different groups can be analyzed on a comparable basis.

Survey research has a high degree of transparency or accountability. Methods and procedures used can be made visible and accessible to other parties (be they professional colleagues, clients, or the public audience for the study report), so that the implementation, as well as the overall research design, can be assessed. With surveys, a standardized language has been developed to describe most of the procedures involved including introductory letters, the survey questionnaire, the code book, analysis of nonresponse, and so on. The transparency of surveys facilitates systematic refinement of survey methods and techniques and the development of theoretical work.

Survey research covers a wide range of topics. Ethical and practical considerations make it difficult to study some topics experimentally, for example, the effect of high insurance premiums and deductibles on access to care and experimental manipulation of patients and organizations. Survey research is often used instead.

Survey research can be an efficient data-gathering technique. While an experiment usually addresses only one research hypothesis, numerous research questions can be included into a single questionnaire instrument. The wealth of data collected through the survey method may help identify new hypotheses. Surveys may be reanalyzed as secondary data or with different theoretical perspectives, thus facilitating the cumulative development of scientific knowledge and methods.

Survey research has a number of difficulties and weaknesses. First, in many instances, the identification of an existing, suitable sampling frame poses problems, particularly if the group of interest is small or widely scattered. Second, the requirement for standardization makes certain questions appear artificial or superficial, particularly in the coverage of complex topics.

Third, certain topics may not be amenable to measurement through questionnaires. A survey cannot measure actual behavior and action; it relies almost exclusively on self-reports of recalled past behavior and action or of prospective or hypothetical behavior and action. As a result, data accuracy may be limited due to respondents' misinterpretation of questions, inaccurate recall, or purposeful misrepresentation of facts. A survey is also susceptible to reactivity, the tendency of respondents to give socially desirable answers to sensitive questions. Thus survey results are generally weak on validity.

Fourth, survey research does not deal with the context of research setting. Although questionnaires can provide information in this area, a brief encounter for the purpose of administering a survey does not afford survey researchers the opportunity to develop the feel for the total situation and background in which respondents are thinking and acting and the context within which behavior may be interpreted over an extended period of time.

Finally, survey research has severe limitations in explanatory analysis. Causal inferences from survey research generally are made with less confidence than inferences from experimental research. The three criteria for inferring causality include substantiating an association between the dependent and independent variables, establishing the time sequence that the independent variable (cause) occurs before the dependent variable (effect), and ruling out alternative explanations. While experiments can satisfy these criteria by design, surveys can only meet one of the criteria with complete confidence: establishing the association between variables. Since surveys collect data at a single point in time, it is difficult to establish the time sequence of variables. While experiments control alternative explanations through randomization and direct control procedures during the experiment, survey research uses statistical and modeling procedures to control these variables during data analysis.

SUMMARY

Survey research uses systematic methods to collect data from respondents. Its characteristics include large and randomly chosen sample, systematic instrument, and quantitative analysis. Its major elements consist of topic selection, literature review, unit of analysis, survey instrument design, choice of survey mode, sampling, pretesting, gaining access, survey administration, follow-up on nonrespondents, data processing, and data analysis. Surveys may be self-administered, administered by others, cross-sectional, or longitudinal. The major strengths of survey research are related to its transparency or accountability, efficiency, and flexibility in terms of topics covered. However, survey research has a severe limitation in explanatory analysis.

Key Terms

survey research	self-administered survey
interview survey	telephone survey
cross-sectional survey	longitudinal survey

Review Questions

1. What purposes does survey research serve?

2. What are the essential elements of survey research?

3. What are the types of survey research? Describe situations that most appropriately fit each of these types.

REFERENCES

Aquilino, W. S., and Losciuto, L. A. (1990). Effects of mode of interview on self-reported drug use. *Public Opinion Quarterly,* 54(3), 362–391.

Babbie, E. (1992). *The Practice of Social Research.* Belmont, CA: Wadsworth Publishing.

Bailer, B., and Lanphier, C. (1978). *Development of Survey Research Methods to Assess Survey Practices.* Washington, DC: American Statistical Association.

Baker, R. P., and Lefes, W. L. (1988). The design of CATI system: A review of current practice. In R. M. Groves, P. N. Biemer, L. E. Lyberg, J. T. Massey, W. L. Nichols II, and J. Waksberg (Eds.), *Telephone Survey Methodology.* New York: John Wiley.

Billiet, J., and Loosveldt, G. (1988). Interviewer training and quality of responses. *Public Opinion Quarterly,* 52(2), 190–211.

Converse, J. (1987). *Survey Research in the United States.* Berkeley, CA: University of California Press.

Cox, B. G., and Cohen, S. B. (1985). *Methodological Issues for Health Care Surveys.* New York and Basel: Marcel Dekker.

Fowler, F. J. (1993). *Survey Research Methods.* Newbury Park, CA: Sage.

Fowler, F. J., and Mangione, T. W. (1990). *Standardized Survey Interviewing.* Newbury Park, CA: Sage.

James, J., and Bolstein, R. (1990). The effect of monetary incentives and follow-up mailings on the response rate and the response quality in mail surveys. *Public Opinion Quarterly,* 54(3), 346–361.

Kalton, G. (1983). *Introduction to Survey Sampling.* Beverly Hills, CA: Sage.

Lavrakas, P. J. (1987). *Telephone Survey Methods.* Newbury Park, CA: Sage.

Miller, D. C. (1991). *Handbook of Research Design and Social Measurement.* Newbury Park, CA: Sage.

Singleton, E. A., Straits, B. C., and Straits, M. M. (1993). *Approaches to Social Research.* Oxford: Oxford University Press.

Suchman, L., and Jordan, B. (1990). Interactional troubles in face-to-face survey interviews. *Journal of the American Statistical Association,* 85, 232–241.

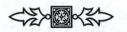

CHAPTER

9

Evaluation Research

LEARNING OBJECTIVES

- To understand the different types of evaluation research.
- To become familiar with the process of evaluation research.
- To be able to apply cost-benefit analysis and cost-effectiveness analysis.

PURPOSE

Evaluation research serves two major purposes: for program monitoring and improvement or for policy application and expansion (Stecher and Davis, 1987; Herman, Morris, and Fitz-Gibbon, 1987). The first purpose is concerned with the program itself. It examines the operations of a program, assesses whether and to what extent the stated program objectives have been fulfilled, summarizes the strengths and weaknesses in the implementation of the program, and identifies areas of improvement that can be made in program operations. Specifically, evaluators are interested in addressing the following questions: How has the program been implemented compared to the plans? What are the essential program components? What are the characteristics of program participants? To what extent has the program served its intended purposes? Are there any impacts of the program that are unintended or unplanned? How satisfied are participants with the program? What is the attrition or dropout rate? How cost-effective and cost-efficient is the program? How can the program be improved in the future?

The second purpose extends beyond the program itself and is concerned with policy application as a result of program implementation. It focuses on the policy implications of the program and assesses whether the program can be adapted in a different setting. Specifically, evaluators are interested in addressing the following questions: What policy implications can be derived from the program? How generalizable are the program findings? How likely could the program be adopted in other settings? What are the conditions or prerequisites for such an adoption? What adaptations, if any, have to be made before the program can be introduced to other settings? What will be the likely costs and benefits of the program to other settings?

The major difference between these two purposes is that the first purpose is limited to assessing and/or improving the effectiveness of a specific program within a particular setting and usually satisfies the needs of the management or administration within that setting. The second purpose serves to enlighten policymakers (federal, state, or local level) and funders by providing pertinent information regarding how to solve particular health and social problems and how to modify and expand the program to other settings.

Both efficacy and resource scarcity provide the impetus for conducting evaluations. Not all new programs are beneficial and conducive to solving the problems encountered. The usefulness of a program needs to be tested and confirmed before the program is expanded or promulgated. Program efficacy is all the more critical in the face of resource constraints. Resources both human and financial are limited at both organizational and governmental levels. Resource constraints make it necessary to prioritize problem areas on which to concentrate and to choose the program(s) that can most effectively and efficiently address these areas. Evaluation research is thus conducted to establish the validity of programs and to dismiss those programs that are ineffective and/or inefficient.

DEFINITION

In health services research, **evaluation research** is the use of one or more research methods in assessing various aspects of a program or policy, including components, operation, impact, and generalizability. The evaluation target may be a particular product (e.g., drug), service (e.g., family planning), or problem (e.g., lack of access). Since evaluation usually focuses on particular programs, evaluation research is sometimes called program evaluation. It can be conducted at the individual, group, institution, community, county, state, or national levels.

Evaluation research has a number of characteristics (Rossi and Freeman, 1993). First, evaluation research is technical. Using established research methods, evaluators design, implement, and examine a program in ways replicable by other investigators. Rigorous application of scientific research methods is necessary for the evaluation results to be valid and legitimate. Thus for evaluation to be successful, evaluators must be knowledgeable about commonly used evaluation methods and capable of applying them.

Evaluation research is applied. In contrast to basic research, evaluation research is undertaken to solve practical organizational and social problems. The growth of evaluation research reflects the increasing desire by health services researchers to actually make a difference in the delivery of health care services. The applied nature of evaluation research is typically reflected in the sponsor and funder of the project, who may be managers or administrators in a business, government, service, or private funding agency. The influence of increased requirements, particularly at the federal level, for evaluation to accompany the implementation of new programs and the set-aside of evaluation funds to fulfill that requirement cannot be neglected. The value of evaluation often depends on its utilization by sponsors and funders. To maximize the use of evaluation research, evaluators should be knowledgeable about the social dynamics of the setting in which they perform the evaluation, as well as the subject matter related to the evaluation.

Evaluation research should maintain objectivity. Results obtained objectively are more valid and useful in the long run for both organizations and society. Funders, sponsors, administrators, and evaluators all have the responsibility of making the evaluation objective. On the part of program funders and administrators, the results of evaluation should not be tied to the current or future reward for the evaluator. If evaluators are personally or financially tied to the project they evaluate, they may be hesitant to report negative findings and become "hired guns" of their sponsors. On the part of evaluators, they should not let the process of gaining trust and rapport affect their rigorous application of scientific research methods or change their perspectives. Regardless of the sponsor's intent, changing policy expectations, resources, and other constraints, evaluators should strive to maintain ethical integrity and scientific objectivity.

TYPES

The field of evaluation is marked by diversity in disciplinary training, perspectives on appropriate method, and evaluation activities and arrangements. Evaluation itself may be classified into various types according to different purposes. The major types include **needs assessment, process evaluation, outcome evaluation,** and **policy analysis** (Patton, 1990; Herman, Morris and Fitz-Gibbon, 1987; Stokey and Zeckhauser, 1978; Rossi and Freeman, 1993).

Needs Assessment

The purpose of needs assessment is to identify weaknesses or deficiency areas (i.e., needs) in the current situation that can be remedied or to project future conditions to which the program will need to adjust (Herman, Morris and Fitz-Gibbon, 1987). The results of a needs assessment can be used to allocate resources and efforts to meet identified, unfulfilled needs.

Needs assessment can be performed at the organization or community level (Kark, 1981; Mullan, 1982; Herman, Morris and Fitz-Gibbon, 1987; Dignan and Carr, 1987; Green and Kreuter, 1991; Farley, 1993; Barker, Bayne, Higgs, Jerkin, Murphy, and Synoground, 1994; Young, 1994). In either case, data are identified and collected from a variety of sources, including available databases, provider and patient/client focus groups, interviews, surveys, and meetings. The objectives are to identify and diagnose organizational or community-wide problems, prioritize them based on their critical nature and complications, and determine desired outcomes to be sought.

In an organizational needs assessment, the following questions may be asked: What are the key components of the current services and programs, including medical, social, and health services? What are the problems for each service or program? What are the possible causes of the identified problems? Examples of problems include services that are absent; inadequate; insufficient; poorly managed, coordinated, or delivered; inefficient; ineffective; incompatible with service objectives; or exceeding capacity or underutilized. What are the possible solutions to identified problems for each service or program? Examples of solutions include adding new services or redesigning and improving current services in terms of management, coordination, and delivery. For each solution identified, what are its organizational consequences on service objectives, management, staff, clients, finance, and service delivery? What optimal course of action can be chosen based on needs assessment? An optimal course of action is one that takes into account all the consequences of all alternatives, both positive and negative, and has the greatest net benefit among all alternatives.

In a community needs assessment, the following questions may be asked: What are the populations at risk or in need within the community? Populations at risk or in need typically include the uninsured, underinsured, minority groups, unemployed, and single mothers and their children. What are the most frequently encountered health problems? What are the most costly health problems? What are the current services and programs, including primary, secondary, and tertiary, that target the population at risk or in need? Examples of services and programs include prenatal care, primary care, vision and hearing screening, dental services, drug and alcohol abuse programs, mental health, counseling, long-term transitional housing for chemically dependent women with children, and low-income housing for displaced mothers. What are the problems and deficiencies of current community services and programs? Examples of problems include lack of effectiveness of current services and programs, gaps between current community services/programs and needs, lack of knowledge of services and programs by providers and patients, lack of coordination, inadequate referral transfer patterns, duplication of certain parts, misinformation, poor information management, poor patient education, and maldistribution of current services and providers. What strategies can be tried to improve current community services and programs? Examples of viable strategies include developing an integrated service system that is consumer focused and addresses their social, medical, and health needs; involving providers, funders, and clients in the planning, development, and implementation of services and programs; coordinating funding sources; regularly evaluating services and programs and their impacts; improving awareness of services and programs; and improving accessibility to services (e.g., relocating services, extending hours, providing transportation services, standardizing service eligibility requirement). How can a course of action be implemented to solve the most pressing community-wide problems?

Process Evaluation

Process evaluation is concerned with how a particular program actually operates. It focuses on the staffing, budget, activities, services, materials, and administration of the program. Process evaluation serves as a monitoring function, assessing whether the program has been implemented as planned and in compliance with legal and regulatory requirements and what problems have been encountered in the implementation stage. Based on process evaluation, changes may be made in certain aspects of the program to address unintended consequences or to resolve unexpected problems.

There are many reasons for monitoring the process of implementing a program. Rossi and Freeman (1993, pp. 35–36), in their comprehensive discussion of evaluation research, have summarized the following. First, program monitoring ascertains that program administrators conduct their day-to-day activities efficiently and, if not, identifies ways to enhance efficiency. Second, program funders, sponsors, or stakeholders require evidence to indicate that the program is being implemented as planned and for the purpose that it was paid for. Third, process evaluation identifies unexpected problems that need to be corrected immediately rather than held for the end of the normal duration of the program. Fourth, process evaluation is often a prelude to outcome evaluation. There is no point in assessing the impact or outcome of a program unless it has indeed taken place in the way intended. Finally, monitoring program costs and resource expenditures provide essential information for estimating whether the benefits of a program justify the costs.

Important questions to be addressed in process evaluation include: What are the critical activities and services and their schedules in the program? How are they operated? How are resources—including staff, budget, and time—allocated and managed? What is the relationship between program activities and program outcomes or objectives? To what extent has the program been implemented as planned? Is the program implemented efficiently? What problems, both anticipated and unforeseen, have been encountered in the implementation stage? What adjustments in program operation and management are necessary to address the problems?

Many of the data elements required for process evaluation are either available or can be incorporated in an organization- or a program-wide management information system that routinely collects information on a client-by-client basis about sociodemographic data, services provided, staff providing the services, diagnosis or reasons for program participation, services and their costs, outcome measures, and satisfaction. The information is essential for program monitoring as well as assessment at a later stage.

Outcome Evaluation

Outcome evaluation focuses on the accomplishments and impact of the service, program, or policy and its effectiveness in attaining the intended results that were set prior to program or policy implementation (Herman, Morris, and Fitz-Gibbon, 1987). Program results may also be compared with the status quo or some competing alternative program or policy with the same goals. The results of outcome evaluation enable sponsors and stakeholders to decide whether to continue or discontinue a program, or whether to expand or reduce it. Examples of outcome measures include health status (e.g., recovered from an illness), behaviors (e.g., primary care visits), performance (e.g., stop smoking), cognitive (e.g., knowledge or skill gained), or affective (e.g., satisfaction level). While evaluation is primarily concerned with explicitly defined goals and objectives, evaluators should also watch for unintended or unanticipated outcomes, both positive and negative.

Due to resource constraints, knowledge of program accomplishments alone is insufficient; the results produced by a program or policy must be compared with the costs incurred in implementing the program. Cost–benefit analysis is conducted and the program's net benefit is compared with some objective standard or that of a competing program with the same goals. Programs that are continued and promulgated are likely to be cost-effective.

Important questions to be addressed in outcome evaluation include: What are the goals and objectives of the program or policy? How are they measured and assessed? What programs are available as alternatives to this program? How are the program's essential components (e.g., activities, services, staffing, budget, and administration) related to achieving program goals and objectives? How successful is the program in accomplishing its intended results? How effective is the program in comparison with alternative programs or some objective standards? How costly is this program in comparison with alternative programs? What are the effects of the program and its components? Which program components best accomplish each of the program goals and objectives? What gaps exist in meeting the program goals and objectives? What changes should be made that might lead to better attainment of the goals and objectives? What are the unanticipated outcomes, both positive and negative, associated with the program? What decisions can be made regarding program continuation, expansion, modification, and promulgation?

Outcomes research conducted at the patient level is called medical outcomes or effectiveness research. Typically, research focuses on the most prevalent, costly medical conditions, for which there are alternative clinical strategies or pathways. Outcomes research involves linking the type of care received by a variety of patients with a particular condition to positive and negative outcomes in order to identify what works best for which patients (Guadagnoli and McNeil, 1994). Type of care refers not only to medical or surgical interventions, such as the use of a particular drug or surgical procedure, but also to diagnostic, preventive, and rehabilitative care.

Generally, outcome measures refer to the health status of patients (Greenfield and Nelson, 1992). They include the traditional outcome measures of mortality and morbidity, as well as assessments of physical functioning, mental well-being, and other aspects of health-related quality of life (Bergner, 1985; Ware, 1986; Steinwachs, 1989; Greenfield and Nelson, 1992). Structured instruments exists for most dimensions of health status and include general health measures (e.g., Nottingham Health Profile, Sickness Impact Profile, and the Medical Outcomes Study Instrument/SF36 that provide global profiles of health including well-being, function, social, and emotional health) (Hunt and McEven, 1980, 1985; Bergner et al., 1976; Bergner, Bobbitt, Carter, and Gilson, 1981; Tarlov, Ware, Greenfield, Nelson, and Perrin, 1989; Riesenberg and Glass, 1989), measures of physical functioning (e.g., the Lambeth Disability Screening Questionnaire which determines levels of disability, impairment, and physical function within general populations) (Patrick et al., 1981), pain measures (e.g., the McGill Pain Questionnaire and visual analogue scale) (Melzack, 1983; Scott and Huuskisson, 1979; Dixon and Bird, 1981), social health measures (e.g., the Social Health Battery) (Williams, Ware, and Donald, 1981), psychological measures (e.g., the General Health Questionnaire that identifies people with psychological or psychiatric morbidity) (Goldberg and Hillier, 1979), quality of life measures (e.g., the Four Single Items of Well-being and the Quality of Life Index, which seek to measure the overall satisfaction and well-being of individuals) (Andrews and Grandall, 1976; Spitzer, Dobson, and Hall, 1981), and the specific disease measures (e.g., the Arthritis Impact Measurement Scale and the Oswestry low back pain questionnaire) (Meenan, Gertman, and Mason, 1980; Fairbank, Couper, Daview, and O'Brien, 1980).

Another important aspect of outcomes research is concerned with costs of medical care. By associating the costs with alternative clinical pathways or strategies, outcomes research contributes to a clear understanding of the costs associated with alternative clinical strategies for the treatment of the most prevalent and costly conditions. Such information will benefit health services managers and medical directors in their efforts to operate efficiently in the managed care environment. Two interrelated health care trends of immediate and critical importance to health services organizations are the movement to managed care, and the organization of previously independent health care providers into integrated networks (Bureau of Primary Health Care, 1994a, b, 1995; Ginzberg, 1994). Managed care organizations combine the organization, financing, and delivery of health care in ways that respond to the demographics and economics that prevail in different regions of the country (Shortell, Gillies, and Anderson, 1994). In a managed care setting, health services organizations will be placed at risk by way of capitation and will be expected to cope with externally imposed controls on utilization.

The interest in the measaurement of health-related outcomes and their predictors has escalated in recent years because of the increasing number of therapeutic options available to patients, the concomitant increase in cost of health care, and the resultant need for health care reform to control these costs (Parkerson, Broadhead, and Tse, 1995). Both the public (e.g., federal and state government) and private sectors are under considerable pressure to control the rapid increases in expenditures for the Medicaid, Medicare, and private insurance programs and at the same time improve the quality of care (Bailit, Federico, and McGivney, 1995). In part, these objectives can be achieved by allocating their limited resources to treatments of established effectiveness (Kitzhaber, 1993). Clinical-based outcome research has increased tremendously with the advent of the Medical Treatment Effectiveness Research Program sponsored by the Agency for Health Care Policy and Research (AHCPR, 1991, 1992a, b, 1994a, b; Bailit, Federico, and McGivney, 1995; Greenfield and Nelson, 1992).

Policy Analysis

Policy analysis lays out goals, identifies alternatives that can meet the goals, uses logical and rational processes to evaluate identified alternatives, and chooses the best or optimal way to reach the goals. Policy analysis is typically performed with constraints on time, information, and resources. Its purpose is to inform policy or decision makers of the options available to them, provide a framework of valuing these options, predict the consequences of these options, and assist them in making rational and informed decisions to solve the problem they face. Policy analysts rely heavily on the techniques developed in economics, mathematics, operations research, and systems analysis.

The five-step framework (Stokey and Zeckhauser, 1978) for policy analysis includes: (1) establishing the context, (2) identifying the alternatives, (3) predicting the consequences, (4) valuing the outcomes, and (5) making a choice. Each of these steps contains important questions and issues to be addressed by the policy analysts. For example, to establish the context of analysis, policy analysts must find out the underlying problem that must be dealt with, and the goals to be pursued in confronting the problem.

To lay out the alternative courses of action, analysts need to be knowledgeable about the particular policy and program and know how to obtain further information for analysis. The alternatives should also be designed to take advantage of additional information as it becomes available, enabling policy and decision makers to change the course of action as they learn more about the real world.

In predicting the consequences or estimating the likelihood of the alternatives, researchers rely heavily on the analytic techniques of the management sciences, in particular economics, and operational research (e.g., forecasting and simulation, cost–benefit analysis, discounting, decision analysis, linear programming, critical path method, and Markov models).

To value the predicted outcomes, analysts try to choose objective (often quantitative) standards or criteria against which policy choices can be evaluated. Since some alternatives will be superior with respect to certain goals and inferior with respect to others, analysts may have to address the goals separately and descriptively.

In selecting the alternative, analysts draw all aspects of the analysis together to identify the preferred course of action. Sometimes, the analysis is straightforward and the best alternative will emerge from the analysis and be selected. At other times, the analysis may be so complex that researchers have to rely on a computer program to keep track of all the options and their possible outcomes. In most situations, the choice among competing policy alternatives is difficult, for the future is uncertain and the trade-offs among viable options are alternatively inevitable and painful.

PROCESS

Before conducting an evaluation, the investigator has to be first designated as an evaluator. The selection of an evaluator often hinges on many considerations including credibility, level of competence, availability, cost, and time, among others. Perhaps the most important consideration is credibility. Evaluation has to be credible to be useful. For evaluation to be credible, the evaluator has to be trustworthy. An evaluator's credibility is enhanced when that person is competent, knowledgeable, personable, and has a good track record.

Competence can be indicated by credentials (degrees, certificates, licenses), reputation, relevant experiences (past projects on similar areas or using similar skills), perceived technical skills that are critical to the project, and the validity and reliability of the evaluation design, data-gathering, and analysis methods adopted. Competence also means that evaluators are articulate about the evaluation methods they are going to use. Since most users or sponsors are not sophisticated in terms of research methodology and people are usually more skeptical of the methods and arguments they do not comprehend, evaluators should try to keep the design, data-gathering, and analysis methods sufficiently simple and straightforward yet valid.

Knowledge of the subject matter is another way to gain credibility. Both research and work experience can enhance knowledge level. Personality is important because conducting evaluation often requires gaining trust and rapport with administrators, participants, and users or audiences. Strong interpersonal skills have to be nurtured. At the same time, evaluators should remain objective in their work and not be constrained by friendship, professional relations, or the desire to land future evaluation jobs. Finally, a good track record on relevant research projects is helpful for establishing evaluators' credibility.

There are many ways to conduct evaluation research. The following is a description of a six-step process to conduct evaluation research: (1) determine the scope of evaluation, (2) get acquainted with the program, (3) choose the methodology for evaluation, (4) collect data, (5) analyze data, and (6) report findings. Evaluators may use this as a framework in their evaluation projects. At the same time, they should be aware that adaptations with respect to components of the framework may be necessary for their unique projects.

Determine the Scope of Evaluation

To determine the scope of evaluation, first the evaluator reviews all pertinent information about the evaluation assignment. Then some background investigation is conducted to find out more about the nature of the assignment. Finally, the evaluator negotiates and reaches agreements with the sponsor about their mutual expectations of the evaluation assignment.

Review Information about the Evaluation

Once selected, in most situations, the evaluator is likely to be presented with a lot of information about the program or project to be evaluated, as well as the scope of work. In other cases, the evaluator may have to help locate any pertinent information related to the program or project to be evaluated. Regardless of how information is collected, the evaluator should review these materials carefully and have a clear sense of the scope or boundaries of the evaluation assignment. After the review, the evaluator should find answers to the following questions: What is the ultimate objective of this assignment?

What is to be evaluated? What issues or questions will the evaluation address? What is the nature of this evaluation? Is it a needs assessment (e.g., planning for the future), process evaluation (e.g., improving an ongoing program or project), outcome evaluation (e.g., making judgments about program results and impact), policy analysis (e.g., evaluating alternatives and making a choice), or a combination of these? What specific tasks must be accomplished? How are these tasks related to the objective of the evaluation? What resources (e.g., budget, data sources, staff, informants, etc.) are made available to the evaluator? What is the duration of the evaluation? What deliverables are expected from the evaluator in the course and at the end of the evaluation project? What is the time schedule of these deliverables? How will the evaluation results be utilized? What additional information will be provided to the evaluator? If some of these questions cannot be answered from the materials provided, the evaluator may contact the host to obtain additional information.

After obtaining answers to these questions, the evaluator then critically assesses the assignment. Does the sponsor require more than someone can possibly deliver both in terms of scope of work and time frame? Does the evaluator serve the role of a researcher or analyst, or is he or she required or expected to be an advocate? Many researchers find it inappropriate to mix research with advocacy. An advocacy role could also have a potential negative impact on the credibility of the evaluation. The evaluator should let the sponsor know this concern. Are resources (e.g., budget, data sources, staff, informants, etc.) sufficient for carrying out the necessary tasks? What additional resources are required? The evaluator should record all the concerns along with missing elements from the previous sets of questions. He or she also considers potential designs to be used for data collection and analysis and develops a preliminary evaluation plan. Such advance preparation will enable the evaluator to be both knowledgeable and sensitive in the first meeting with the sponsor and enable him or her to use that meeting productively to probe and clarify the intended scope of the assignment.

Conduct Background Investigation

Next, the evaluator conducts some background investigation to find out more about the program and evaluation, and reviews related literature about the subject area and the evaluation methods relevant for this type of assignment. If the evaluator is not already familiar with this type of program or project, he or she should contact someone who is familiar with this or similar programs or projects. Conversation with such a person can help the evaluator know more about the program, its context and setting, the political nature of the evaluation, the problems in the program, and potential pitfalls in evaluating the program. Such information is valuable to conduct the evaluation work effectively.

Background investigation should help the evaluator assess the extent important stakeholders are likely to be affected by either the program or the evaluation. Possible stakeholders include policy and decision makers, program sponsors, evaluation sponsors, program target population, program participants, program managers and staff, and competitors. The evaluator should understand the relationships among the various stakeholders.

Meanwhile, the evaluator will find it beneficial to examine the literature of the subject to see what has been written about this type of programs or about specific components of the program. Access to earlier evaluations of this or similar programs will also be valuable. The review of evaluation methods will assist the evaluator in refining the approach to conduct the evaluation and improving the evaluation plan.

Negotiate the Contract

Having become familiarized with the scope of work and identified areas of missing information or concerns, the evaluator meets with the project sponsor. The sponsor may be the funder or primary users of the evaluation. The primary purpose of this meeting is to reach a common understanding about the exact scope and nature of the evaluation. Failure to reach a common understanding about the exact scope of the evaluation could lead to wasted money and effort, frustration, and acrimony if sponsors or evaluators feel they do not get what they expected. The evaluator and sponsor should go over the scope of work and reach a common understanding about all the stipulations. The evaluator should raise questions or concerns for any areas unclearly or unsatisfactorily addressed in the scope of work. At the end of the session, after negotiation, both sides should be clear about:

- The general purpose of the evaluation assignment.
- The users and audiences for the evaluation.
- The program or project components to be evaluated.
- A description of the evaluation questions or issues to be addressed.
- The respective roles, tasks, or responsibilities of the evaluator and sponsor or staff in the evaluation process. For example, for the evaluator, the specific tasks to perform, the assignments to turn in, and the time frame for accomplishing these. For the sponsor or staff, what kind of access (e.g., data, informants, assistant, coordinator, program records, files, computer, copy machine, fax machine, telephone), commitment of required resources (e.g., persons assigned to the project or staff time to administer instruments), and what types of cooperation, collaboration, and assistance (e.g., random assignment possibility, pilot test feasibility) will be provided.
- A set of criteria to be used to judge the successful completion of the evaluation.
- Determination of the acceptable methodology or general approach to be used for the evaluation, including evaluation design (e.g., experiment, time series, case control, case study), data collection methods (e.g., tests, observations, interviews, questionnaires), types of instruments (readily available or to be designed) and

measurements used (particularly those related to outcome), criteria of judging success or failure, and data analysis methods. The administrative requirements underlying the proposed methodology should also be considered and laid out. If certain methods are not feasible, the potential trade-offs between administrative feasibility and technical quality should be made clear and well understood to both sides.

- Choice of a reporting style. This may include the major sections of the report, the extent to which quantitative or qualitative information is to be reported, whether the evaluator will write technical reports, brief notes, or confer with the staff, and whether revisions will be necessary and under what condition.
- A budget for evaluation. The budget is prepared based on the specific tasks and schedules for conducting the evaluation. It includes both fixed and variable cost items. Examples of cost items include personnel (the evaluator and assistants, including the time spent reviewing the project; outside consultants; statisticians), travel and transportation, subcontracting (e.g., the collection of both primary and secondary data), postage (for questionnaires, draft reports, etc.), photocopying, printing, computer hardware and software (and/or computing time, when access is to a mainframe computer), and phone calls (including long-distance). If in-kind support is provided for certain items, this should be so indicated.
- A schedule of all the major activities, meetings, and assignment(s) due dates.
- A plan for utilizing the evaluation results.
- A contingency plan that specifies the conditions under which the evaluation plan may be changed, who will make decisions about changes, and who will implement the changes. Examples of conditions include unexpected illness, delay in data collection, change of policy, and so forth.

The agreement that has been reached as a result of this meeting should be documented, reviewed, and signed by both parties. The meeting between the evaluator and sponsor will result in a formal contract on terms agreeable to both parties. The final contract will include the following: a description of the evaluation questions to be addressed by the evaluator; the methodology to be used, including design, data collection and analysis methods; a timeline for these activities; list of the tasks and responsibilities program staff or others are expected to undertake in support of the evaluation; schedule of reports and meetings, including tentative agendas where possible; and a budget estimating anticipated costs.

Get Acquainted with the Program

Once the contract has been signed, the evaluator officially proceeds with the evaluation. The first task is to get fully acquainted with the program or project to be evaluated. Specifically, the evaluator should find out about the program's goals and objectives, its principal activities, organizational arrangements, staffing, roles, and responsibilities, relationships between program operations and outcomes, profiles of the clients and services provided, financial performance, and its primary problem(s). The level of understanding at this phase should be more specific than during the background investigation phase. In addition, some contextual information about the organization that administers the program will be useful. Such information includes the organization's mission, history, services, characteristics of staff and clients, and so on.

Often, the evaluator's organizational collaborators or coordinators are the best source of such information. They can at least suggest places to obtain the information. Some common sources from which this information may be obtained include the proposal written to obtain funding for the program, the request for proposals (RFPs) written by the sponsor or funding agency, brochures of the program, program curriculars or other materials, program implementation directives and requirements, administrative manuals, annual reports, an organizational chart, description of the administrative and service roles assumed by different people in the program, patient or client records, daily schedules of services and activities, the program's budget and actual spending reports, memos, meeting minutes, newspaper articles, document describing the program's history or the social context that it has been designed to fit, legislation, administrative regulations, completed evaluation studies, and perspectives and descriptions from program managers, participants, sponsors, or users. If feasible, the evaluator may want to personally experience some or all of the program components and activities. At a minimum, he or she should conduct one site visit to obtain firsthand impressions of how the program actually operates.

The evaluator then directs attention to the goals, objectives, and outcomes of the program and their measurements. The goals and objectives specified for the program will be used as a benchmark. Program staff and planners will be consulted with to make sure these indeed are the goals and objectives of the program. They may be asked to write a clear rationale describing why the particular activities, processes, materials, and administrative arrangements in the program will lead to the goals and objectives specified for the program. The evaluator may look for additional sources for program goals and objectives. For example, are there written federal, state, or local guidelines about program processes and goals to which this program must conform? What are the needs of the community or constituency that the program is intended to meet? Utilizing this information, the evaluator can recreate a detailed description of the program, including statements identifying program goals and objectives, cross-classifying them with program components, and comparing how the program is supposed to operate with how it actually does.

Information about the outcomes of the program may be obtained from the program's published documents, performance records, productivity indicators, patient or client database, and cost data such as financial performance records, insurance claims records, and workers' compensation claims records. Often it may be necessary to conduct additional studies to find out more about the program and its performance. For example, participant and/or staff surveys or interviews may be conducted to obtain additional or supporting data to back up the description of program events, operations, and outcomes. Past evaluations of this or a similar program, if available, will provide insight into how measurements can be constructed. Books and articles in the evaluation literature that describe the effects of programs similar to this one are also valuable. If feasible, the evaluator should personally observe or monitor the program outcomes.

Finalize the Methodology for Evaluation

Although the evaluation plan must be thought of at the start, now that the evaluator has become acquainted with the program, it is time to finalize the method(s) of evaluation. Specifically, the evaluation design, data instruments and measures, data collection methods, and data analysis techniques should be decided upon. It is encouraged to involve the primary potential users in the planning for the evaluation to facilitate their ownership of the study and enhance trust and cooperation. A detailed time schedule should also be drawn indicating when each activity will be performed, by whom, using what types of resources, and the duration of these activities. The schedule will be used to monitor the progress of the tasks so that the evaluation can be completed in a timely fashion.

Evaluation Design

Evaluation design is concerned with choosing the appropriate research method(s), including both quantitative and qualitative methods, and deciding on the unit of analysis and sampling methods (Rossi and Freeman, 1993; Fitz-Gibbon and Morris, 1987; Alkin, Kosecoff, Fitz-Gibbon, and Seligman , 1974; Campbell and Stanley, 1966; Cooke and Campbell, 1976).

Many research methods can be used in evaluation research including surveys, experiments, case studies, and so on. The choice depends mainly on the objectives of the evaluation and the constraints of the situation. The evaluator should choose the best possible design from a methodological and practical standpoint, taking into account the potential importance of the program, the practicality and feasibility of each design, the resource constraints, and whether the results produced will be valid or generalizable.

In choosing evaluation methods, the evaluator may incorporate both quantitative and qualitative approaches. Quantitative approaches (such as surveys, experiments, longitudinal research, secondary analysis) are necessary to measure, summarize, aggregate and compare program outcomes and effects, attribute their causes, and generalize program results to the population as a whole.

Qualitative approaches (such as focused group interviews, observation, case studies, fieldwork) are important to understand the meaning of a program and its outcomes from the participants' perspectives. The emphasis is on detailed descriptions and on in-depth understanding as it emerges from direct contact and experience with the program and/or its participants. Qualitative approaches are appropriate when the evaluator is interested in detailed descriptive information about the program, the dynamics of program processes and implementation, specifics of its problem areas, and unanticipated outcomes and side effects. Qualitative approaches add depth, detail, and meaning to empirical findings.

The combination of both quantitative and qualitative methods may be needed for the purpose of evaluation. If the program components, operations, and outcomes are well defined, a quantitative approach can easily be used to determine program effectiveness. If these elements are poorly defined, a qualitative approach may be used first to identify critical program features and potential outcomes before employing a quantitative approach to assess their attainment. A quantitative approach can be used to assess whether program objectives have been reached. A qualitative approach can be used to understand how program objectives have or have not been reached. A quantitative approach can show the breadth of information about the program. A qualitative approach can add depth and sensitivity to program information.

The design of an evaluation also considers the unit of analysis and sampling procedures. The choice of unit of analysis depends on program objectives and is related to the target the program or intervention is designed to affect. If the objective is to see progress made at the individual level, then individuals are the unit of analysis. If the objective is to see progress at the organizational level, then the organization is the unit of analysis. Other examples of unit of analysis include groups, communities, associations, neighborhoods, hospitals, companies, districts, counties, states, or nations. Some times, multiple units of analysis are necessary.

A sampling plan specifies how the unit(s) of analysis will be selected for study. Sampling is used when it is too expensive and time-consuming to study every unit. Sampling is a good way to increase the kinds of information to be collected given limited budget and time. If interviews or surveys are to be conducted, a random sampling method should be used to select subjects. If a focus group is to be conducted, participants should be selected based on their representativeness of different organizational units and responsibility as well as personal demographic characteristics. Chapter 11 provides detailed discussion of the frequently used sampling methods.

Evaluation Instrument and Measures

Once the evaluation method has been chosen, the evaluator then looks for or designs instruments that contain measures of the variables to be studied. The principal advantage of using an existing instrument is that the validity and reliability of the measures may be available. However, if no relevant instrument is available or accessible, or only portions of the measures are available, a new instrument has to be developed.

The instrument, whether available or newly constructed, should include all important measures related to the evaluation objectives and, if possible, to advancing the development of scientific theories related to the subject matter of interest. When possible, the program sponsor and staff are invited to participate in the selection or design of the research instrument. At minimum, the draft instrument should be circulated to them for inputs and changes. The involvement of potential users is important to gain their trust and cooperation. The completed instrument should be pilot-tested and revised, and the validity and reliability of the measure, documented. In general, the following measures are usually examined as part of an evaluation:

- participant characteristics (e.g., age, sex, race and ethnicity, education, income, occupation, attitudes and beliefs, experience, and baseline data on performance to be affected by the intervention);
- characteristics of program structure or context that might affect the intervention (e.g., staff characteristics, organizational setting, and environmental impact);
- characteristics of program implementation or processes (e.g., type of intervention, activities, services including materials, staffing, and administration);
- characteristics of program outcomes, both long-term and short-term (e.g., measures of program goals and objectives including health status, condition, knowledge, attitude, satisfaction level, behavior changes, and unanticipated outcomes— both positive and negative); and
- costs associated with the program (personnel, materials, equipment, facilities, and indirect opportunity costs) and benefits associated with program outcomes (e.g., improved health status, reduced use of costly services, and savings on opportunity costs).

Data Collection Methods

Data for evaluation research may be obtained through surveys, interviews, administrative records, observations, or content analysis. The evaluator should first try to find useful information that has been or is being collected routinely in the setting. Some data elements may already exist in the agency's files, reports, journals, logs, service records, provider records, participant records, and information system, which can be copied and processed to provide information for the evaluation. Computer-based management information systems are becoming more popular and sometimes indispensable for health and other human services programs. They produce tables and reports periodically containing information regularly used by staff and management. Service records can be narrative reports or highly structured data forms on which project staff check which services were given, how they were received, and the observable results. Provider data may cross-list services delivered to clients as well as provider's characteristics. Participant data may record services received as well as participants' characteristics.

Other data elements may be developed and incorporated into the system or collected firsthand. When there is no record-keeping system, the evaluator may suggest its establishment to collect needed information. He or she might persuade program staff to establish record-developing systems that will benefit both the evaluation and the program. A good way to increase the amount of information collected is by involving assistants and program staff in data collection. Not only should the evaluator specify which data collection method(s) to use, and when to use them, the evaluator must also understand whose responsibility it is to collect or provide different data elements.

Data Analysis

The types of data analyses conducted are related to the evaluation design (Patton, 1987, 1990; Fitz-Gibbon and Morris, 1987). When designs consist of control groups or nonbiased comparison groups, the analysis is quite straightforward. Comparisons can be made between the outcomes of the experimental and control groups, together with statistical procedures for determining whether observed differences are likely to be due to chance variations. For programs with nonuniform coverage, evaluators may take advantage of variations in intervention in order to approximate quasi-experimental designs, and program effect can be assessed in the same way as with experimental designs. However, variables measuring program intensity should be included in the analysis.

When no control groups are built into the design, as in the case of full-coverage programs, the impact of intervention is difficult to assess with confidence. Designs without control groups generally are evaluated by using before–after, time-series designs in which there are multiple measurements before and after the program is introduced. Specifically, preprogram and postprogram outcome measurements are compared to see if the differences are significant.

More sophisticated multivariate statistical procedures are available for causal analyses and for providing statistical controls. For example, a regression analysis that includes both the program and other competing measures can be conducted to test whether the program is a significant predictor of outcome. A number of procedures can be performed, including modeling all but the program variable against the outcome measure and then adding the program measure to the regression equation to assess its impact on the overall variance explained, over and above the variance explained by the other measures included in the analysis. Chapter 14 examines the statistical methods that can be used in data analysis.

Collect Data

Once the evaluation methodology has been finalized, the evaluator then proceeds to perform the tasks as scheduled. Much of the initial research will involve implementing the planned methodology, including design, sampling, and data collection and processing. Usually, there will be different kinds of data and different ways of collecting them. Data may be collected cross-sectionally or longitudinally. They may be collected from program staff and/or participants themselves. Staff surveys might indicate that services have been delivered. Participants' surveys are valuable for a number of reasons. First, they provide evidence to corroborate the staff's response. If not, different perspectives can be obtained. Second, securing participant data enables providers and program planners to find out recipients' comprehension of and satisfaction with the program, as well as their self-perceived important elements of the program. Finally it is an important way to find out, not only whether services were delivered, but what was actually delivered and whether they were utilized as intended. Collecting a variety of information enables the evaluator to gain a broad and thorough perspective of the program and to obtain more indicators of program effects.

The evaluator should make sure that the instruments are administered, interviews and observations conducted and coded, secondary data gathered and processed, and the scheduled deadlines met. If necessary, the investigator should see to it that proper training has been given to those responsible for data collection (sending out questionnaires and monitoring their return, or conducting telephone or face-to-face interviews, observations, fieldwork, etc.).

Analyze Data

Data analyses are conducted according to the techniques specified in the methodology section. The major objective is to find out the net outcome of the program, that is, whether or not a program produces desired levels of effects, reflected by the outcome measures, over and above what would have occurred either without the program or with an alternative program. Net outcome may be expressed as gross outcome subtracting the effects from nonprogram related, extraneous confounding factors and design effects. The net outcome may then be compared with that from other programs or some objective standards. In this section, we review the literature concerning some commonly used approaches to analyze evaluation data: measuring program coverage, cost–benefit analysis, cost-effectiveness analysis, and modeling. Readers should consult Chapter 14 for statistical techniques useful for evaluation analysis.

Measuring Program Coverage

Often, one of the program goals is related to program coverage or exposure. The program sponsor and administrators are interested in the extent of program coverage because they want to be accountable for the spending. Program coverage is also a precondition for achieving program effect. After all, how can the intervention be expected to work without first being implemented?

Rossi and Freeman (1993, p. 179) have discussed a number of measures of program coverage based on program participants' characteristics. The overcoverage rate may be expressed as the number of program participants who are not in need, compared with the total number of participants in the program or with the total number not in need in a designated population, if this number is available:

$$\text{Overcoverage rate} = 100 \times \frac{\text{number of program participants not in need}}{\substack{\text{total number of program participants} \\ \text{or those not in need in a designated population}}}$$

The program coverage rate refers to the proportion of the target population in need of the program who actually participate in it. This may be expressed as:

$$\text{Program coverage rate} = 100 \times \frac{\text{number of program participants who are in need}}{\text{total target population who are in need}}$$

The undercoverage rate refers to the proportion of the target population in need of the program who have not participated in it. This may be expressed as:

$$\text{Undercoverage rate} = 100 \times \frac{\text{number of nonparticipants who are in need}}{\text{total target population who are in need}}$$

or

$$\text{Undercoverage rate} = 100 - \text{program coverage rate}$$

The efficiency of a program depends on both maximizing the number served who are in need and minimizing the number served who are not in need. This may be expressed as:

$$\text{Coverage efficiency rate} = 100 \times \left(\frac{\text{number of program participants who are in need}}{\text{total target population who are in need}} - \frac{\text{number of program participants not in need}}{\text{total number of program participants or those not in need in a population}} \right)$$

The coverage efficiency rate ranges from +100 to −100 with +100 indicating total coverage of people in need of the program and −100 indicating total coverage of those not in need.

Cost–Benefit Analysis and Cost-Effectiveness Analysis

Purpose

Both **cost–benefit analysis (CBA)** and **cost-effectiveness analysis (CEA)** are means of analyzing or judging the efficiency of programs (Stokey and Zeckhauser, 1978; Pearce, 1981; Drummond, 1987; Blaney, 1988; Department of Veterans Affairs, 1989; Veney and Kaluzny, 1991; Patrick, 1993; Rossi and Freeman, 1993; Tolley, 1995). Efficiency analyses provide a framework for relating program costs to program results.

Significance

Efficiency analysis, as provided by CBA and CEA, is crucial for decisions related to the planning, implementation, continuation, and expansion of health services programs. Since programs are usually conducted under resource constraints, only programs that are effective in achieving the intended goals and/or are efficient in terms of resource consumption deserve to be continued or expanded. Funders and decision makers often make decisions regarding continuing program support based on a consideration of the "bottom line" (i.e., financial benefits, or the equivalent, outweigh costs). CBA and CEA help identify and compare the actual or anticipated program costs with the known or expected program benefits and provide valuable information for efficiency analysis.

Definitions

Cost–benefit analysis compares the benefits of a program with its costs. Both direct and indirect benefits and costs are identified and included in the analysis. Both benefits and costs are quantified and translated into a common monetary unit. Both benefits and costs may be projected into the future to reflect the lifetime of a program, or the future benefits and costs may be discounted to reflect their present values. Certain assumptions may be made in order to translate certain program elements (both inputs and outputs) into monetary figures. The basis for the assumptions that underlie the translation and analysis must be specified and discussed. Different analyses may be undertaken based on different sets of assumptions. The net benefits are typically used to judge the efficiency level of the program, or they may be compared with those of other competing programs.

Cost-effectiveness analysis also compares the benefits of a program with its costs, but it requires monetizing only the costs of programs and not the benefits of them. CEA expresses program benefits in outcome units. The efficacy of a program in attaining its goals or in achieving certain outcomes is assessed in relation to the monetary value of the resources or costs spent in the implementation of the program. CEA is more appropriate than CBA when there are controversies about converting outcomes into monetary values (e.g., human lives saved).

Differences

The difference between CBA and CEA is related to how program outcomes or effects are expressed. Program outcomes are expressed in monetary terms in CBA but in nonmonetary or substantive terms in CEA. For example, a cost–benefit analysis of a health promotion program to reduce cigarette smoking would focus on the difference between the dollars spent on the antismoking program and the dollars saved from reduced medical care for smoking-related diseases, days lost from work, and so on. A cost-effectiveness analysis of the same program would estimate the dollars spent to convert each smoker to a nonsmoker, or a heavy smoker to a moderate smoker. Whereas CBA compares benefits to costs in monetary terms, CEA compares costs expressed in monetary terms to units of substantive goals achieved. CBA is mainly concerned with cost relative to output. CEA first assesses the degree to which a program achieves its goals and then examines the efficiency level in goal attainment.

Use

CBA or CEA can be used during all phases of a program including planning, implementation, and evaluation. In the planning phase, CBA may be undertaken to estimate a program's anticipated costs and benefits. Assumptions must be made of the magnitude of a program's potential positive net impact, and its costs. CBA conducted before program implementation is particularly appropriate for programs that are expensive, time-consuming, resource intensive, or difficult to abandon once they have been put into place. In the implementation phase, CBA and CEA can be used to monitor the progress of a program toward anticipated benefits and costs. Program adjustments may be needed if great variations between anticipated and actual benefits or costs are noted. CBA and CEA are most commonly undertaken after program completion as part of the evaluation strategy to assess the net impact of a program. The efficiency of a program may be assessed in either absolute or comparative terms. CBA and CEA are particularly valuable when decision makers are considering alternative programs, rather than whether or not to continue the existing program.

Method of Cost–Benefit Analysis

Specify the Accounting Perspectives

In CBA, the costs and benefits may be considered from different perspectives, such as program participants, program sponsor, or society as a whole (Rossi and Freeman, 1993). Program participants are individuals, groups, or organizations that receive the program or services. The program sponsor is the funding source of the program intervention or services and may be a private, for-profit firm; a community, nonprofit agency; a foundation; or a government agency. Society's perspective takes the point of view of the community affected either directly or indirectly by the program intervention or services.

A CBA based on the program participants' perspective often produces higher net benefits than those using other perspectives because much of the program costs may be borne or subsidized by the program sponsor or society. A CBA based on the program sponsor's perspective resembles a profitability analysis conducted by private firms. It may be used by private firms sponsoring a program for the employees or constituents, or by sponsors who must make choices between alternative programs in the face of limited financial resources. The social perspective is the most comprehensive one, taking into account all identifiable costs and benefits. However, it is usually the most complex, largely because of the difficulty in obtaining all relevant information for analysis. Different accounting perspectives may not only cause differences in the choice of cost and benefit items; they may also value those items in varying ways. For example, the social perspective differs from individuals' or sponsor's perspective in valuing or monetizing costs and benefits (Stokey and Zeckhauser, 1978).

The decision of which accounting perspective to use is generally made by the evaluation sponsor. The evaluator has the responsibility to make clear to the sponsor the choices available and their implications. It may also be possible to conduct the analysis based on different or all perspectives. As a minimum, the evaluator needs to specify which perspective(s) has been chosen and the rationale for such a choice.

Identify Costs and Benefits

After the accounting perspective(s) has been selected, the next step is to identify all costs and benefits of the program. Those whose accounting perspectives were chosen may be surveyed to identify their costs and benefits related to the program. Other useful sources include program documents and previous literature. All relevant cost and benefit components must be included to ensure CBA results are valid. Identifying program costs and benefits is typically more difficult before than after the program because the anticipated program costs and benefits are merely speculations and may over- or underestimate the true effects of the program. Information is also more limited before than after the program.

Measure Costs and Benefits

After program costs and benefits are identified, the next step is to measure them in terms of a common monetary unit. Measuring program costs and benefits is typically more difficult before than after the program because the hypothetical measurements may be inaccurate when compared with true program results. There are various ways of measuring program costs and benefits. The most straightforward approach is to use the actual monetary costs and benefits. Another approach is to value program costs and benefits at their fair market prices, that is, how much the current market would charge for certain program inputs or outputs. When market prices are not readily available, program or service providers or recipients may be asked to provide a value to them for providing or receiving a particular service.

In measuring cost, the evaluator should not neglect **opportunity costs.** Opportunity costs reflect alternative ways resources can be utilized. For example, if the resources were not spent on a particular program, they might be used for alternative choices. Therefore, the costs of a program may be estimated by the worth of the foregone options these resources might be used for. Sick leave is another example of opportunity cost in that the time spent in receiving treatment and recuperating cannot be used for earning income. Even when sick leave is part of the employment benefit, it represents an opportunity cost for the employer who may have to hire a replacement, pay overtime to existing employees to perform the additional work, or reschedule program activities.

In measuring benefits, the evaluator should not neglect measuring program externalities, or the unintended, "spillover" consequences due to the program. Program externalities may be beneficial or harmful. The beneficial externalities should be added to the program benefits total and the harmful externalities to the costs total. Because such effects are not the intended outcomes, they may be inappropriately omitted from cost–benefit calculations if special efforts are not made to include them.

The evaluator should try to measure or monetize all identified cost and benefit components and specify the measurement methods. When cost items are omitted, the program will seem more efficient than otherwise. When benefit items are omitted, the program will seem less efficient than otherwise. Either situation would likely produce biased results. However, sometimes it may be impossible or unethical to measure certain elements or there is considerable disagreement on the monetary values to be placed on a particular element (such as the value of a human life). The general approach for the evaluator is to produce elements that can be valued and then list those that cannot. If essential elements or too many elements cannot be valued, CBA may not be the appropriate evaluation method to use. Cost-effectiveness analysis might be a preferred alternative.

Value Costs and Benefits

After costs and benefits have been measured in the monetary unit, the evaluator then conducts the actual valuation. Often, a computer spreadsheet program is used to facilitate the valuation. In setting up the spreadsheet, the evaluator may need to choose the relevant time periods and associated discounting factors for noncurrent time periods. The inclusion of different time periods may be required because (1) the program is long and overlaps different time periods; (2) there are several programs to be compared and they take place in different time periods with each period reflecting a particular monetary value; and (3) the program produces benefits that may also be derived in the future, sometimes long after the intervention has taken place. Indeed, holding everything else equal, the longer the time horizon chosen, the more a program would appear beneficial.

To facilitate analysis, costs and benefits occurring at different time periods are brought into the same time period. If the chosen common time period is the present, present values must be calculated for all costs and benefits that are expected in the future. If the chosen common time period is some future time period, future values must be calculated for all costs and benefits that are expected for that future time period. Discounting is the technique to reduce costs and benefits that are spread out over time to their present values or to their common future values.

The results of discounting, and the whole cost–benefit analysis, are particularly sensitive to the discount rates applied. Why particular discounting rates are selected needs to be explained. Often, to resolve the controversies surrounding the choice of discount rates, evaluators conduct cost–benefit analysis using several different rates. One of the discount rates chosen might be the internal rate of return of the program, that is, the discount rate the program would have to obtain for its benefits to equal its costs. Another rate might be the prevailing lending rate at a local bank. Not only different discounting rates may be used, different assumptions may be applied. Indeed, such sensitivity analyses using varying discounting rates and assumptions to estimate their consequences on program results are often considered signs of a well-conducted cost–benefit analysis.

Another factor that needs to be taken into account when comparing costs and benefits at different time periods is inflation (or deflation, which is much less common). Inflation factors are often published for different years, and adjustments can accordingly be made to reflect the true value of money for different periods of time.

The final step in valuing costs and benefits is to compare total program costs to total program benefits by subtracting costs from benefits. If the result is positive, then the program has a net benefit. If the result is negative, then the program has a net loss. The net result of one program may be compared with that of another program or some objective standard to have a sense of the relative success of a particular program.

Method of Cost-Effectiveness Analysis

The identification, measurement, and valuation of costs, including assumptions and discounting factors, are similar between CBA and CEA (Guttentag and Stuening, 1975; Stokey and Zeckhauser, 1978; Rossi and Freeman, 1993). Cost-effectiveness analysis, however, does not require program benefits to be reduced to a monetary unit. Instead, program benefits are measured in terms of whether the program has reached its substantive goals, or at least significant portions of these goals. If the goals have been reached, or substantially reached, then the program is considered effective. CEA is often used to compare the efficiency (i.e., the monetary value of program costs) of programs that share the same or similar goals and outcome measures. The key is to compare which program components are more efficient. Programs may be ranked in terms of their costs for reaching given goals. If different programs have different degrees of goal achievements, CEA can be used to describe the various inputs required for achieving different degrees of goals. CEA may be used both before and after the program.

Limitations

In spite of their values, there are also limitations in the use of CBA and CEA. First, the identification of costs and benefits may be incomplete or subject to controversies. Even though efficiency analyses are largely quantitative and rigorous, there is no single "right" analysis. Different costs and outcomes may be taken into account, depending on the perspectives and values of sponsors, stakeholders, targets, and evaluators themselves. Second, the valuation of costs and benefits may also be problematic. Controversies may result from placing economic values on particular input or outcome measures. Different ways of valuing costs and outcomes may be used, depending on the perspectives and values of sponsors, stakeholders, targets, and evaluators themselves. Third, complete use of CBA or CEA may not be feasible, practical, or wise in many evaluation projects. The required data elements for undertaking cost–benefit calculations may not be fully available.

CBA and CEA may be appropriately performed when the program has independent funding, not when program costs or benefits cannot be separated from those related to other nonprogram activities. It may be too expensive or time-consuming to collect all the data needed. Some measures of inputs or outcomes cannot be meaningfully converted into monetary terms. CBA and CEA cannot be performed when program impact and magnitude of impact are not known or cannot be validly estimated.

Modeling

Models are constructed to reduce the complexity of the problem to be solved by eliminating trivial and noncritical elements so that attention can be focused on the essential features of the program. They are the abstraction of the real world designed to capture the essential elements of the problems. One major advantage of modeling is that it helps a person think rationally before action. Consider, for example, the common notion that we should improve access to physicians in medically underserved areas. However, providing rural people with access to doctors and other health care providers is merely a means to an end. The goal, frequently overlooked, is to improve people's health. It is possible for a decision maker to be so involved with access that the health of the population becomes a side issue.

Another advantage of modeling is that it forces us to focus on fundamental principles rather than nonessential elements. Models convert a complex situation into one that clearly lays out the critical elements. The process of constructing a model forces us to find out about the situation and the types of information needed to construct the model. The difficulty experienced in constructing a model may indicate how little we know about the problem and how much more we need to understand about all aspects of the system to be modeled. Understanding the system is not simply a matter of finding out the relationships among variables; it is also a matter of obtaining accurate information. The effective analyst should not only talk to those knowledgeable about the system but look for independent corroboration before relying on the information obtained.

Modeling is also less expensive and more feasible than experimenting with the system itself. For example, in designing the construction of a hospital, planners need to find out the impact of many variables on design, including patient load, intensive care load, emergency rate, to name a few. To experiment with an actual hospital would be prohibitively expensive in terms of time and money, and dangerous to patients' health. Modeling, on the other hand, allows us to gain insights into the potential impact of various combinations of the essential variables of interest.

There are many examples of models. Graphs and charts are a type of model. Flow charts that draw boxes and show the connections between them are a type of diagrammatic model. Decision trees that identify distinct stages in a complex process are another type of model.

Models may be classified as deterministic or probabilistic, and descriptive or prescriptive (Stokey and Zeckhauser, 1978, pp. 13–16). Deterministic models describe or predict outcomes that are assumed to be certain. Probabilistic models refer to situations where the result following a particular action is not a unique outcome but consists of a range of possible outcomes with associated probabilities of happening. When confronted with uncertain consequences of a policy choice, and in particular if the possible consequences differ widely from one another, the analyst can construct a decision tree and estimate the probability of each outcome.

Descriptive models attempt to describe or explain how variables of interest operate, predict how they will respond to changes in other parts of a system, or show what outcomes will likely result from choices or actions. Prescriptive models encompass elements of descriptive models that delineate the choices available to decision makers and predict the outcome of each. They further include procedures that help decision makers choose among alternative choices of action, taking into account decision makers' preferences among alternative choices and outcomes. Prescriptive models are so named because they help prescribe courses of action. They may also be termed normative or optimizing models.

Report Findings

Evaluators have many ways to report the findings of their evaluation, including informal meetings with program and evaluation sponsors, memos, newsletters, formal presentations, formal written reports, and scholarly publications (Morris, Fitz-Gibbon, and Freeman, 1987). To program sponsors, a formal written report is perhaps the most important product of evaluation and is required from the evaluator. To enhance their utility, evaluation results should be presented in a way that nonresearchers can easily understand. The evaluator may share any draft reports with the clients for review before turning in the final product.

The formal evaluation report typically starts with an executive summary that presents the highlights of the major sections of the report, with particular emphasis on the major findings of the evaluation. In the introduction section of the report, the purposes of the evaluation and the major evaluation questions to be discussed are briefly reviewed.

In the evaluation methods section, the design of the evaluation, sources of data, and techniques for data analysis are described. Their limitations, if any, should be discussed along with other constrains of the evaluation (e.g., limited budget and time, political and organizational constraints, etc.).

In the program implementation section, the evaluator summarizes the major features of the program, how the program is operating, whether it is being implemented as planned, major problems encountered during the program, and external and internal factors that have influenced the program. When a program includes more than one site, the evaluator should also compare similarities and differences in program staffing, administration, targets, implementation, or surrounding environments among the sites.

In the evaluation results section, the results of the analysis are presented with particular emphasis on the effects of the program, that is, to what extent the goals and objectives of the program have been achieved. The presentation should be organized to address all the objectives of the evaluation. Both quantitative and qualitative results should be presented. Tables and graphs may be used to summarize major quantitative analysis results. Qualitative results may be presented as cases, anecdotes, and quotes. While quantitative analysis reveals the outcomes of the program, qualitative analysis explores how the outcomes have been achieved.

In the discussion and recommendations section, the evaluator first delineates the major findings of the evaluation (both statistical and substance significance should be taken into account), summarizes the major strengths and weaknesses of the program, assesses to what extent program goals and objectives have been achieved, and discusses the generalizability about program effectiveness in other similar setting. Then, specific recommendations are made to indicate areas for further improvement related to the program, its staffing, activities, and administration.

STRENGTHS AND WEAKNESSES

The principal strength of evaluation research is its potential for making an impact on policy. Evaluation research can contribute to the improvement of the design and implementation of health programs and interventions aimed at improving the health status of the population. Compared with other types of research, evaluation has greater policy-making relevance and significance and practical utility to policy and decision makers who are looking for research evidence for policy input. The evaluators' challenge is to get the best possible information to policy and decision makers and then to get those people to actually use the information for policy purpose.

There are many ways evaluation results may be utilized. Evaluation results may be directly used in program development and modification. Evaluation research may have an indirect impact on policy and decision makers who are conceptually influenced by evaluation results in their future policy and program planning.

Evaluation research frequently encounters some potentially limiting factors. For example, the internal validity of evaluation may be limited by the unfeasibility of random assignment as a result of resistance from subjects, sponsors, administrators, or staff. The resulting selection bias and the later differential attrition rates could enhance or mask the true impact of the program.

The external validity of evaluation may be threatened by other commonly encountered features of health programs. For example, the program may be effective in a particular geographic setting where external factors are crucial to its implementation. When the effectiveness of a program is dependent on the personal qualities and interests of the staff who administer it, program results might not be generalizable to widespread application of the program by staff who may be less capable, committed, or interested in program success. The knowledge that one is a participant in an experimental health program can generate enthusiasm and cooperation that might not be there when the program is no longer novel or being evaluated. These potential threats to external validity should be watched carefully, or the extension of a program or policy to other participants or beneficiaries may be problematic.

Time, financial limitations, and political climate are important constraints affecting the scope and depth of program evaluation. The amount of time evaluators can devote to the project may determine the choice of evaluation methods and affect the ultimate breadth and quality of an evaluation. The amount of time and effort the evaluator will devote to the project is also dependent on available budget. The political climate could affect an evaluation in several ways. It might place constraints on evaluation design and data collection. The use of research results may be influenced by political considerations. When evaluation results contradict deeply held beliefs, or vested interests, they may not be taken very seriously. After all, an evaluation is only one ingredient in a political process of balancing interests and making decisions.

SUMMARY

Evaluation research serves the purposes of program monitoring and refinement or policy application and expansion. It is the systematic application of scientific research methods for assessing the conceptualization, design, implementation, impact, and/or generalizability of organizational or social (including health services) programs. Evaluation research is technical, applied, and should be objective. The major types of evaluation consist of needs assessment, process evaluation, outcome evaluation, and policy analysis. The process to conduct evaluation research consists of determining the scope of evaluation, getting acquainted with the program, choosing the methodology for evaluation, collecting data, analyzing data, and reporting findings. The principal strength of evaluation research is its potential of making an impact on policy. However, the validity of evaluation is often limited due to impractical application of strict scientific design.

Key Terms

evaluation research	needs assessment
process evaluation	outcome evaluation
policy analysis	cost–benefit analysis (CBA)
cost-effectiveness analysis (CEA)	opportunity costs

Review Questions

1. What is evaluation research? What are the different types of evaluation? What kinds of questions are usually asked for each type of evaluation?

2. How does a researcher conduct an evaluation? What are the elements to be considered in designing an evaluation?

3. Draw the distinctions between cost–benefit analysis and cost-effectiveness analysis. Use an example to illustrate their differences.

4. What are the potential limitations of an evaluation? How can researchers guard against them?

REFERENCES

AHCPR (Agency for Health Care Policy and Research). (1992a). Health Services research on rural health. *NIH Guide for Grants and Contracts,* 21(16, May 1).

AHCPR (1992b). *National Medical Expenditure Survey: Questionnaires and Data Collection Methods for the Medical Provider Survey.* (AHCPR Pub. No. 92-0042) Rockville, MD: U.S. Department of Health and Human Services.

AHCPR. (1994a). Medical treatment effectiveness research: Part II. *NIH Guide for Grants and Contracts,* 23(18, May 13).

AHCPR. (1994b). Medical treatment effectiveness research: Summary. *NIH Guide for Grants and Contracts,* 23(22, June 10).

AHCPR. (1991). Rural health care research: Impacting vulnerable populations. *NIH Guide for Grants and Contracts,* 20(6, Feb. 8).

Alkin, M. C., Kosecoff, J., Fitz-Gibbon, C., and Seligman, R. (1974). *Evaluation and Decision-Making: The Title VII Experience.* (CSE Monograph Series in Evaluation no. 4). Los Angeles: Center for the Study of Evaluation.

Andrews, F., and Grandall, R. (1976). The validity of measures of self-reported well-being. *Social Indications Research,* 3, 1–19.

Bailit, H., Federico, J., and McGivney, W. (1995). Use of outcomes studies by a managed care organization: Valuing measured treatment effects. *Medical Care,* 33(4), AS216–AS225.

Barker, J. B., Bayne, T., Higgs, Z. R., Jenkin, S. A., Murphy, D., and Synoground, G. (1994). Community analysis: A collaborative community practice project. *Public Health Nursing,* 11, 113–118.

Bergner, M., Bobbitt, R., Carter, W. B., and Gilson, B. S. (1981). The sickness impact profile: A development and final revision of a health status measure. *Medical Care,* 19(8), 787–805.

Bergner, M., Bobbitt, R., Kressel, Pollard, W., Gilson, B., and Morris, J. (1976). The sickness impact profile: Conceptual formulation and methodology for the development of a health status measure. *International Journal of Health Services,* 6, 393–415.

Bergner, M. (1985). Measurement of health status. *Medical Care,* 23, 696–704.

Blaney, D. R. (1988). *Cost-Effective Nursing Practice: Guidelines for Nurse Managers.* Philadelphia: Lippincott.

Bureau of Primary Health Care. (1994a). *BPHC-Supported Primary Care Centers Directory.* Bethesda, MD: Health Resource Service Administration, U.S. Public Health Service, U.S. Department of Health and Human Services, October.

Bureau of Primary Health Care. (1994b). *Community Health Centers' Performance under Managed Care.* Bethesda, MD: Health Resource Service Administration, U.S. Public Health Service, U.S. Department of Health and Human Services, December.

Bureau of Primary Health Care. (1995). *Integrated Service Networks and Federally Qualified Health Centers.* Bethesda, MD: Health Resource Service Administration, U.S. Public Health Service, U.S. Department of Health and Human Services, February.

Campbell, D. T., and Stanley, J. C. (1966). *Experimental and Quasi-experimental Designs for Research.* Chicago: Rand McNally.

Cooke, T. D., and Campbell, D. T. (1976). The design and conduct of quasi-experimental and true experiments in field settings. In M. Dunnette (Ed.), *Handbook of Industrial and Organizational Psychology.* Chicago: Rand McNally.

Department of Veterans Affairs (1989). *Cost–Benefit Analysis Handbook.* Washington, DC: Department of Veterans Affairs, Assistant Secretary for Finance and Planning, Deputy Assistant Secretary for Planning and Management Analysis.

Dignan, M., and Carr, P. (1987). *Program Planning for Health Education and Health Promotion.* Philadelphia: Lea and Febiger.

Dixon, J. S., and Bird, H. A. (1981). Reproducibility along a 10cm vertical visual analogue scale. *Annual of Rheumatic Diseases,* 40, 87–89.

Drummond, M. F. (1987). *Methods for the Economic Evaluation of Health Care Programmes.* New York: Oxford University Press.

Fairbank, J., Couper, J., Daview, J., and O'Brien, J. (1980). The Oswestry low back pain disability questionnaire. *Physiotherapy,* 66, 271–273.

Farley, S. (1993). The community as partner in primary health care. Nursing and Health Care, 14, 244–249.

Fitz-Gibbon, C. T., and Morris, L. L. (1987). *How to Analyze Data.* Newbury Park, CA: Sage.

Fitz-Gibbon, C. T., and Morris, L. L. (1987). *How to Design a Program Evaluation.* Newbury Park, CA: Sage.

Ginzberg, E. (1994). Improving health care for the poor. *JAMA,* 271(6), 464–466.

Goldberg, D., and Hillier, V. (1979). A scaled version of the General Health questionnaire. *Psychology Medicine,* 9, 139–145.

Green, L., and Kreuter, M. (1991). *Health Promotion Planning: An Educational and Environmental Approach.* Mountain View, CA: Mayfield.

Greenfield, S., and Nelson, E. C. (1979). Recent developments and future issues in the use of health status assessment measures in clinical settings. *Medical Care,* 30(Supplement), MS23–MS41.

Guadagnoli, E., and McNeil, B. J. (1994). Outcome research: Hope for the future or the latest rage. *Inquiry,* 31 (Spring), 14–24.

Guttentag, M., and Struening, L. (Eds.). (1975). *Handbook of Evaluation Research,* vol. 2. Beverly Hills, CA: Sage.

Herman, J. L., Morris, L. L., and Fitz-Gibbon, C. T. (1987). *Evaluator's Handbook.* Newbury Park, CA: Sage.

Hunt, S., and McEven, J. (1985). Measuring health status: A new tool for clinicians and epidemiologists. *Journal of R. Col. Gen. Practice*, 35, 185–188.

Hunt, S., and McEven, J. (1980). The development of a subjective health indicator. *Social Health and Illness*, 2(3), 231–246.

Kark, S. L. (1981). The Practice of Community-Oriented Primary Health Care. New York: Appleton-Century-Crofts.

Kitzhaber, J. A. (1993). Prioritizing health services in an era of limits: The Oregon experience. *BMJ*, 307, 373.

Meenan, R., Gertman, P., and Mason, J. (1980). Measuring health status in arthritis. *Arthiritis and Rheumatism*, 23(2), 146–152.

Melzack, R. (Ed.). (1983). *Pain Measurement and Assessment.* New York: Raven Press.

Morris, L. L., Fitz-Gibbon, C. T., and Freeman, M. E. (1987). *How to Communicate Evaluation Findings.* Newbury Park, CA: Sage.

Mullan, F. (1982). Community-oriented primary care: An agenda for the '80s. *New England Journal of Medicine*, 307, 1076–1078.

Parkerson, G. R., Broadhead, W. E., and Tse, C. J. (1995). Health status and severity of illness as predictors of outcomes in primary care. *Medical Care*, 33(1), 53–66.

Patrick, D. L. (1993). *Health Status and Health Policy: Quality of Life in Health Care Evaluation and Resource Allocation.* New York: Oxford University Press.

Patrick, D., Darby, S., Green, S., Horton, G., Locker, D., and Wiggins, R. (1981). Screening for disability in the inner city. *Journal of Epidemiology Community Health*, 35, 65–70.

Patton, M. Q. (1987). *How to Use Qualitative Methods in Evaluation.* Newbury Park, CA: Sage.

Patton, M. Q. (1990). *Qualitative Evaluation and Research Methods.* Newbury Park, CA: Sage.

Pearce, D. W. (1981). *The Social Appraisal of Projects: A Text in Cost–Benefit Analysis.* London: Macmillan.

Riesenberg, D., and Glass, R. M. (1989). The medical outcomes study. *JAMA*, 262(7), 943.

Rossi, P. H., and Freeman, H. E. (1993). *Evaluation: A Systematic Approach.* Newbury Park, CA: Sage.

Schulman, K. A., Rubenstein, L. E., Chesley, F. D., and Eisenberg, J. M. (1995). The role of race and socioeconomic factors in health services research. *Health Services Research*, 30, 179–193.

Scott, J., and Huuskisson, E. C. (1979). Vertical or horizontal visual analogue scales. *Annual of Rheumatic Disease*, 38, 560.

Shortell, S. M., Gillies, R. R., and Anderson, D. A. (1994). The new world of managed care: Creating organized delivery systems. *Health Affairs*, Winter, 46–64.

Spitzer, W. O., Dobson, A. J., and Hall, J. (1981). Measuring quality of life of cancer patients: A concise QL-Index for use by physicians. *Journal of Chronic Disease*, 34, 585–597.

Stecher, B. M., and Davis, W. A. (1987). *How to Focus an Evaluation.* Newbury Park, CA: Sage.

Steinwachs, D. M. (1989). Application of health status assessment measures in policy research. *Medical Care*, 27(Supplement), S12–S26.

Stokey, E., and Zeckhauser, R. (1978). *A Primer for Policy Analysis.* New York,: W. W. Norton and Co. Inc.

Tarlov, B. R., Ware, J. E., Greenfield, S., Nelson, E. C., and Perrin, E. (1989). The medical outcomes study. *JAMA,* 262(7), 925–930.

Tolley, K. (1995). *Evaluating the Cost-Effectiveness of Counseling in Health Care.* London, New York: Routledge.

Veney, J. E., and Kaluzny, A. D. (1991). *Evaluation and Decision Making for Health Services.* 2nd ed. Ann Arbor, MI: Health Administration Press.

Ware, J. E. (1986). The assessment of health status. In L. H. Aiken and D. Mechanic (Eds.), *Applications of Social Science to Clinical Medicine and Health Policy.* New Brunswick, NJ: Rutgers University Press.

Williams, A., Ware, J., and Donald, C. (1981). A model of mental health, life events and social supports applicable to general populations. *Journal of Health and Social Behavior,* 22, 324–336.

Young, K. R. (1994). An evaluative study of a community health service development. *Journal of Advanced Nursing,* 19, 58–65.

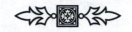

CHAPTER

10

Design in Health Services Research

LEARNING OBJECTIVES

- To summarize the characteristics of commonly used research methods.
- To understand the guidelines in choosing appropriate research methods.

Research design is concerned with the planning of research and specifies the hypotheses or questions to be studied, the data to be collected, the methods of data collection, and analysis. It is the "blueprint" of research that lays out the strategy and framework for the conduct of research, integrating different phases of the research activities and providing the basic direction (Miller, 1991; Keppel, 1991; Creswell, 1994). Even though research design is a distinctive stage in itself, it is built upon knowledge of many previous and subsequent stages of the research process. The conceptualization stage (Chapter 2) lays the foundation of research questions to be studied. If the research is based on available data, the groundwork stage identifies the sources of relevant available data (Chapter 3). If the research is based on a primary source of data, the sampling stage (Chapter 11) provides the appropriate sampling method, and the data collection stage (Chapter 13) indicates the best method of data collection. The data analysis stage (Chapter 14) selects the most appropriate and efficient method(s) of data analysis. Please consult those related chapters for relevant issues when designing a study.

Another important decision, often considered simultaneously when choosing specific design for the study, is the selection of an appropriate research method. **Research method,** or *methodology,* consists of a body of knowledge that reflects the general philosophy and purpose of the research process, the assumptions and values that serve as rationale for research, the general approach of data collection and analysis, and the standards used for interpreting data and reaching conclusions.

Chapters 4 through 9 have presented the major types of research methods useful for health services research. These include research review, meta-analysis (Chapter 4), secondary analysis, research analysis of administrative records (Chapter 5), qualitative research, case study (Chapter 6), experiment, quasi experiment (Chapter 7), survey research, longitudinal research (Chapter 8), and evaluation research (Chapter 9). Each of these methods has its own unique characteristics, strengths, and weaknesses. In choosing the type of method suitable for a particular study, researchers need to compare the characteristics between these methods and their particular studies and select the method(s) that optimally matches the study requirements and constraints. In this chapter, the characteristics of the major types of research methods will be summarized, and an approach to choosing the method(s) most suitable for the investigator's intended study will be suggested.

CHARACTERISTICS OF RESEARCH METHODS

There are various ways to consider the characteristics of research methods (Creswell, 1994). Research methods may be classified as primary or secondary, quantitative or qualitative, cross-sectional or longitudinal. The purposes of research methods may be exploratory, descriptive, or causal. Research methods may be considered in terms of their cost, time, sample, depth of information provided, design, and analysis. In this section, we examine how the research methods differ in terms of these characteristics. Table 10–1 summarizes the results of the comparisons.

TABLE 10.1 Characteristics of major types of health services research methods

Research Methods

Characteristics	Research Review	Meta-analysis	Secondary Analysis	Administrative Records	Qualitative Research	Case Study	Experiment, Quasi Experiment	Survey Research	Longitudinal Research	Evaluation Research
Primary	x	x	x		x	x	x	x	x	x
Secondary	x	x	x	x	x	x		x		x
Quantitative	x	x	x	x		x	x	x	x	x
Qualitative		x	x		x	x				x
Cross-sectional	x	x	x		x	x		x		x
Longitudinal	x	x	x	x	x	x	x	x	x	x
Exploratory	x	x	x	x	x	x		x		x
Descriptive	x	x	x	x		x	x	x	x	x
Causal		x	x				x	x	x	x
Cost: high	x	x			x	x	x		x	x
moderate							x	x		x
low	x	x	x	x	x	x				x
Time: long	x	x	x	x	x	x	x	x	x	x
moderate							x	x		x
short	x	x	x	x	x	x				x
Sample: large	x	x	x			x	x	x		x
moderate	x	x								
small		x			x	x				
Depth: great	x	x			x	x			x	
moderate	x				x	x				x
low		x	x	x			x	x	x	x
Design: hard	x	x			x	x	x	x	x	x
moderate					x	x				x
easy	x	x	x	x		x		x		x
Analysis: hard	x	x	x	x	x	x		x	x	x
moderate	x	x	x	x	x	x		x	x	x
easy	x		x	x	x	x	x	x		x

Primary versus Secondary Research

Research is considered primary when the data originate with the study. Research is considered secondary when the data were collected for some other purposes. In general, compared with secondary research, primary research tends to produce data more relevant for the study. However, it is also more costly and time-consuming to collect data in primary than secondary research.

Among the research methods discussed, experiment, quasi experiment, survey, and longitudinal research are primary research methods. Research review, meta-analysis, secondary analysis, and research analysis of administrative records are secondary research methods. Qualitative research and case study are mainly primary methods although they may also include elements of secondary analysis. Evaluation research can be either primary or secondary.

Quantitative versus Qualitative Research

Quantitative research focuses on using numbers in the analysis. Qualitative research focuses on using statements in the analysis. Compared with qualitative research, quantitative research is able to cover more people and hence presents broader and more generalizable findings. By contrast, qualitative research tends to produce more depth and detailed information, and hence its findings tend to be more valid.

Among the research methods discussed, meta-analysis, research analysis of administrative records, experiment, quasi experiment, survey, and longitudinal research are quantitative research methods. Research review and qualitative research are qualitative research methods. Evaluation research, case study, and secondary analysis can be either quantitative or qualitative.

Cross-Sectional versus Longitudinal

Cross-sectional research refers to using data collected at one point in time. Longitudinal research refers to using data collected at two or more points in time. Collecting cross-sectional data is cheaper and less time consuming than collecting longitudinal data. Longitudinal data tend to be more extensive and better suited for causal research than cross-sectional data. However, attrition is a potential problem when designing longitudinal studies.

Among the research methods discussed, research review, meta-analysis, research analysis of administrative records, experiment, quasi experiment, and evaluation research tend to be longitudinal. Secondary analysis, qualitative research, case study, and survey research can be either cross-sectional or longitudinal.

Exploratory, Descriptive versus Causal Research

Exploratory research is conducted when little is known about the subject matter. The purpose is to gain an initial insight into the subject matter, finding out its critical issues and concepts. Descriptive research provides a more detailed account of the distributions of the major characteristics of the subject matter. Causal research explains subject matter of interest, testing hypotheses and examining relationships, including cause and effect, among variables. Generally, the design of causal research is most rigorous, followed by descriptive and exploratory research. There is often a time sequence among the three research purposes. Exploratory research is conducted first to provide categories and concepts of characteristics important to a subject. Descriptive research is performed next to understand the distributions of these characteristics. Causal research then is carried out to assess the relationships among these characteristics.

Among the research methods discussed, qualitative research and case study tend to be exploratory. Research review and research analysis of administrative records tend to be descriptive. Experiment, quasi experiment, meta-analysis, evaluation, and longitudinal research tend to be causal. Secondary analysis and survey research are mostly descriptive, although they can be causal if proper statistical methods are used.

Cost

The cost of research is primarily concerned with the cost of data collection and analysis. It usually costs more for primary research than secondary research, because data have to be collected firsthand; longitudinal research than cross-sectional research, because data have to be collected at multiple points in time; and causal research than exploratory or descriptive research, because the design is typically more difficult to implement.

Among the research methods discussed, generally longitudinal research and experiment tend to be most costly, followed by survey research. Methods of relatively low cost include research review, meta-analysis, secondary analysis, and research analysis of administrative records, primarily due to savings in data collection. Qualitative research and case study tend to be of moderate to low cost depending on the scope of investigation. Evaluation research perhaps has the greatest variations in terms of cost, ranging from very low to very high, depending on the scope of the evaluation, the methods used, and the time permitted.

Time

The time spent in conducting research is primarily concerned with data collection and analysis. Like cost, more time is usually spent in primary research than secondary research, longitudinal research than cross-sectional research, and causal research than exploratory or descriptive research. Indeed, there is a close correlation between research time and cost.

Among the research methods discussed, longitudinal research and experiments tend to be lengthier than other methods, followed by survey research. Research review, meta-analysis, secondary analysis, and research analysis of administrative records usually require less time. The time spent for qualitative research and case study tend to be moderate. Evaluation research has the greatest variations in terms of time spent, depending on the scope and urgency of the evaluation.

Sample

The sample is drawn from the population of interest and its characteristics may be used to generalize to the population of interest. The size of the sample depends on many factors. Research purpose is related to sample size in that exploratory research typically requires a smaller sample than causal or descriptive research. The homogeneity of population characteristics is also associated with sample size. A smaller sample size is needed for a more homogeneous population. Research budget and available time also influence sample size. A larger sample requires more time and money than a smaller sample. Chapter 11 provides a more systematic review on how to determine the sample size for a study.

Among the research methods discussed, the less costly quantitative methods such as survey research, secondary analysis, and research analysis of administrative records generally use large sample sizes. More costly quantitative methods such as experiment, quasi experiment, and longitudinal and evaluation research generally use moderate sample sizes. Qualitative methods such as qualitative research, case study, and research review tend to use moderate to low sample sizes. Meta-analysis uses moderate to low samples because of the difficulty of locating relevant research articles for secondary analysis.

Depth

The depth of research has to do with how much detailed information can be collected from the subjects. Given the same research budget, there is a trade-off between the scope of coverage (i.e., how many respondents can be surveyed as reflected by the sample size) and the depth of coverage. Generally, qualitative research sacrifices scope in favor of depth and quantitative research sacrifices depth in favor of scope. Exploratory research emphasizes depth whereas descriptive and causal research emphasize scope. The depth of coverage is also more limited for longitudinal than for cross-sectional studies due to greater amount of missing data.

Among the research methods discussed, qualitative methods such as qualitative research and case study provide great depth of coverage. Quantitative methods such as survey research, secondary analysis, experiment, quasi experiment, research analysis of administrative records, and longitudinal research provide moderate to low depth of coverage. Meta-analysis usually has low depth due to lack of common variables from all relevant studies. Research review has moderate to low depth depending on how much research has been conducted on a particular subject. The depth of evaluation research varies based on the method(s) used and the extent of evaluation.

Design

As stated at the beginning of this chapter, design is the planning phase of research, specifying research questions and data sources and determining the methods for data collection and analysis. Research design is usually more complex for causal research than exploratory or descriptive research, for longitudinal than cross-sectional studies, and for quantitative than qualitative research. The complexity of design is also positively correlated with time and cost.

Among the research methods discussed, experiment, quasi experiment, and longitudinal research generally have the most complex design, since much of the research effort goes into improving and implementing the design. Specific tasks include refining the number of conditions, measuring key variables, providing instructions to subjects, pretesting, introducing intervention, and collecting data. The design for survey research, qualitative research, and case study is of moderate difficulty. Research review and meta-analysis have relatively easy designs. The design for secondary analysis and research analysis of administrative records depends on available designs and is therefore easy for the current investigator. The design of evaluation research relies on the method chosen for the evaluation. Many health services are intended to cause things to happen, for example, by improving health status, increasing utilization, and so forth. Evaluation research that aimed at determining whether health services (or other interventions) actually accomplish their purposes is typically related to experiment or quasi experiment.

Analysis

Data analysis involves applying statistical methods to data collected from the research and generating results to be used to answer the research questions. Data analysis is generally more difficult for quantitative than qualitative research, longitudinal than cross-sectional studies, and causal than exploratory or descriptive research. The difficulty of analysis positively influences the time and cost of research.

Among the research methods discussed, longitudinal research, secondary analysis, research analysis of administrative records, meta-analysis, and survey research generally require more complex data analysis. In contrast, the analysis of experiment and quasi experiment data is relatively easy and straightforward. The analysis of data from qualitative research, case study, and research review is of moderate difficulty. The difficulty of analyzing data from evaluation research depends on the type and number of methods chosen for the evaluation.

CHOOSING APPROPRIATE RESEARCH METHODS

The comparison of the major research methods indicates that each method offers particular strengths and weaknesses and contributes in different ways to some particular purposes. For example, research review, meta-analysis, secondary analysis, and research analysis of administrative records all have the principal advantages of speed and relatively low costs compared to other types of study methods. Their principal disadvantage is that the scope and depth of the study is constrained by available studies or data. Further, when the data were collected for another purpose, gaining familiarity with the data elements and evaluation of data quality become difficult and may be time-consuming. Experiment and longitudinal research have the principal advantage of validity in study design. However, these methods are usually very costly and sometimes not appropriate. Survey research is the most widely used method because it is the most efficient research design capable of obtaining a larger sample size per dollar spent than any other methods. However, data analysis requires great effort and skill, especially when causal relationships are studied.

Because research methods involve differing strengths and weaknesses, they constitute alternative, rather than mutually exclusive, strategies for research. In many situations, a combination of methods can be used in the same study. The first task in choosing a research method should be to sort out the various methods and their relative merits, deciding whether choices must be made or two or more methods should be combined. In this section, we suggest some guidelines for choosing the appropriate method(s) for investigation. These guidelines should be evaluated based on the investigator's particular research situation, and used carefully.

Research Purpose

The type of research methods chosen is closely related to the purpose of the investigator's research. If researchers are conducting an exploratory research in which they had little prior knowledge of the subject matter, a qualitative research method—such as case study, fieldwork, or observation—is generally more appropriate. If they are conducting a descriptive study in which their primary interest is to provide a detailed description of the major characteristics related to the subject matter, then survey research is preferred. If they are conducting a causal or explanatory research in which they want to find out the relationships among various factors related to the subject matter, experiment, quasi experiment, or longitudinal research may be considered. Secondary analysis and research analysis of administrative records may be selected for both descriptive and causal research if available data are relevant to the research purpose. When researchers are asked to perform an evaluation of a program or project, evaluation research comes into play. If there are large numbers of prior studies on a subject matter, researchers may want to conduct a research review or meta-analysis (when study results are published quantitatively) before undertaking their own study.

Available Resources

The type of research methods chosen is also related to the available resources for conducting the research. Valuable resources include knowledge, money, time, support, and analytic skills. Investigators' knowledge and familiarity with research methods play a significant role in the method chosen for the study. Some researchers are limited in their research training and experience. The options available to them are correspondingly limited only to the ones with which they are most familiar and comfortable. An interdisciplinary research team can sometimes overcome this problem by including people from different scientific disciplines and research backgrounds.

The available budget is critical for decisions about the type of methods to be used and the scope of study. Qualitative research is generally cheaper than quantitative research. Survey research is cheaper than experiment research. Cross-sectional study is cheaper than longitudinal study. Research population, data sources, sample size, data collection, and analysis methods are all tied to monetary consideration. Like money, time plays an essential role in the choice of research method. For example, the time allowed for evaluation often dictates which method and how many methods can be chosen.

Staff support is important because given the same amount of time, more staff support usually means more data collected. The interview survey perhaps is the best example. After subjects have been identified and located, the more qualified interviewers researchers have available to them, the sooner they can collect information from the subjects. Finally, analytic skills are crucial for data analysis. After all, data have to be analyzed to address important research questions. Analytic skills often involve statistical skills and computer skills. They are especially important for large-scale studies or studies using data from multiple sources. Indeed, absence of those skills may limit the investigator to generally descriptive analysis, which does not make full use of the data collected.

Access

Access to research subjects or available data is an important determinant to selecting research methods. Subjects' willingness may dictate whether experimental techniques can be used or a quasi experiment has to be used instead. Subject attrition is a critical concern for longitudinal research designs. The data collection methods chosen for survey research—whether mail questionnaires or telephone or face-to-face interviews—may depend on the characteristics of the subjects. Qualitative research relies heavily on the subjects' compliance and willingness to be studied, observed, or interviewed. The availability of, and accessibility to, relevant data sources may determine whether secondary research can be conducted in lieu of primary research. Access to available data and subjects also determines the type of methods chosen for evaluation research.

Combining Research Methods

In choosing methods for study, investigators should not be confined to finding only one method for a particular study. Often, a combination of methods can more effectively fulfill the research purpose (Greene, Caracelli, and Graham, 1989; Creswell,

1994). For example, research review is typically conducted before any study is conceptualized and often included in the final research report. Meta-analysis can be performed as an independent study as well as an integral, preliminary part of a primary research. Secondary data may be used in combination with primary data sources, collected to make up for the missing elements. Qualitative research can be used in combination with quantitative research, with the former laying the groundwork as well as providing interpretations for data drawn from large-scale quantitative research. Many more examples may be cited about various configurations of combining research methods. Table 10–2 summarizes those combinations.

Specifying the Limitations

Finally, investigators should explicitly specify the limitations or constraints facing their study, as well as be clear about what can, and what cannot, be tackled by the study. Frequently, investigators have to scale down the design, modify the research question, or select alternative methods because of uncontrollable factors. The specification of study constraints is important for the reader or other researchers who may not be limited by the identified constraints. When faced with budgetary or other constraints, researchers should sacrifice scope of study to maintain validity and reliability of study findings. For example, costs can typically be reduced by having smaller sample sizes, more clustered or narrowly defined samples, and shorter questionnaires.

TABLE 10–2   Combining different types of health services research methods

Primary Types	*Possible Additional Types*
Research review (Chapter 4)	Meta-analysis
Secondary analysis (Chapter 5)	Research review, Meta-analysis, Survey research, Longitudinal research
Qualitative research (Chapter 6)	Research review, Case study, Observation, Focused interview
Experiment (Chapter 7)	Research review, Meta-analysis, Quasi experiment, Longitudinal research, Survey research
Survey research (Chapter 8)	Research review, Meta-analysis, Qualitative research, Secondary analysis, Longitudinal research
Evaluation research (Chapter 9)	Research review, Experiment, Quasi experiment, Survey research, Secondary analysis, Longitudinal research, Qualitative research

SUMMARY

Research methods may be classified as primary or secondary, quantitative or qualitative, cross-sectional or longitudinal. Their purposes may be exploratory, descriptive, or causal. They may be considered in terms of their cost, time, sample, depth of information provided, design, and analysis. In choosing appropriate research method(s) for a study, researchers should consider such factors as the purpose of the research, the available resources for conducting the research, access to research subjects or available data, and the possibility of using a combination of methods. The limitations or constraints of the design should also be specified.

Key Terms

research design   research method

Review Questions

1. What are the commonly used types of research methods? Differentiate their major characteristics.
2. What factors need to be considered in choosing the appropriate research method(s)?

REFERENCES

Creswell, J. W. (1994). *Research Design: Qualitative and Quantitative Approaches.* Thousand Oaks, CA: Sage.

Greene, J. C., Caracelli, V. J., and Graham, W. F. (1989). Toward a conceptual framework for mixed-method evaluation designs. *Educational Evaluation and Policy Analysis,* 11(3), 255–274.

Keppel, G. (1991). *Design and Analysis: A Researcher's Handbook.* 3rd ed. Englewood Cliffs, NJ: Prentice-Hall.

Miller, D. C. (1991). *Handbook of Research and Social Measurement.* 5th ed. Newbury Parks, CA: Sage.

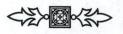

CHAPTER

Sampling in Health Services Research

LEARNING OBJECTIVES

- To understand the logic of sampling and commonly used sampling terms.
- To describe the major types of probability and nonprobability sampling.
- To identify factors considered in determining sample size.

DEFINITION

Sampling is the process of selecting a subset of observations from an entire population of interest so that characteristics from the subset can be used to draw conclusions or make inferences about the entire population of interest (Babbie, 1992; Henry, 1990).

Logic of Sampling

The logic of sampling is that a large population of interest can be studied efficiently and accurately through examination of a carefully selected subset or sample of the population. Efficiency has to do with obtaining information at an acceptable cost. Accuracy is concerned with minimizing sampling error or the differences between sample estimates and population parameters.

Sampling is a familiar activity to most people. Few would consume the whole pot of soup just to determine whether it was properly seasoned. Often, a sample of a spoonful of soup would be sufficient. Likewise, sampling is an efficient way to study a population. Rather than observing every individual unit within the population, sampling selects a subset of the units, thus saving money and time that would have been incurred if all units within the population were observed.

Since the purpose of sampling is to make generalization about the whole population of interest—that is, make estimates and test hypotheses about population characteristics based on data from the sample—a sample must be carefully selected to adequately represent population variability and make statistically valid inferences about the population. In the physical and medical sciences, because sampling elements often share a high degree of homogeneity, not many units would be needed to adequately represent the properties of the elements. One test tube of blood, for example, will be quite similar to another. In the social sciences, including health services, sampling elements often involve humans and are far less homogenous than physical or chemical elements. Thus, the sample must be carefully selected to make sure that all major population variations are adequately represented. When the population of interest is large, a well-selected sample can generate more accurate and informative results about the population than information from the entire population. This is because the quality of data collection can be im-proved and there are less opportunities for introducing clerical and measurement errors that may arise from collecting, processing, and analyzing data for a large population.

The central limit theorem provides the theoretical foundation for sampling. It states that sample means are normally distributed (i.e., the bell-shaped curve) around the population mean, and sample distribution will approximate population distribution as the sample size increases. Therefore, carefully used, sampling will enable us to generate information about the population. Specifically, given sufficient sample size, 68 percent of the sample observations will fall within one standard deviation of the population

◈

mean, 95 percent within two standard deviations of the population mean, and 99 percent within three standard deviations of the population mean.

In addition to efficiency and accuracy considerations, sampling is sometimes necessary due to access problems. Not all sampling elements are known, or if identified, accessible. When there is no **sampling frame** or a list of the study population, it may be too time-consuming, let alone costly, to enumerate all the population elements. A stratified sampling plan that enumerates elements within selected strata might be more reasonable and preferred. Sometimes, even when investigators intend to study every member of the population, some members may refuse to be studied. Research ethics dictates that informed consent is a prerequisite of research participation. Some individuals are considered ethically at risk, including minors (those under 18), prisoners, mentally disabled, and institutionalized or hospitalized people. When these people are included in the population being considered, special efforts should be given to ensure informed consent. These efforts include seeking permission from parents or guardians, and conducting reviews through institutional review boards (IRBs).

Sampling Terms

Before describing the different types of sampling methods commonly used in health services research, we first define some frequently used terms in sampling (Rubin, 1983; Henry, 1990; Babbie, 1992; Fowler, 1993). These include **unit of analysis, sampling element, sampling unit, observation unit, population, sampling frame, design,** variable, **statistics,** and **parameters.**

Unit of Analysis

Unit of analysis refers to the object about which the researcher wishes to draw conclusions based on the study. The purpose of the study typically dictates what or who is to be studied and hence what the appropriate unit of analysis is. A variety of units may be studied, including individuals (e.g., patients, doctors), groups (e.g., families, couples, census blocks, cities, geographic regions), institutions (e.g., hospitals, nursing homes, group practices), or events (traffic accidents, diseases). Units of analysis in a study are typically also the sampling elements and the units of observation. When aggregate data are used, conclusions may only be drawn at the aggregate level but not at the individual level to avoid making an ecological fallacy.

Sampling Element

Sampling element refers to the unit of sample to be surveyed, and provides the information base for analysis. The sampling element must be specified before sampling can be undertaken. The choice of a particular sampling element depends on the unit of analysis to be used for a study. The unit of analysis, in turn, depends on the purpose of the study and the target population about whom study results are to be generalized. In applied research, practical policy-related considerations, such as the level at which legislation becomes operative, often determines the relevant unit of analysis. It is important to understand the concept of ecological fallacy: information collected at the aggregate level, such as organizations, counties, or states, may not be generalized to the level of individuals.

In health services research, typically sampling units are individuals, households, or organizations. Social group, industry, or nation state can also be used as sampling element. When individuals are used as the sampling element, they can be further specified in terms of individual characteristics to be included or excluded from a study such as age, sex, race, occupation, income, education, as well as other characteristics pertinent to the study such as those with a particular disease or receiving a particular service. When households are used as the sampling element, they may be further defined in terms of family characteristics, such as presence of children or elderly members, intact or single-parent, number of generations, and the like. When organizations are used as the sampling element, they can be further described in terms of organizational characteristics, such as profit status, services provided, size, and so forth.

Sampling Unit

Sampling unit is the actual unit that is considered for selection. Sampling unit and sampling element are the same in single-stage sampling but different in multistage sampling. An example of multistage sampling would be when one wants to select a sample of counties, then a sample of hospitals within the selected counties, and finally, a sample of patients within the selected hospitals. In this example, the sampling units are county, hospital, and patient, but only the last (patient) is the sampling element because individual patients will be the unit of analysis.

Observation Unit

Observation unit is the unit from which data are actually collected. Observation unit and sampling element may be different when, for example, heads of households (observation unit) are surveyed about all household members (sampling element), or administrators (observation unit) are questioned about characteristics of organizations or their clients (sampling element).

Population

Population refers to the target to which investigators generate the study results. Population may be defined as universe or study relevant. A universe population consists of a theoretically specified aggregation of sampling units. A study population includes only the aggregation of sampling units from which the sample is to be selected. A study population is usually less than a universe population, because some sampling units may be omitted from the sampling frame available. Investigators should find out which types of sampling units are likely to be omitted or inadequately represented in the study population so that generalization about the universe population can be adjusted accordingly.

Sampling Frame

Sampling frame is a list of sampling units from which the sample is actually selected. Examples include telephone directories, membership lists, student rosters, patient records, and the like. Although researchers hope that the sampling frame represents the entire universe population, this is seldom the case, because the sampling frame is typically incomplete and not up-to-date. Sampling frame determines the scope of the study population.

Sampling Design

Sampling design refers to the method used to select the sampling units, and may be classified into probability and nonprobability sampling methods. In **probability sampling,** all sampling units in the study population have a known, nonzero probability of being selected in the sample, typically through a random selection process. Random does not mean haphazard or arbitrary; rather, an unbiased probability method is used to select the sample. Specifically, all sampling units have an equal or known chance of being selected in the sample, and the selection of one unit will not affect the chance of selecting another unit. Random selection produces unbiased sample whose results may be validly generalized to the population of interest.

In **nonprobability sampling,** the probability of selecting any sampling unit is not known because units are selected through a nonrandom process. A nonprobability sample may be biased, because certain units may be more or less likely included in the sample. A biased sample will produce results that cannot be validly generalized to the population of interest.

Variable

A variable is a set of mutually exclusive attributes. Variables are collected with an instrument (e.g., questionnaire, interview guide) from observation units about sampling elements. For example, hospital administrators (observation unit) may be asked about the age, sex, racial, and insurance characteristics (variables) of their patients (sampling element).

Statistics and Parameters

Statistics refer to the summary numerical description of variables about the sample. Parameters refer to the summary numerical description of variables about the population of interest. Statistics are combined from information collected from the sample and used to provide estimates of the population parameters. The accuracy of the estimation may be assessed by the confidence intervals of the sample statistics.

PROBABILITY SAMPLING

Probability sampling requires the specification of the probability that each sample element will be included in the sample. The process of probability sampling consists of using a sampling frame and some random procedure of selection that makes probability estimation and the use of inferential statistics possible. Random sampling, however, does not guarantee that any single sample will be representative of the population. The extent that a sample represents the population depends on the variability within the population and the sample size. If the investigator is certain that a random sample produces unusual and nonrepresentative cases, based on previous experience of the population, he or she should not replace the atypical cases with more typical ones. Rather, the entire sample may be discarded and a new sample drawn instead. Sometimes, it may be necessary to increase the sample size.

Probability sampling methods are generally used at later rather than exploratory phases of research, when accuracy of samples is critical so that sample finding may be validly generalized to the population. Commonly used probability sampling methods include **simple random sampling, systematic sampling, cluster sampling,** and **stratified sampling.** The choices among these methods are typically based on the nature of the population under study, the purpose of the study, and available resources to conduct the study. If the population is homogeneous, simple random and systematic sampling methods are more likely to be used. If the population is heterogeneous, stratified sampling is more likely to be used. If the population is scattered, cluster sampling would be the method of choice. The purpose of the study will determine how accurate the data collected need to be and the types of strata that need to be sampled and analyzed. Resource constraints in terms of time and money will favor cluster over simple random or systematic sampling when face-to-face interviews are planned. The availability of a sampling frame will also affect the choice of a particular method.

Simple Random Sampling

Simple random sampling means that every unit in a population has an equal probability of being included in the sample. The procedure for conducting simple random sampling is:

1. Define the population of interest that constitutes the complete set of units or elements of the universe under study.
2. Establish the sampling frame that lists all units or elements in the population of interest. The sampling frame represents the study population. Whether simple random sampling method is feasible or preferred depends largely on whether or not there exist accurate and complete lists of the population elements from which the

sample is to be drawn. It would be prohibitively expensive and time-consuming to compose such a sampling frame.

3. Assign a number to each element in the sampling frame from 1 to N.
4. Decide upon the desired sample size (n).
5. Select n different random numbers between 1 and N using a table of random numbers. The sample elements corresponding to the selected n random numbers become the sample.

Appendix 5 contains a table of random numbers. Suppose researchers want to sample 400 (n) patients from one year's patient records that include 5000 patients (N). The patient records system may already have assigned codes to patients, say from 0001 to 5000. Since the numbers in Appendix 5 are completely random, it makes no difference where one starts or whether one chooses numbers by moving down columns or across rows. However, in order to remain random, researchers need to decide how to start before they start. Once researchers start using the numbers, they should not use the same numbers again. Say the researcher closes his or her eyes and points a finger at the sixth number down in the second column: 74717. Since the population of patients total 5000, or four digits, only four digits of numbers will be needed and the researcher may choose either to use the first or latter four numbers. Say the researcher chooses to use the latter four digits; the first sampled patient is number 4717. Moving down the column, the second patient becomes 0805. The next number 7602 is beyond the total population size (5000) and hence should be ignored. The next patient selected is 2135. This procedure is used until all 400 sample elements or patients are selected. When researchers come across the same number they have already selected, they should simply ignore it and move on. When the numbers on one page are used up, those on the next page are then used.

6. Collect information from the selected sampling elements. See Chapter 13 for data collection methods.

Systematic Sampling

Systematic sampling selects every kth element from the sampling frame after a random start. The procedure for conducting systematic sampling is:

1. Define the population of interest.
2. Establish the sampling frame that contains a complete list of the population.
3. Decide upon the desired sample size (n).
4. Calculate the sampling interval, which is the distance between elements to be selected for the sample. The sampling interval may be calculated by dividing the population size N (total elements in the sampling frame) by the sample size n, or

N/n. For example, if there are 5000 patients and the researcher wishes to select 400, then the sampling interval is 12.5 (5000/400).

5. For a random start, randomly choose a number from 1 to *k*, with *k* being the sampling interval. In our example, a number from 1 to 13 will be selected. This can be accomplished by drawing a number from a hat containing 13 pieces of paper numbered 1 to 13.

6. Select every *k*th number until the total sample is selected. In our example, since a patient cannot be divided by half, researchers may alternately sample every 12th and then every 13th patient until the total 400 patients are selected. Suppose the randomly selected number is 10, the sample then would include patients numbered 10, 22, 35, 47, 60, . . . , 4998.

Systematic sampling is easier to draw than simple random sampling because the investigator does not have to read from the random numbers all the time to draw the sample or have to number all the list of elements if they are not prenumbered. Therefore, it is often used in lieu of simple random sampling particularly if the sampling list is long or the desired sample size is large. Systematic sampling is commonly used when choosing a sample from city or telephone directories or other preexisting but unnumbered lists.

However, researchers should be cautious about the existence of periodicity or cyclical patterns that may correspond to the sampling interval. For example, if a household survey decides to select every 10th housing unit from the block and the 10th unit happens to be at the corner of the block, then all corner houses would be selected. If there are systematic differences between corner houses and other houses (for example, in terms of size, expensiveness, etc.), then the sample would be biased. In sampling months from a large number of years, if the sampling interval happens to be 12, the investigator will end up selecting the same month within each year, a month that might coincide with a peak patient volume or the worst bad debt ratios. To guard against periodicity, the investigator should carefully examine the sampling frame. If periodicity is detected, systematic sampling can still be used simply by having a random start on every page of the sampling list.

Cluster Sampling

Cluster sampling first breaks the population into groups or clusters and then randomly selects a sample of clusters. In single-stage cluster sampling, all elements of selected clusters are studied. In multistage cluster sampling, two or more stages of sampling are performed and elements from the selected clusters of the last stage sampling may be randomly selected. The sampling units in the first stage of sampling are called primary sampling units (PSUs); those in the second stage of sampling are called secondary sampling units, and so on. Clusters are usually natural groupings, such as organizations, associations, or geographic units, such as regions, states, counties, census tracts, towns, cities, neighborhoods, and blocks. The procedure for conducting cluster sampling is:

1. Define the population of interest.
2. Identify the clusters within the population. For example, if researchers are interested in studying the individual households within a state (i.e., population of interest) in terms of their use of medical services, they may use such clusters as counties (i.e., primary sampling units), residential areas (i.e., secondary sampling units), and street blocks (i.e., tertiary sampling units).
3. Decide upon the desired sample size (n). Knowledge of the total population size and population elements at different clusters will be useful to determine how many units to be selected for each stage of cluster sampling. In our example, the numbers of households within state and county are readily available from the census data, but those within residential areas and street blocks may have to be estimated with the help of staff from the Census Bureau.
4. Establish the sampling frame that contains a complete list of the population elements within the clusters selected at the last stage of sampling. In our example, researchers only need to compile lists of households for all the selected blocks, rather than preparing lists for all state households.
5. Either select all the elements within the clusters selected at the last stage of sampling or randomly select a sample of these elements. In our example, researchers may either interview one owner or adult resident from all the households from the blocks selected, or randomly select the households from the block and then interview one owner or adult resident.

The decision of whether to study all elements within the cluster or randomly select the elements for study usually depends on the heterogeneity (or variations) of the elements within the clusters. The more heterogeneous (or various) the elements, the greater proportion of them should be studied. Since usually there are more variations between clusters than within clusters, researchers sample more clusters and select fewer elements within clusters to generate more representative samples. The downside of this practice, however, is that it is more expensive both in terms of sample frame preparation and data collection. Population lists have to be compiled for more clusters and, if interview is the method of data collection, people have to be sent to more places to conduct the interview. When natural clusters are not of the same size, researchers may sample clusters with probabilities proportional to population size so that the equal probability requirement is not violated.

The principal advantage of cluster sampling lies in its efficiency, particularly when the populations of interest are unlisted or widely dispersed. Considerable amounts of money and time can be saved because cluster sampling does not require that complete lists of each and every population unit be constructed. Only the population elements in the last-stage clusters need to be listed so that a sample of elements can be drawn from these lists. Data-gathering costs may be reduced significantly particularly when face-to-face interview is the method of choice. Individuals within clusters are obviously much less dispersed than individuals within the entire population. Therefore, travel related time and costs for the purpose of conducting interviews are greatly reduced.

The potential drawback of cluster sampling is its representativeness. If significant differences exist among clusters in terms of the important variables being studied, then cluster sampling may be biased if particular clusters are not sampled. Increasing the sample size of clusters will improve the probability that different clusters are sampled, but this will increase sampling costs at the same time, therefore defeating the major benefit of cluster sampling.

Stratified Sampling

In stratified sampling the population is divided into nonoverlapping groups or categories, called strata, and then independent simple random samples are drawn for each stratum. It may be used either for the purpose of making comparisons among subgroups of the population or for making estimates of the entire population. Stratified sampling may be proportional or disproportional, depending on the probability of each sampling element to be selected. In proportional stratified sampling, all population strata are sampled proportional to their composition in the population, so that all sampling elements will have an equal probability of being selected. Proportional stratified sampling allows direct generalization from sample to population without any statistical adjustments.

In disproportional stratified sampling, different probabilities are used to sample different population strata, so that sampling elements will have an unequal probability of being selected. Typically, more units are sampled from the strata with a smaller proportion of the population. Disproportional stratified sampling is used when one or more strata within the population are underrepresented and would not otherwise appear in sufficient numbers in simple random sampling. In general, disproportional sampling is used whenever a simple random sample would not produce enough cases of a certain type to support the intended analysis.

Disproportional stratified sampling does not affect analysis within each stratum. However, if researchers want to combine different strata, disproportional stratified sampling does not allow direct generalization from sample to population because the probability of selection varies from stratum to stratum. In generalizing from sample to population, estimates must be weighted by the inverse of the *sampling fraction* to compensate for oversampling in some strata and reflect the proportion that each stratum represents in the population. The sampling fraction reflects the proportion of subjects to be sampled for the study. For example, if 10 percent of black patients were selected versus 5 percent of white patients, then, to generate population estimates, the proper weighting for black patients would be 10, or the inverse of the sampling fraction 10/100, and for white patients 20, or the inverse of the sampling fraction 5/100. The weighting procedure may be simplified by giving every white patient a weight of 2 (20/10) and no weighting for black patients, or by giving every black patient a weight of 0.5 (10/20) and no weighting for white patients. Statistics software (e.g., SPSS, SAS) usually has detailed description on how weighting can be performed and analyzed. The procedure for conducting stratified sampling is:

1. Define the population of interest.
2. Identify the strata within the population. Strata could be demographic characteristics such as sex, age, race; socioeconomic status such as income, education, occupation; or any types of variables that have significant bearing on the dependent variables. One or more strata may be used at the same time.

   For example, if researchers want to find out the relationship between certain patient characteristics such as race, sex, and insurance status, and medical treatment procedures for one particular illness, the strata of interest will be race (white, black, other), sex (male, female), and insurance (private insurance, Medicare only, Medicaid only, no insurance).
3. Decide upon the desired sample size (*n*). Knowledge of the total population size and population elements at different strata will be useful to determine how many units to be selected for each strata. In our example, total population size refers to all patients admitted for the particular illness of interest. Population elements at different strata refer to patient distributions according to race, sex, and insurance status, that is, the number of patients who are white, male, and have private insurance; white males with Medicare only; white males with Medicaid only; white males with no insurance; the number of patients who are black, male, and have private insurance, and so on.
4. Establish the sampling frame that contains a complete list of the population elements within the strata selected. In our example, each patient is classified into groups or strata based on race, sex, and insurance. Therefore, researchers will have a list of white male patients with private insurance, a list of white male patients with Medicare insurance only, and so on. Preparing sampling frames that classify elements into strata may be difficult if the information needed is not readily available or too costly to obtain.
5. Apply a simple random sampling method to select elements from each stratum using the sampling frame prepared for this purpose. Either a proportional or a disproportional sampling method may be used. In proportional sampling, patients from all strata have the same probability of being selected. In disproportional sampling, they have different probability of being selected. Disproportional sampling is used when certain strata have relatively few patients so that an insufficient num-

ber of them will be selected if proportional sampling is used. Indeed, the principal advantage of stratified sampling is to increase representation particularly for strata with small proportions of elements in the population.

NONPROBABILITY SAMPLING

Nonprobability sampling does not require the specification of the probability that each sample element will be included in the sample (Henry, 1990; Patton, 1990; Babbie, 1992). Typically, nonrandom procedures are used to select sampling elements. Nonprobability sampling may not be representative of the population of interest and hence may not be generalized to the population. Sampling error cannot be calculated and selection biases are not controlled. However, it is much more convenient, less expensive, and less time-consuming than probability sampling and may be useful when probability sampling methods cannot be used. For example, when there are very few population elements (e.g., cities, hospitals in the region, etc.), random sampling may not generate a representative sample and sampling based on expert judgment may be more reliable.

Nonprobability sampling methods are frequently used in the early or exploratory stage of a study where the purpose is to find out more information about the topic under study, discover interesting patterns, and generate hypotheses for later, more formal investigation. It is also used when data accuracy is not very important, when resources such as time and money are very limited, or when certain subjects are difficult to locate or access. Commonly used nonprobability sampling methods include **convenience sampling, quota sampling, purposive sampling**, and **snowball sampling**.

Convenience Sampling

Convenience sampling relies on available subjects for inclusion in a sample. Available subjects may be people encountered in the streets, volunteers who answered an advertisement, or a captive audience such as students in classrooms, patients in hospitals, employees in organizations, and the like. Convenience sampling is quick and easy but generally does not represent the population of interest. It may be used at an early stage of research when a mere feel for the subject matter is needed.

Quota Sampling

Quota sampling specifies desired characteristics in the population elements and selects for the sample appropriate ratios of population elements that fit the characteristics. The desired characteristics may be age, sex, race, income level, education, occupation, or geographic region. Quota sampling is similar to stratified random sampling in that both methods divide the population into relevant strata. However, the two methods are fundamentally different because unlike stratified random sampling, quota sampling does not provide all population elements an equal or known probability for being selected. Investigators may use any methods to select population elements to fulfill their assigned quota. Quota sampling is cheap, easy, convenient, and saves time in terms of data collection. Its representativeness is often questionable, particularly when investigators select subjects who are most conveniently available.

Purposive Sampling

Purposive sampling selects sampling elements based on expert judgment in terms of the representativeness or typical nature of population elements and the purposes of the study. Purposive sampling may be used when sample size is small and simple random sampling may not select the most representative elements. It is an economical way of generating a "representative" or "typical" sample using few elements. However, considerable prior knowledge of the population is required before the sample is selected.

Snowball Sampling

Snowball sampling relies on informants to identify other relevant subjects for study inclusion. Those other subjects may in turn provide leads to additional relevant subjects. The term snowball is used because, like a snowball that starts small but becomes bigger and bigger as it rolls downhill, sampling based on chain referrals starts with a small number of subjects but expands as subjects refer additional people for inclusion. Snowball sampling is particularly useful for studying populations who are difficult to identify or access, for example, persons with HIV/AIDS or drug abusers. Since the sample depends heavily on the referrals by investigators' informants, its representativeness is limited to the investigators' network of informants.

SAMPLE SIZE DETERMINATION

Sample size is determined by a number of factors including the characteristics of the population, the nature of the analysis to be conducted, the desired precision of the estimates the researcher wishes to achieve, the resources available, the study design used, and the anticipated response rate. Often these factors have to be considered simultaneously and trade-offs made before the final sample size is decided upon.

Population Characteristics

Since the sample is drawn to represent a population, certain population characteristics, such as its heterogeneity and size, have a significant impact on the size of a representative sample. In general, the more heterogeneous a population, the larger the sample size required. On the other hand, the less heterogeneous a population, the smaller the sample size required. In the extreme case, where all population elements are different, a census of every element is required. When there is no heterogeneity or variability among population elements, a sample of one is sufficient. In health services research, as in other social sciences research, the populations of interest are generally much more heterogeneous than they are in most other disciplines.

The accuracy of a sample estimate may be indicated by its standard error, calculated with the standard deviation divided by the square root of the sample size ($\sigma/\sqrt{N}$). The standard error reflects the magnitude of differences on the measured variable among study subjects. The formula indicates that the standard error of the sample estimate is directly related to the standard deviation or heterogeneity of the population and indirectly related to the sample size. In other words, the more heterogeneous the population, the larger the sample size required to minimize the standard error. Specifically, because of the square root function, in order to reduce the standard error by one-half, researchers must increase the sample size by four times. It can be seen that at a certain point, for example after 2,000, there is a diminishing return in the reduction of standard error by sample size increases. As a rule of thumb, a minimum sample of 100 is preferred for the purpose of statistical analysis.

In addition to heterogeneity, the size of the population also affects the sample size. Given the same heterogeneity, a larger population requires a larger sample size than a smaller population. However, contrary to intuition, sample size does not need to increase in proportion to population size. An examination of the complete formula for the standard error makes this clear. According to Kish (1965), the complete formula for the standard error for finite populations is $SE = (\sigma/\sqrt{N})(\sqrt{1-f})$, where f is the sampling fraction. For a large population, the sample fraction is generally so small that the correction factor $\sqrt{1-f}$ is very close to $\sqrt{1}$ or 1, having negligible impact on the standard error. Only when the population is small does the sampling fraction have a significant impact on standard error.

Analysis

The sample size is also determined by the nature of the analysis to be performed. Specifically, the number of comparisons that will be made and the number of variables that have to be examined simultaneously have a significant influence on the sample size. In general, the more comparisons or subgroup analyses to be performed, the larger the sample size should be. For example, before surveying the patients population, researchers need to decide how many levels of analyses or breakdowns they will have. Possible breakdowns include age (under 65 or 65 and above), sex (male and female), race (white, black, and other), insurance status (Medicare, Medicaid, private, none), and so on. If they are interested in insurance status of black male under age 65, they need to have relatively large sample to make sure sufficient cases will be included. Sometimes, the population elements that fit into a particular category may be too few to be selected in simple random sampling. Then, stratified sampling may be considered as a method to sample the subcategories or strata separately.

The number of variables to be analyzed at one time also influences the sample size. Typically, in nonexperimental research, relevant variables have to be controlled statistically because groups differ by factors other than chance. The more variables that need to be analyzed simultaneously, the larger the sample size should be to make sure the investigator will have sufficient cases representing the variables considered. Therefore, before deciding upon the sample size, researchers should also know the type of analysis they are going to conduct with the data. A rule of thumb is to include at least 30 to 50 cases for each subcategory.

Precision of Estimates

The precision of the estimates the investigator wishes to achieve also influences sample size. As has been shown before, the precision, or accuracy, of a sample estimate may be indicated by its standard error, the standard deviation divided by the square root of the sample size ($\sigma/\sqrt{N}$). The more precise the estimates, the larger the sample size is required. Generally, the level of accuracy of estimates hinges on the importance of the research findings. If important decisions, those that have serious and costly consequences, are going to be based on research findings, then decision makers demand a very high level of confidence in the data and estimates. A larger sample size would be needed. On the other hand, if there are few, if any, major decisions to be based on the research findings or only rough estimates are required by the sponsor, then the sample size would be correspondingly small.

Available Resources

Resources available to the researcher also influence sample size. Important resources include money, time, and staff support. Sometimes, the sample size is prespecified by the sponsor through available funding. Regardless of the theoretical sample size decided upon, the amount of budget may dictate the upper limit of a sample. The budgeted research funding is not merely for data collection. It is also needed for research preparation, data analysis, and reporting. The time element is important if decisions based on the research have to be made at a certain time. Then research activities have to be planned around this deadline. Compromises have to be made that may include having a smaller sample size. Staff support is particularly important in interview surveys where the number of interviewers available is directly correlated with the number of subjects that can be studied given a particular time period, or how soon data can be collected given the number of interviews to be conducted.

Study Design

Different study designs tend to have different demands for sample size. In experiments where variables are controlled, researchers can use relatively smaller sample size. In nonexperimental designs, a larger sample size is generally required to statistically control for extraneous factors. For the same reason related to control, stratified, cluster, and quota sampling methods generally require a smaller sample size than simple random or systematic sampling methods.

Response Rate

Often, the ideal and the actual sample sizes are different because of less than perfect response rate. Respondents may refuse to be studied. They may turn in illegible or unusable questionnaires. It may not be possible to locate them. Even among usable questionnaires, not all questions are answered. Some items may be left blank or answered improperly. Therefore, the final sample size, especially relevant to a particular questionnaire item, is always smaller than the initial plan. Researchers need to anticipate these factors and make necessary adjustments at an early stage. For example, if the ideal sample size is 500, and past experience indicates that the average response rate for this questionnaire is 65 percent plus a 5 percent ineligible questionnaires (e.g., those with too many missing values), then, to achieve the target sample size of 500, researchers may need to start with 810 [500/(0.65 − 0.05 × 0.65)].

Response rate also has an impact on the validity of research. If a systematic bias exists that affects response, then the results of the study may not be generalizable to the whole population. To evaluate the extent of nonresponse bias, researchers should gather information about nonrespondents (e.g., demographics, geographic locations) so that comparisons can be made between respondents and nonrespondents. These comparisons and possible bias are then included in reports of the study.

SUMMARY

In sampling, researchers select a subset of observations from the population and make inferences about the population based on sample characteristics. Sampling is necessary due to efficiency, accuracy, and access consideration. Commonly used probability sampling methods, where all sampling units in the study population have a known, nonzero probability of being selected in the sample, include simple random sampling, systematic sampling, cluster sampling, and stratified sampling. Nonprobability sampling methods, where the probability of selecting any sampling unit is not known because units are selected through nonrandom processes, include convenience sampling, quota sampling, purposive sampling, and snowball sampling. In determining the sample size required for the study, researchers consider such factors as the characteristics of the population, the nature of the analysis to be conducted, the desired precision of the estimates the researches wish to achieve, the resources available, the study design used, and the anticipated response rate.

Key Terms

sampling	sampling frame
unit of analysis	sampling element
sampling unit	population
observation unit	sampling design
sampling	nonprobability sampling
probability	statistics
parameters	simple random sampling
systematic sampling	cluster sampling
stratified sampling	sampling fraction
convenience sampling	quota sampling
purposive sampling	snowball sampling

Review Questions

1. Why is sampling used?

2. What are the differences between probability and nonprobability sampling? When is one more appropriate than the other?

3. Among probability sampling methods, what kind of research conditions are more appropriate for each sampling method?

4. Among nonprobability sampling methods, what kind of research conditions are more appropriate for each sampling method?

5. How does a researcher decide on the appropriate sample size for a given study?

REFERENCES

Babbie, E. (1992). *The Practice of Social Research.* Belmont, CA: Wadsworth Publishing Co.

Fowler, F. J. (1993). *Survey Research Methods.* 2nd ed. Newbury Parks, CA: Sage.

Henry, G. T. (1990). *Practical Sampling.* Newbury Parks, CA: Sage.

Kish, L. (1965). *Survey Sampling.* New York: Wiley.

Patton, M. Q. (1990). *Qualitative Evaluation and Research Methods.* 2nd ed. Newbury Park, CA: Sage.

Rubin, H. J. (1983). *Applied Social Research.* Columbus, OH: Charles E. Merrill Publishing Co.

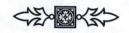

CHAPTER

12

Measurements in Health Services Research

LEARNING OBJECTIVES

- To identify the ways concepts can be measured and the levels of measurement.
- To understand the ways to improve measurement validity and reliability.
- To construct a research instrument for data collection.

DEFINITION

Health services researchers and practitioners often talk about health status, quality care, patient satisfaction, access to care, and so on. These are concepts that cannot be observed directly. We cannot see health status or quality care in the same sense that we can see a house or tree. They need to be specified or operationalized before research can be conducted on these concepts. **Measurement,** then, is the process of specifying and operationalizing a given concept.

In specifying a concept, we identify its particular dimensions and their indicators. For example, we may identify four dimensions of quality care: structure, process, outcome, and satisfaction. For each dimension, we can further specify a series of indicators. The structural indicators may be facility licensure, certification of physicians, availability of certain medical equipment, and the like. Process indicators include diagnostic procedures, laboratory tests, drugs prescribed, operations, and so forth. Outcome indicators consist of readmission rate, recovery rate, death rate, infection rate, and the like. Satisfaction indicators may contain patients' attitudes towards physician, hospital, treatment outcome, and so on.

The indicators need to be operationalized to complete the measurement process. Specifically, researchers need to specify the procedures for measuring indicators, deciding upon the questions to ask, the response categories, and instructions on how to ask questions and assign answers to particular response categories. For example, the structural indicator facility licensure may be measured by asking administrators to submit a copy of the license certificate. The response categories can be yes (referring to those who submit a license) and no (referring to those who are unable to submit a license). The process indicator diagnostic procedures may be measured by examining patient records. The specific diagnoses may be coded into International Classifications of Diseases categories or their relevant DRG groupings. The outcome indicator readmission rate can also be assessed through an examination of patient records, say after 60 days of patient discharge. The readmission diagnoses can be compared with the previous diagnoses. If there is a match, researchers may define this as an admission for the same condition. If the diagnoses are different, researchers may define this as an admission for different conditions. The patients' attitudes towards physician, a satisfaction indicator, may be measured by asking patients directly about their overall satisfaction level. The answer categories may be coded as very satisfied, somewhat satisfied, somewhat dissatisfied, and very dissatisfied.

All concepts should and can be measured. They should be measured because without so doing we cannot conduct empirical studies. They can be measured because measurement is simply a process of defining and describing the dimensions or categories of concepts and their related indicators or variables (Babbie, 1992). To the extent people can talk about and describe a concept, they should be able to measure it. To claim that all concepts are measurable is not to say that they can all be measured with comparable ease, accuracy, or in the same way. Some concepts are certainly more difficult to measure than others. Many researchers, going through the conceptualization and measurement phases of research, find a great deal of confusion within their mental images. Since research is cumulative, before designing our own measures, we typically review the measures used by those who have previously conducted similar research, and use them as references. The final measures adopted are frequently the result of countless revisions.

Although ideally we would like to agree on how a particular concept should be best measured, in practice this is seldom accomplished. One reason for differences in measurement has to do with whether the research community has some explicitly agreed-upon criteria for certain measurements. Few of us would argue about the proper measures for body weight, temperature, height, and blood pressure because the measures are explicitly established and accepted, whether it be a scale, a thermometer, a ruler, or a monitoring device. We have little concern about using these measures because when properly used, they generally produce accurate results that are almost universally accepted.

The difficulty of reaching commonly agreed-upon criteria may be due to the different situations researchers face and to the evolving nature of certain concepts. Research is often conducted in specific settings with specific expectations for certain concepts. Research on quality care at a long-term care facility probably emphasizes the caring aspect rather than treatment. Research on quality care in an acute care setting may emphasize the treatment aspect more than the caring aspect. Different cultures may also have different interpretations of quality. Concepts themselves may evolve over time in accordance with changing social values, expectations, and technological advancements. To the extent that society is highly medicalized, the public's demand for medical services will rise and expectations increase. The rapid advancement of medical technology and highly publicized miracles in medicine further raise the level of expectation and correspondingly provide impetus to the expansion of quality indicators. However, difficulty in reaching commonly acceptable measurement criteria should not prevent the research community from trying to develop new and better ways to measure conceptual dimensions. At a minimum, core dimensions and indicators of concepts should be decided upon, reviewed, and revised every now and then. Consistent measurement is needed to ensure that accurate or valid studies are performed and that different studies based on the same concepts can be compared.

Another reason that researches may use different measures for the same concepts has to do with the constraints different types of research methods face. Secondary study, for example, is limited by available variables. If certain dimensions of a concept are not represented by existing variables, researchers may have to work without them. It is also possible that certain indicators, although important, are difficult, expensive, or too time-consuming to collect.

The choice of measures is also dictated by the research population. Can research subjects supply the information researchers are requesting? Are the measures compatible with their levels of literacy? The range of response categories is also influenced by the expected distribution of attributes among the subjects under study.

Despite differences and incompleteness in measures, the measurement process is still valuable because while investigators may disagree on the dimensions used, indicators chosen, and the operational procedures, they are at least clear about the measures used. The measures are specific and unambiguous, even though incomplete or imprecise. At least investigators know how to interpret the results and criticize the study based on the measures used.

There are various procedures a researcher can use to operationalize indicators or variables of interest. These include relying on existing measures, observations, and self-reports. Often, the type of research method used plays a significant role in the choice of a particular procedure. Existing measures refer to commonly agreed-upon or frequently used measures. Using existing measures is intrinsic to secondary analysis. It is also common in primary research. If the research community has already agreed upon certain measures, then investigators should try their best to use or at least adapt them in their studies. To find out whether those measures exist, they may need to conduct a thorough literature review of relevant studies and consult with experts on the topic. Researchers can also approach organizations specializing in health-related research for available instruments. For example, the Medical Outcomes Trust distributes a number of surveys related to health outcome, including the SF-36 Health Survey, the medical Outcomes Study (MOS) Outpatient Visit Short Form, the NEMC Outpatient Visit Form, the HCA Patient Judgments of Hospital Quality Form, the HCA Patient Hospital Report Card, the GHAA Consumer Satisfaction Form, the Patient Satisfaction Questionnaire, and HCA Medical Staff Judgments of Hospital Quality Form. Another example is the National Committee for Quality Assurance.

Sometimes, even if there are no explicitly agreed-upon criteria for measuring certain concepts, researchers should still try to find existing measures from available, similar studies. There are many advantages to using existing measures. In addition to savings in time and money, using existing measures is consistent with the cumulative nature of scientific inquiry and gives investigators the benefit of other people's experience. Existing measures have already been tried out and their **reliability** and **validity** may have been documented.

Observation is a direct way researchers may use to examine indicators or variables of interest. Targets that can be observed include behavior, attitude, clothing, conversations, relationship, feelings, events, surroundings, and the like. Qualitative research methods, and field research in particular, generally favor observation. Observations can also be used to complement quantitative research methods such as structured face-to-face interviews by noting the demeanor of the interviewee as a measure of personality and the type of household and neighborhood as a measure of social class. An experiment can also include observations to assess the impact of interventions.

Self-report refers to respondents' answers to questions in questionnaires or interviews. Self-report can be used to measure both objective and subjective variables including demographics (age, sex, race), socioeconomic indicators (income, education, occupation), knowledge (awareness of certain concepts, facts, events, people), behaviors (frequency of doctor visits and hospitalization), attitudes (opinions about health care reform), feelings (satisfaction with care received), and beliefs (viewpoint about life events). With certain limitations, self-reports can include both past events and future intentions. Self-report is most commonly used in survey research. Qualitative research can also include self-report in the form of focus group studies or in-depth interviews.

Regardless of the operational procedures used, each measure should satisfy two important qualities: it should be exhaustive and mutually exclusive. The response categories that represent each indicator should be exhaustive so that all observations or sampling elements can be classified using the response categories. If, at the initial stage, researchers are uncertain about the variations among the subjects, they may want to design more categories than are eventually needed. Later, in analyzing the data, if needed, they can always combine precise attributes into more general response categories. Response categories should also be mutually exclusive so that each observation or sampling element can be classified into only one of the response categories.

LEVELS OF MEASUREMENT

Once the dimensions and indicators have been specified, and the procedure to collect data determined, as part of the operationalization process, researchers need to decide what level of measurement to use for the response categories of the indicators or variables. The four levels of measurement are nominal, ordinal, interval, and ratio (Babbie, 1992; Singleton, Straits, and Straits, 1993).

Nominal measures classify elements into categories of a variable that are exhaustive and mutually exclusive. The categories represent characteristics or attributes of a variable. For example, sex can be classified into two categories, male and female, which are both exhaustive (there can be no other categories of sex) and mutually exclusive (being classified as a male precludes one from being classified as a female). Nominal measures are the lowest level of measurements. There is no rank-order relationship among categories and the investigator cannot measure the distance between categories. When numbers are assigned to the categories, they mainly serve as codes for the purpose of data collection and analysis but have no numerical meanings. In other words, Category 2 is not twice as many as Category 1.

Ordinal measures refer to those indicators or variables whose attributes may be logically rank-ordered along some progression. For example, the variable "satisfaction with the medical treatment" may be categorized as very satisfied, somewhat satisfied, somewhat dissatisfied, and very dissatisfied. There is an obvious rank order among those categories, with very satisfied ranked first and very dissatisfied ranked last. Another use of ordinal measures is respondents' ranking of certain items in terms of their preference. For example, patients may be asked to indicate their preference by rank-ordering insurance options such as high premium and no deductible, low premium and low deductible, and

◙

no premium and high deductible. Ordinal measurement is more advanced than nominal measurement. In addition to the rank-order function, it contains all the characteristics of a nominal measure including classification, exhaustiveness, and exclusiveness.

Interval measures refer to those variables whose attributes are not only rank-ordered but are separated by equal distances. The often-used example is the Fahrenheit or the Celsius temperature scale. The difference, or distance, between 65 degrees and 75 degrees is the same as that between 35 degrees and 45 degrees, which is 10 degrees. We can feel not only that 35 degrees is cooler than 45 degrees (rank-order function) but how much cooler it is (interval function). Interval measure is more advanced than both nominal and ordinal measures and contains all the properties of the latter two measures. Interval measures do not have a true zero, and zero is merely arbitrary. For example, zero degrees does not indicate no temperature. (In fact, it is a very cold temperature.) Because of this arbitrary zero condition, there are very few interval measures in health services research. Very often, interval measures are mixed together with ratio measures, called *interval-ratio measures,* and the arbitrary-zero requirement is ignored.

Ratio measures are similar to interval measures except that ratio measures are based on a nonarbitrary or true zero point. For example, the variable "number of years of education" is a ratio measure because zero years of education has a true meaning: no education whatsoever. The true-zero property of ratio measures makes it possible to divide and multiple numbers meaningfully and thereby form ratios. Other examples of ratio measures include age (measured in years), income (measured in dollars), hospitalization (measured in days), among others. Like interval measures, ratio measures are a higher level of measurement than nominal and ordinal measures and contain all their properties.

To the extent possible, researchers should try to measure their indicators or variables at a higher level rather than a lower level. The level of measurement chosen has significant implications for analysis. Most statistical techniques, including the most powerful ones, are designed for interval-ratio variables. Therefore, to make full use of statistical techniques and improve data analysis, researchers should construct interval-ratio measures whenever possible. Of course, some variables are inherently limited to a certain level. Another reason that interval-ratio measures are preferred is that even if later on the investigator decides to analyze the variable in different ways, the interval-ratio measure can always be recoded into ordinal and nominal measures. For example, age can be recoded into old, middle age, and young (an ordinal measure); or working population (18–64) and nonworking population (less than 18 or greater than or equal to 65) (a nominal measure). You will not be able to convert measurements in the other direction, from a lower-level measure to a higher-level one.

MEASUREMENT ERRORS

After an operationalization of a concept has been applied with sampling elements, we notice that there are certain differences or variations among sampling elements with respect to the response categories. Part of the observed differences are true differences among elements that we wish to observe through the measurement process. Indeed, a valid measure should account for most of the variations in observed differences.

In addition to "true" differences, certain portions of the observed variations may be the results of **measurement errors.** Measurement errors, then, refer to sources of differences observed in the elements that are not caused by true differences among elements. Researchers classify measurement errors into two types: systematic and nonsystematic, or random, errors. Systematic errors refer to certain biases consistently affecting the measurement process. Nonsystematic or random errors refer to certain biases affecting the measurement process in haphazard, unpredictable ways.

Systematic errors may be caused by inaccurate operationalization of the concept of interest. Important dimensions or categories of the dimensions of the concept may be missing so that there is only a weak link between the categories used and the concept they try to measure. Sometimes, too few items are used to measure one particular concept so that it is difficult to assure their accuracy. For example, when only one item is used to measure an attitude, it is open to errors of interpretation and formulation of a response. When questions are improperly or ambiguously formulated, they may induce biased responses.

Systematic errors may also occur because of the research experience itself. When respondents act differently in front of researchers from their usual behavior, then observations may be biased. For example, when the data collection process is nonanonymous and/or nonconfidential, people may give socially desirable but not necessarily truthful responses. They may give inaccurate responses to sensitive questions or simply leave them blank. Certain people may choose not to participate in the research or drop out in the middle of the research. Low response or high attrition may present significant distortions to the study outcome because participants and nonparticipants or dropouts are typically different.

Random errors occur when certain characteristics of individuals, respondents, or investigators affect the measurement process. Respondents may have fluctuations in mood as a result of illness, fatigue, or personal experiences. Certain individuals may not understand the wording of a questionnaire item or may wrongly interpret the item. Certain questions may be too complicated for some respondents. Sometimes, individuals may not know the contents of the item being asked and either ignore the item or give a spontaneous response. This is particularly common with attitude and opinion questions. Not everyone has formed an opinion about everything. In addition, respondents may be too tired to think through the question, or their responses may be affected by the people, noises, and other distractions present.

Random errors originating from investigators may include improper interview methods such as not following instructions, changing the wording of questions or the order they are asked, asking leading questions or making subjective interpretations of respondents' answers. These biases are especially common when certain results are likely to benefit the investigators or are consistent with their beliefs. Investigators may also omit instructions due to fatigue or lack of interest.

Both respondents and investigators may be turned off by each other due to their demographics, attitudes, or demeanor. The lack of trust by either side could affect how the questions are asked, responded, or recorded. Both are also prone to make classification errors. Respondents may erroneously choose a category or select a rating. Interviewers may check off the wrong boxes. Key punchers may strike the wrong key while inputting data into the computer. Programmers and analysts may make mistakes in modeling and calculation.

Systematic errors are serious threats to study validity and reliability. Researchers should spend great efforts to reduce sources of systematic errors. In contrast, unsystematic or random errors do not present a great threat to research, although they may also affect study reliability. Their impacts are unpredictable and tend to cancel each other out with sufficient sample size. There are so many sources of measurement errors that they are almost impossible to eliminate. Researchers should take into account those sources and try their best to reduce or minimize their impacts. At a minimum, their impacts should be studied so that measurement validity and reliability can be assessed.

VALIDITY AND RELIABILITY OF MEASUREMENT

Measurement validity refers to the extent that important dimensions of a concept and their categories have been taken into account and appropriately operationalized. In other words, a valid measure has response categories truly reflecting all important meanings of the concept under consideration. For example, a measure of quality care that includes the structure, process, outcome, and satisfaction dimensions is more valid than one that only includes one of these dimensions.

Measurement reliability refers to the extent that consistent results are obtained when a particular measure is applied to similar elements. Thus, a reliable measure will yield the same or very similar outcome when it is repeated to the same subject or subjects sharing the same characteristics being measured. For example, estimating a person's age or weight by checking his or her birth certificate or weighing him or her is more reliable than asking directly, which is more reliable than asking others.

A valid measure is usually also reliable, but a reliable measure may not be valid. For example, checking a birth certificate is both a valid and reliable measure of one's age but is not a valid measure of work experience since current age reflects not only a person's work experience but also includes years not spent in the labor force. An unreliable measure cannot be valid; when the results fluctuate significantly, how can the measure capture the true meaning of a concept? The credibility of one's research will be influenced by the perceived validity and reliability of the measures used. Therefore, researchers, as a common practice, include in their report an assessment of the validity and reliability of their measures.

Validity Assessment

Even though there is no direct way of confirming the validity of a measure—otherwise there would be no need for the measure—there are many indirect ways researchers use to establish the validity of their measures. These include **construct validity,** content validity, **concurrent validity,** and **predictive validity.**

Construct Validity

Construct validity refers to the fact that the measure captures the major dimensions of the concept under study. For example, a measure of quality care should include questions about each of the major dimensions of quality, structure, process, and outcome (which includes satisfaction). Construct validity may be strengthened in a number of ways. If agreed-upon criteria exist in terms of measuring a particular concept, then those criteria should be reflected in the measures. Literature review and checking with experts are ways to find out whether there are established ways of measuring certain concepts. The construct validity of a measure can also be enhanced by establishing a high significant level of correlation with other measures of the same concept, or other theoretically related variables, or a low correlation with measures of unrelated concepts. If investigators know for sure that some elements possess the construct of interest, they can enhance construct validity by including those elements in their measurement.

Content Validity

Content validity refers to the representativeness of the response categories used to represent each of the dimensions of a concept. For example, to sufficiently represent the outcome dimension of quality care, the researcher may have to include questions about recovery rates, functional status, complication rates, morbidity, mortality, disability, mental well-being, and so on. After establishing construct validity, taking into account all major dimensions of a concept, the constructs or dimensions have to be translated in terms of specific categories that reflect how things actually work. Content validity is strengthened when all facets of a dimension have been taken into account. Again, experts' knowledge, prior literature, and existing instruments are good sources to help identify different facets or components of a particular dimension.

Concurrent Validity

Concurrent validity may be tested by comparing results of one measurement with those of a similar measurement administered to the same population and at approximately the same time. If both measurements yield similar results, then concurrent validity can be established.

Concurrent validity may be tested with items included in the same instrument. For example, to check the validity of a certain scale (e.g., items related to satisfaction), the investigator may hypothesize the relations of the scale with other variables (e.g., a question directly asking satisfaction level) in the instrument. Confirmation of the hypothesis (e.g., when the scale and the question are highly correlated) produces evidence in support of the validity of the scale.

Predictive Validity

Predictive validity may be examined by comparing the results obtained from the measurement with some actual later-occurring evidence that the measurement aims at predicting. When there is a high degree of correspondence between the prediction and the actual event—the predicted event actually takes place—then predictive validity is established. The predictive validity of Graduate Record Examination or Graduate Management Admission Test, for example, lies in the extent of correlation between higher scores attained and better graduate school performance.

Reliability Assessment

While validity is related to systematic errors, reliability has to do with random errors. When a measure yields consistent or similar results from time to time, then we know it does not have too many random errors and we become more comfortable about its reliability. Reliability assessment mainly involves the examination of the consistency level of the measurement. There are many indirect ways researchers use to establish the reliability of their measures. Commonly used methods for reliability assessment include **test–retest reliability**, **split-half reliability,** and **interrater reliability.**

Test–Retest Reliability

Test–retest reliability involves administering the same measurement to the same individuals at two different times. If the correlation between the same measures is high (usually above .80), then the measurement is believed to be reliable. However, in using test–retest approach, researchers should beware about the potential impact of the first test on the second test. If the first test can potentially affect responses on the second test, then the second test result will be different from that of the first test. Sufficient time should elapse before the second test so that memory of the first test is no longer good. At the same time, researchers should not wait for too long before administering the second test lest real changes might take place during the interval. The general procedure is to wait for one to two months before the second test. Of course, the applicability of this method and the actual time spacing depend on the particular measurement under study.

Split-Half Reliability

Split-half reliability involves preparing two sets (or two halves) of measurement of the same concept, applying them to research subjects at one setting, and comparing the correlation between the two sets of measurement. To the extent the correlation is high, then the measurement is reliable. The advantage of split-half method over test–retest method is that it avoids problems with "real changes" between tests. The disadvantage or challenge is that two very similar sets of the measures have to be created.

Interrater Reliability

Interrater reliability involves using different people to conduct the same procedure, whether it be interview, observation, coding, rating, and the like, and comparing the results of their work. To the extent that the results are highly similar, interrater reliability has been established. Interrater reliability is particularly useful when subjective judgments have to be made, for example, in inspecting and rating a health care facility.

Measures to Improve Validity and Reliability

To improve the validity and reliability of measurement, researchers can proactively take a number of measures, including using established measures, a pretest, or a pilot study; ensuring confidentiality; improving research instrument design; and training the research staff. When possible, efforts should be made to obtain existing measures that are well established. Only when no relevant measures are available or accessible may investigators then construct their own measures.

Before formally using one's own measures, a pretest or a pilot study will help identify those words, phrases, terms, sentences, response categories, and definitions that are ambiguously worded, unknown, or irrelevant to the respondents. Revisions can be made accordingly, and the final measures should be sufficiently clear, relevant, and understood.

Confidentiality will help reduce biases associated with questions that are embarrassing, sensitive, or have a response set (e.g., social desirability). To ensure confidentiality, investigators should assure anonymity where possible and, in the case of interviews, establish rapport with the subjects so that the promise of confidentiality can be trusted. The names of the interviewees should be replaced by codes when inputting data and the original instrument should be locked away and only accessible to core research staff. The interviews should be conducted in private, quiet settings.

Improving instrument or questionnaire design is important to reducing many response biases. Not only should investigators avoid asking leading, loaded, ambiguous, or too complex questions, sometimes in dealing with sensitive topics, they may have to use indirect questions. The sequence of questions and response categories within questions may also affect how they are answered. Greater care should be given to questionnaire arrangement, by varying the arrangement and the ways questions are asked. To avoid response set, the tendency for respondents to be very agreeable or stick to a particular pattern of response, investigators can use two different items opposite in meaning to measure the same concept, and compare responses to these items to see whether they were answered differently. Questionnaire construction will be considered in detail in the next section.

Training research staff is crucial to ensure the proper conduct of research so that a high level of reliability can be reached. Items of training include how to conduct an interview, make observations, follow instructions, record data, and input data. In addition to training, close supervision is necessary in the course of all phases of research activities. For example, in telephone interviews, the supervisor may either listen in or call a subsample of respondents to verify selected items in the questionnaire. In field research, the supervisor may accompany the new investigators to the settings or interviews at an early stage of the research. The supervisor can routinely check at the inputted data against the original instrument.

RESEARCH INSTRUMENT DESIGN

When no relevant measurement exists or is accessible, researchers will have to construct their own measurement. Sometimes there is access to some existing measurement but not others. Then the remaining measures will still need to be constructed. A research instrument contains the operational definitions of all measures related to the research and is primarily used to collect data. When a research instrument contains only questions and statements to be answered by respondents, it is called a questionnaire. Beware the term *questionnaire* implies a collection of questions but in reality may contain statements as well.

Before putting together the research instrument, investigators should have already identified the study objective(s), the major concepts to be investigated, the major dimensions of these concepts, and their representative categories. If they are still unclear about any of these elements, they should conduct more research to find out about them before constructing the instrument. In the process of designing the research instrument, researchers make decisions about frame of reference, time, response format, composition of questions, instrument assembling, and pretesting.

Frame of Reference

Frame of reference is related to the respondents' particular perspectives. Before writing up the questions, investigators must find out about the general characteristics of their respondents. What is their general educational level? What words, phrases, terms, or languages are familiar to them? How well informed are they about particular issues? What kind of general experience do they have? Do they have a particular perspective that must be taken into account? Knowledge about these questions will help choose the right words and ask the relevant questions. If investigators do not have prior knowledge of the frame of reference of the research population, they have to conduct a pilot test of their instrument before finalizing it. More definitions and examples may be given to make sure respondents understand exactly what is meant by each question and how they are supposed to answer these questions.

Time Frame

In designing an instrument, researchers can ask questions about the past, current, or future. Current questions generally produce more accurate answers than either past or future questions, and the longer the time span from the present, the less accurate the answers become. Asking questions about the past is affected by memory problems. Significant differences exist among people in terms of memory. In addition, the ability to remember things is also influenced by the importance of the event. People are more likely to remember their hospitalization experience than doctor visits presumably because hospitalization is usually related to a more serious health event, which is a rare occurrence. Even when we remember an important event, we may still place it on a wrong date. A common memory problem is what Sudman and Bradburn (1986) have termed "telescoping," the tendency to recall the timing of an event as having occurred more recently than it actually did. Asking questions about the future involves guesswork on the part of respondents and tends to be even less reliable than recalling past events. When the time frame is improperly extended into the past or future, the responses are likely to be inaccurate.

A variety of methods exist to improve the accuracy of responses related to memory problems. Where possible, respondents should be encouraged to check with the records they possess before answering certain questions. Examples include hospital bills (when asking questions about hospital costs), birth certificates (when asking about the ages of children), payroll stubs (when asking questions about income), school records (when asking questions about time of education, courses taken, and degrees obtained), financial records (when asking questions about expenditures), diaries (when asking questions about health events or other activities), and so forth.

Another method to aid recall is to provide a list of response categories so that subjects have some references to think about. For example, patients may be presented a list of services and asked which ones they have received, or a list of illnesses and asked which ones they have had. Providing lists is not only useful for recalling past events but also helpful for remembering current events. For example, to find out the insurance coverage of patients, investigators can list all the insurance programs available in the region to aid patients in identifying the programs to which they subscribe.

Paying attention to question formulation will also reduce memory problems. In addition to detailed lists of items, questions can be worded more specifically and include specific contexts. Where possible, visual aids may be used in either interviews or mailed questionnaires. Recall periods should be reduced to reasonable level, usually within two weeks. For example, while it may be reasonable to ask patients about their hospitalization history during the past year, it may be necessary to ask about their physician visits during the past few weeks or months. In general, the importance and frequency of the events dictate how long a period a person can reasonably recall.

Response Format

In terms of response format, the researcher must make the choice between open-ended questions and close-ended questions. Open-ended questions require the respondents to provide their answers using their own words. Open-ended questions can have quantitative as well as qualitative answers. Quantitative open-ended questions require respondents to provide numerical answers that are often categorized as interval ratios. Since interval-ratio measures provide the most advanced measurement and are most suitable for statistical analysis, researchers should try their best to include as many quantitative open-ended questions as feasible in their instruments. Examples include questions about age, income, years of education, number of children, and the like, which can be analyzed directly. Table 12–1 provides some commonly used examples. Qualitative open-ended questions require respondents to answer the questions using their own words.

Close-ended questions provide answer categories for the respondents to choose based on their own characteristics. The following is an example of a question asked in both open-ended and close-ended ways.

- What type(s) of health insurance plans do you have? *[Qualitative open-ended]*

- What type(s) of health insurance plans do you have? *(Check all those that apply.)*
  ( ) Medicare
  ( ) Medicaid
  ( ) Blue Cross/Blue Shield
  ( ) HMO/Prepaid Plan
  ( ) Other Private Insurance (Specify _____)
  ( ) Other Public Insurance (Specify _____)
  ( ) No Insurance
  ( ) No Charge   *[Close-ended]*

While quantitative open-ended questions should be used wherever possible, the choice between qualitative open-ended and close-ended questions is based on many factors including knowledge of subject matter, depth of information required, sample size, desired response and completion rates, desired level of standardization, length of questionnaire, data analysis techniques, and the amount of time to complete the research.

Knowledge of the subject matter is critical for close-ended questions. If the researcher does not know the subject area well enough, he or she cannot identify the important dimensions, their associated categories, and the range of possible answers. A qualitative open-ended format will have to be used, as in qualitative research, to explore the dimen-

TABLE 12–1 Commonly used quantitative open-ended questions

- How old are you now? _____ years of age

- How many years of education have you received from educational institution(s)? _____ years

- What is your annual salary or wage plus bonus? $ _____

- How many children do you have? _____ number of children

- How often did you visit the doctor during the past 3 months? _____ times

- How often were you hospitalized during the last 2 years? _____ times

- What is the number of licensed beds in your hospital? _____ beds

- What was the occupancy rate in your hospital last year? _____ %

- How many patients with congenital heart failure (ICD-9 Code 42800) did your hospital have last year? _____ number of patients

- What is the average length of stay for patients with congenital heart failure (ICD-9 Code 42800) in your hospital? _____ days

sions, categories, and range of answers. Therefore, an open-ended, qualitative or pilot study may be conducted prior to large-scale, close-ended survey. Even in close-ended questions, researchers cannot always be sure that the response categories are exhaustive. Often, an "Other (Specify _____)" category is included after the listing of known items.

The depth of information required also plays a significant role in the choice between qualitative open-ended and close-ended questions. Open-ended questions provide greater depth than close-ended questions, giving respondents the opportunity to describe their unique experiences, rationale, anecdotes, opinions, feelings, attitudes, beliefs, logic, and thought processes. Frequently, unanticipated things may be revealed and the strength of the feeling detected. These results, often in respondents' own words, provide a rich context for the research description and supporting evidences for summary statistics. Therefore, open-ended questions are not only necessary in a qualitative study to explore research issues and categories but also useful in a quantitative study to support and expand on summary findings. It is common to include both open-ended and close-ended questions in survey research.

Expected sample size affects the choice between qualitative open-ended and close-ended questions. Open-ended questions are more appropriate for small sample size and close-ended questions for large sample size. Since open-ended questions generally have to be recoded before analysis, it would be too time-consuming to recode many open-ended questions in large-scale surveys. Furthermore, the results of recoding may be biased. The fact that some respondents have not mentioned certain categories does not necessarily mean they are not relevant to them. They may not have thought about them at the moment and, if provided with these choices, they could well have them checked off. Other sources of bias include the difficult task of analyzing responses and classifying them into different categories, dealing with ambiguous responses, and missing data.

There are also differences in response and completion rates between qualitative open-ended and close-ended questions. Response rate has to do with the proportion of research subjects who actually send back the questionnaire or participated in the interviews. Completion rate refers to the proportion of questions within the research instrument, whether it be questionnaire or interview guide, that gets answered by the responding subjects. Open-ended questions demand greater effort and time on the part of the respondents and are likely to cause relatively low response and completion rates. Moreover, respondents are likely to be different from nonrespondents in that they tend to be more interested in the research topic than nonrespondents. Completion rate has an educational bias. Those with higher levels of education are likely to complete more questions and write more per question than those with lower levels of education. Because of the extra demand on time, effort, and educational level, open-ended questions can turn off potential respondents who are either busy, find the topic less interesting or relevant, or have less education.

Respondents are not the only people affected by open-ended questions. Interviewers who administer open-ended questions need to be trained so that appropriate probing can be used to draw out responses. The interview time for open-ended interviews tends to be much longer than for close-ended interviews. In order to achieve higher response and completion rates, it is recommended that a very limited number of open-ended questions be used and placed near the end of the instrument so that even if they were not answered the earlier close-ended questions would have been completed.

Qualitative open-ended and close-ended questions also differ in the level of standardization in responses. Close-ended questions, by providing the same frame of reference and options to all respondents, generate more standardized responses than open-ended questions, in which individuals differ in terms of their interpretation of questions, perspectives, experiences, and ability to put their thoughts into words.

There is a close relationship between the choice of qualitative open- versus close-ended questions and the length of questionnaire. Open-ended questions, due to their difficulty and time demand, require the questionnaire to be relatively short. Close-ended questions, because of their ease of use, enable the questionnaire to be relatively long. While the length of a questionnaire is inversely related to the response and completion rates, a longer questionnaire with many open-ended questions has a significantly lower response and completion rates than a longer questionnaire with mostly close-ended questions.

The methods of data analysis also determine the choice between qualitative open- and close-ended questions. Most of the statistical techniques are used for quantitative data elements derived from quantitative open-ended or close-ended questions, which can be transferred directly into computer format. Qualitative open-ended questions have to be converted or recoded into close-ended categories before quantitative analysis can be performed.

Finally, the amount of research time may dictate how many qualitative open-ended questions to be included. Open-ended questions take longer to answer, code, and analyze. More interviewers are required to complete the surveys on time. Methods of coding and analysis cannot be predetermined and have to be thought out after data collection. More time is spent on training interviewers and coders to ensure validity and reliability of the results. If research time is very limited, a close-ended format will be more appropriate than an open-ended one.

Once researchers have decided to use close-ended questions, they need to make additional decisions about specific close-ended formats that are most suitable for the research. These formats include contingency questions, two-way questions, multiple-choice questions, ranking scale questions, fixed-sum scale questions, agreement scale questions, Likert-type format questions, semantic differential scale questions, and adjective checklist questions.

Contingency Questions

Contingency questions are those questions whose relevance depends on responses to a prior question. The use of contingency questions makes it possible for some respondents to skip questions that do not apply to them. Special care should be given to the design of contingency questions and clear instructions provided for the skip pattern. Below are two examples of the use of contingency questions.

- Example 1:
  Have you ever been hospitalized?
  ( ) Yes *(Please answer questions 8–11.)*
  ( ) No *(Please skip questions 8–11. Go directly to question 12 on page 3.)*

- Example 2:
  Do you currently smoke cigarettes?
  ( ) Yes ────────────────────┐
  ( ) No   │
                              ▼
  ┌──┐
  │ *If yes:* About how many cigarettes do you smoke a day? │
  │   ( ) Less than 5 a day   │
  │   ( ) 5–10 a day   │
  │   ( ) 11–20 a day   │
  │   ( ) Greater than 20 a day   │
  └──┘

Two-Way Questions

Two-way questions include a question or statement followed by two dichotomous, realistic alternatives. Terms used to designate the alternatives include yes/no, agree/disagree, for/against, approve/disapprove, true/false, favor/oppose, like/dislike, and so on. Sometimes, a third alternative, "don't know" or "no opinion," is included to make the choices more realistic. The following are two examples of two-way questions.

- Example 1:
  Have you had a mammogram in the past 12 months?
  ( ) Yes
  ( ) No
  ( ) Don't Know

- Example 2:
  What is your attitude toward universal coverage for health care?
  ( ) Agree
  ( ) Disagree
  ( ) No Opinion

Multiple-Choice Questions

Multiple-choice questions are among the most frequently used formats in close-ended questions. There are two types of multiple-choice questions, multiple-choice, single-response questions, and multiple-choice, multiple-response questions. In multiple-choice, single-response questions, respondents are presented with a question or statement followed by a list of possible answers from which they are asked to select the one most appropriate to their situation. In multiple-choice, multiple-response questions, respondents are presented with a question or statement followed by a list of possible answers from which they are asked to select as many as relevant or applicable to their situation. Multiple response questions are also called checklist questions, because a list of all relevant items are provided for respondents to check off. In constructing multiple-choice questions, the investigator should make sure that each alternative answer contains only one idea (mutually exclusive), the alternatives are balanced, and convey all important ideas of the question (all inclusive). Often, an "other "category is included to let respondents fill in information not available in the items listed. The following are two examples of multiple-choice questions.

- Example 1:
  Please check *one* race or ethnic origin you belong to.
  ( ) White
  ( ) Black

( ) Asian/Pacific Islanders
( ) American Indian/Eskimo/Aleut
( ) Other   *[Single-response]*

• Example 2:
In which following settings do you currently provide services to your patients?
(Please check all those that apply.)
( ) Hospital Inpatient
( ) Hospital Outpatient
( ) Group Practice Office
( ) Solo Practice Office
( ) Public Health Department
( ) Community/Migrant Health Center
( ) Free Clinic
( ) Other   *[Multiple-response]*

Ranking Scale Questions

Ranking scale, also called forced ranking scale, asks respondents to rank a number of items in relation to one another. A forced ranking scale generally provides more information than multiple-choice questions because it not only allows multiple selections (as in multiple-choice, multiple-response questions) but also obtains the sequence of the ranking in terms of importance or relevance to the respondent. It parallels many life situations where choices among programs, services, treatments, decisions, ideas, and so forth have to be made. However, ranking scale is more difficult to respond to than most other scales because respondents have to assess all items relative to one another. Therefore, in order to facilitate ranking, researchers should limit the number of items to be ranked, generally no more than five items, unless they are easy to compare. The following are two examples of ranking scale questions.

• Example 1:
The following are conditions listed alphabetically that are often cited as influential to the provision of care to patients with HIV/AIDS. Please rank them in the order of preference to *you* that *you* would like to see improved. Assign the number 1 next to the one you prefer most, number 2 to your second choice, and so forth.
( ) Additional Training
( ) Better Community and Social Services Support
( ) Higher Reimbursement
( ) Limited Liability
( ) Specialty Backup

- Example 2:
  The following are sources where a person may obtain knowledge about AIDS. In your situation, please rank these sources in terms of relevance to you. Put the number 1 next to the source most relevant to you, number 2 next to the second most relevant source, and so forth.
  (   ) Newspaper
  (   ) Radio
  (   ) T.V.
  (   ) Book
  (   ) Workplace/School
  (   ) Friends
  (   ) Relatives
  (   ) Family Members
  (   ) Other

Fixed-Sum Scale Questions

Fixed-sum scale asks the respondents to describe what proportion of resource (e.g., time, money, efforts, activities) has been devoted to each of the listed items. In designing fixed-sum scale questions, the researcher should clearly state the total sum when all proportions have been added. To facilitate response and calculation, the researcher should limit the number of items to be considered, generally no more than ten, and the activities described should be very familiar to the respondents. Below are two examples of fixed-sum scale questions.

- Example 1:
  Among your current patients with health insurance, what percent of them have the following insurance?
  (Please be sure to make the total equal to 100%.)

Medicare Only	_____	%
Medicaid Only	_____	%
Medicare plus Medicaid	_____	%
Private Third-Party Insurance	_____	%
HMO/Prepaid	_____	%
Other Insurance	_____	%
Total	__100__	%

- Example 2:
  As a nursing home administrator, how much time do you spend per week on the following activities?

Resident Care	_____	hours/week
Personnel Management	_____	hours/week

Financial Management	_____ hours/week
Marketing/Public Relations	_____ hours/week
Physical Resource Management	_____ hours/week
Laws/Regulatory Codes/Governing Boards	_____ hours/week
Quality Assurance	_____ hours/week
Family Relations	_____ hours/week
Other	_____ hours/week
Other	_____ hours/week
Total	_____ *hours/week**

(*< 35 part-time, 35–45 full-time, > 45 overtime)

Agreement Scale Questions

An agreement scale presents a statement and asks respondents to indicate their level of agreement or disagreement. When a series of such statements are used, it is called the Likert scale, named after its creator Rensis Likert. The agreement scale differs from the two-way dichotomous question in that it has more gradations of agreement and hence is more detailed. There are typically five ordinal response categories: "strongly agree," "agree," "undecided," "disagree," and "strongly disagree." The following are two examples of agreement scale.

- Example 1:
  How much do you agree or disagree with health care reform that stresses universal coverage?
  ( ) Strongly Agree
  ( ) Agree
  ( ) Uncertain
  ( ) Disagree
  ( ) Strongly Disagree

- Example 2:
  The following statements describe your experience as a physician in the community. Please indicate your degree of agreement with each of these statements by circling the number most applicable to your condition.

	Strongly Agree	Agree	Undecided	Disagree	Strongly Disagree
1. I am a valuable contributor to the community's health.	5	4	3	2	1
2. I appreciate what the community offers me.	5	4	3	2	1

3. The local physicians accept me as "one of them."	5	4	3	2	1
4. I was well prepared for the realities of living in this community when I first came.	5	4	3	2	1
5. I am pleased with the backup support or referral system in the community.	5	4	3	2	1

[Likert scale]

Likert-type Scale Questions

The Likert-type format can be used not only for agreement questions but for many other types of questions by modifying the ordinal response categories. For example, the response categories for verbal frequency scale are "always," "often," "sometimes," "seldom," and "never." When using the frequency scale, the researcher should provide some indication about how to interpret the terms in the scale, such as once a day means often, once a month means seldom, and so on, so that respondents have a common frame of reference. The response categories for an evaluation scale are "excellent," "good," "fair," and "poor." The response categories for a satisfaction scale are: "very satisfied," "somewhat satisfied," "somewhat dissatisfied," and "very dissatisfied." As can be seen, the middle neutral category may be omitted to force respondents to make a choice. The decision to include or omit the neutral category should be based on a consideration about reality. If respondents truly might not have an opinion or attitude, the middle neutral category should be included. Another variation of Likert-type scale is the number of response categories used. Although five is most frequently used, one may choose to use fewer (e.g., three) or more (e.g., seven) categories to obtain the most appropriate level of gradations. The following are two examples of Likert-type scales.

- Example 1:
  How would you rate your general health status?
  ( ) Excellent
  ( ) Good
  ( ) Average
  ( ) Fair
  ( ) Poor
  ( ) Don't Know

- Example 2:
  On average, about how often do you visit a doctor, HMO, or clinic?
  ( ) Less than once a year
  ( ) Yearly

( ) More than once a year, but less than once a month
( ) Monthly
( ) More than once a month, but less than once a week
( ) Weekly
( ) More than once a week

Generally, when Likert-type scale is used, a series of statements or items are included that measure different dimensions of a particular concept. Each item should express only one idea. Jargon and colloquialism should be avoided. A total score for a scale is calculated by adding the numerical numbers associated with responses to each item. Negatively worded items are reverse scored so that two opposite items will not cancel out in the total score. The formula used for reversed scoring is: $(H + L) - I$, where H is the largest number, L smallest number, and I a particular response to an item. For example, when a respondent circles 2 for the following question, the reverse score becomes 4 $[(5 + 1) - 2 = 4]$.

	Strongly Agree	Agree	Undecided	Disagree	Strongly Disagree
The pay is inadequate for my job.	5	4	3	2	1

Semantic Differential Scale Questions

The semantic differential scale uses a series of adjectives and their antonyms listed on opposite sides of the page and asks the respondents to indicate their positions about a statement using the adjectives provided. Semantic differential scale questions are often related to measuring people's attitudes, opinions, impressions, beliefs, or feelings about certain events, organizations, behaviors, and the like. The adjective pairs used must truly be antonyms. Table 12–2 lists some of these examples. Below are two examples of semantic differential scale questions.

- Example 1:
  Below are a number of adjectives used to describe a person's feeling toward his or her job. Please pick a number from the scale (1 to 7) to indicate *your* feeling about *your* job.

Boring	1	2	3	4	5	6	7	Exciting
Difficult	1	2	3	4	5	6	7	Easy
Insignificant	1	2	3	4	5	6	7	Significant
Low paying	1	2	3	4	5	6	7	High paying
Risky	1	2	3	4	5	6	7	Safe
Stressful	1	2	3	4	5	6	7	Pleasant

◈

TABLE 12–2 Commonly used adjective pairs for constructing semantic differential scale

negative	*positive*
angry	calm
bad	good
biased	objective
boring	interesting
brave	cowardly
closed	open
cold	warm
confusing	clear
dirty	clean
dull	lively
irrelevant	relevant
old	new
passive	active
prejudiced	fair
reactive	proactive
sad	happy
sick	healthy
slow	fast
static	dynamic
superficial	profound
tense	relaxed
ugly	pretty
uninformative	informative
weak	strong
worthless	valuable
wrong	right

- Example 2:

How important do you think each of the following characteristics is to a successful hospital administrator? Please circle the *one* number that best represents your feeling.

	Least Important						*Most Important*
Analytical Skills	1	2	3	4	5	6	7
Business Skills	1	2	3	4	5	6	7
Communication Skills	1	2	3	4	5	6	7
Decision-Making Skills	1	2	3	4	5	6	7
Entrepreneurial Skills	1	2	3	4	5	6	7

Financial Skills	1	2	3	4	5	6	7
Human Resource Skills	1	2	3	4	5	6	7
Goal Oriented	1	2	3	4	5	6	7
Health Care Background	1	2	3	4	5	6	7
Leadership Skills	1	2	3	4	5	6	7
Networking Skills	1	2	3	4	5	6	7
Planning Skills	1	2	3	4	5	6	7

Adjective Checklist Questions

The adjective checklist questions present a statement about a topic followed by a list of adjectives and ask respondents to check off as many as relevant to their situations related to the topic. Unlike the semantic differential scale, adjectives in the checklist do not have to be antonyms, although some representation of both positive and negative expressions will facilitate the response process. These questions can provide more descriptive information about a topic of interest and can be used to reinforce or illustrate quantitative findings. Simplicity, directness, and economy are the major strengths of this type of questions. Below are two examples using the adjective checklist.

- Example 1:
  Please check off in front of any words or phrases below that describe your current job.

  ( ) Boring   ( ) Dead end   ( ) Difficult   ( ) Easy
  ( ) Exciting   ( ) High paying   ( ) Insignificant   ( ) Low paying
  ( ) Pleasant   ( ) Rewarding   ( ) Risky   ( ) Safe
  ( ) Satisfying   ( ) Significant   ( ) Stressful   ( ) Technical

- Example 2:
  Below are words and phrases describing a person's possible experience at the hospital. Please check off those most appropriately reflecting *your* own experience as a patient along each of the aspects measured.

	Physicians	*Nurses*	*Other (Specify* _____ *)*
caring	( )	( )	( )
effective	( )	( )	( )
inconsiderate	( )	( )	( )
indifferent	( )	( )	( )
ineffective	( )	( )	( )
responsive	( )	( )	( )
tardy	( )	( )	( )
timely	( )	( )	( )

Questionnaire Composition

A research instrument or questionnaire may contain a variety of questions such as background, knowledge, experience, behavior, feeling, opinion, attitude, values, intentions, or plans. Background questions are generally related to the demographic characteristics of the individual being studied. Examples include age, sex, race, education, occupation, and residence. Knowledge questions are asked to find out what factual information the respondent has. Examples include respondent's income, awareness of a particular event, term, issue, law, and the like. Experience questions are related to what a respondent has gone through or is still going through. Examples include being sick, tired, stressful, and so forth. Behavior questions are concerned with what a respondent does or has done. Examples include visiting a doctor, hospitalization, undergoing an operation, and the like. Feeling or attitude questions aim at understanding the emotional state of the respondent with respect to particular issues. Examples include satisfaction, anxiety, happiness, and so on. Opinion, attitude, or value questions try to find out what a respondent thinks about some particular issue. Examples include attitude toward health care reform, values about universal coverage, opinion about managed care plans, and so on. Intentions and plans are generally future-oriented questions. Since they contain a high degree of speculation, their reliability is generally less than questions about the past and present. Examples include number of nurse practitioners to be hired by community health centers in the next three years, conditions necessary to quit smoking, and so forth.

In writing specific questionnaire items, researchers should avoid biases wherever feasible and pay special attention to certain types of questions. Below are a number of popular reminders for questionnaire formulation.

Avoid Loaded Questions

Investigators use words and phrases that reflect their perception of a particular issue or event in **loaded questions.** They are biased because they suggest certain beliefs that could influence respondents' answers. An example of a loaded question is: "What is your opinion toward a socialist one-payer system for health care reform?" The question is loaded because it implies that the one-payer system is necessarily the product of socialism. Respondents may be negatively or positively influenced by their attitude toward socialism regardless of the merit of a one-payer system.

Avoid Leading Questions

Particular wording to suggest or demand a particular answer is used in **leading questions.** They are biased because they hint at a "desired" answer rather than finding out what the respondent feels. An example of leading question is: "The U.S. president believes that universal access to care is an essential element of health care reform. Do you agree that universal access should be mandated?" The question is leading because it uses the president to establish the legitimacy of the claim of universal access. Then, only presenting "Do you agree . . ." may suggest that respondent ought to agree with the statement.

Avoid Double-Barreled Questions

Two separate questions in one statement occur in **double-barreled questions.** They are biased because respondents may have different answers toward different questions. An example of a double-barreled question is: "Do you think the treatment you received from the doctor was costly and ineffective?" Respondents may agree that the treatment was costly but disagree that it was ineffective. The question is also leading because only negative concepts are conveyed.

Use Appropriate Words

The words used to form questions should be appropriate to the respondents. If the respondents have little education, then researchers should use very simple vocabulary. If the respondents do not know a particular event or term, a definition should first be provided so that they understand what is being asked. Providing definitions is also important for words that have different meanings to different people. For example, respondents often have varying interpretation of the words "often," "frequently," "seldom," "occasionally," "a lot," "a few," "rarely," and the like. They should be defined so that everyone can have the same frame of reference.

Appropriate words further means the words used should be very specific rather than abstract. Their meanings are clear to the respondents. Finally, appropriate wording is crucial for sensitive questions. For example to ask about socially undesirable conduct such as smoking, alcohol consumption, and drug abuse, researchers may want to start with a statement that implies that these behaviors are somewhat common before asking respondents to reveal their experiences.

Write Short Questions

If possible, the researcher should try to keep each question under 20 words. Short questions are usually easier to read and answer than longer questions, which tend to become ambiguous and confusing. Indeed, both well educated and poorly educated people prefer short questions to longer ones. Respondents are usually unwilling to study a question or statement for too long before answering it. Short questions are also less likely to be double-barreled.

Write Simple Questions

To write simple questions, researchers should try to limit the number of complex concepts in one question and use words with three or less syllables unless they are certain the vocabulary is familiar to the respondents. They should try to ask questions directly and positively. Indirect questions may confuse some respondents. Negative words in questions may be overlooked. If the researcher must ask negative questions, the negative word can be underlined to draw the respondents' attention. Investigators should always avoid asking double-negative questions, that is, having two negative words in one sentence. An example of a double-negative question is: "Do you disagree with the statement that the United States does not have a coordinated health care system?" Instead, one could ask: "Do you agree with the statement that the United States has a coordinated health care system?"

Item Analyze the Scale

Item analysis is essential when several statements are used to produce one scale. The purpose is to ensure that items included in the instrument form an internally consistent scale, and to eliminate those that do not. By internal consistency, we mean the items measure the same construct. If several items reflect the same construct, then they should also be interrelated empirically. Internal consistency may be tested by administering the scale with a sample of respondents (100–200) and examining the intercorrelations among items representing the scale. Items that represent a common underlying construct are significantly intercorrelated. A given item that is not related to other items should be dropped from the scale. On the other hand, if a very strong relationship is found between two items, then only one may be needed in the scale that also conveys the meaning of the other.

According to Spector (1992), an item–remainder coefficient can be calculated for each item. It is the correlation of each item with the sum of the remaining items. For example, for a scale with 10 items, the item–remainder coefficient for Item 1 can be calculated by correlating responses to Item 1 with the sum of responses to Items 2 through 10. The item–remainder coefficient for Item 2 can be calculated by correlating responses to Item 2 with the sum of responses to Item 1 and Items 3 through 10. Only items with sufficiently high item–remainder coefficients (e.g., > .40 and < .95) are retained. If this criterion leaves too many items, then those with the largest coefficients are chosen. If the number of items is insufficient, then new items need to be constructed and reexamined. Researchers should beware of an inherent trade-off between number of items and the magnitude of item–remainder coefficients. The more items included, the lower the coefficients can be and still yield a good, internally consistent scale. Another important concern in selecting items is to make sure that they can produce sufficient variations in responses.

In addition to item–remainder coefficients, Cronbach's coefficient alpha can be calculated, which measures the internal consistency of a scale. Cronbach's coefficient alpha ranges from 0 to 1.0 and is a direct function of both the number of items and their magnitude of intercorrelations. It is available in most computer statistical programs. For a scale to reach a sufficient level of internal consistency, the coefficient alpha should reach at least 0.7. Further revisions of items may be needed if the coefficient alpha is too low.

After the best items have been selected, researchers then decide whether to assign different weights to the items in the scale. Generally, all items are weighted equally unless there are strong reasons to believe certain items should be given greater weights. One reason is the lack of balance in the items included. If there are fewer items chosen to represent one than other aspects of the concept, then these items may be given higher weights to make the results more balanced. For example, for a scale with three items, if Items 1 and 2 represent the same dimension and Item 3 represents a different dimension, then Item 3 may be assigned a weight of two and the other items a weight of one each. Weighting can also be based on the relative importance of the different dimensions of a particular concept.

Another issue in summarizing scale items is to deal with missing values. When the sample size is large and only few cases have missing values, the researcher may simply exclude these cases from analysis. When the sample size is small, the researcher may want to replace the missing values with the sample average values. This is usually a conservative approach and works against significant findings.

Assembling

Assembling a questionnaire is like packaging a product. The quality of the paper and appearance of the pages all create impressions on potential respondents and may affect the response rate. In general, white-colored paper is used to facilitate reading. Type is recommended that can produce a mimeographed instrument that resembles a printed copy. The appearance of pages of the questionnaire should not be too crammed. Questions and statements should be spread out and uncluttered. Sufficient space should be available for answering every question, particularly open-ended ones. Cramming many questions on fewer pages is not the way to shorten the length of a questionnaire. In addition to paper and appearance, assembling the questionnaire also involves the sequencing of questions and writing instructions that facilitate questionnaire administration.

Sequencing

Questionnaire sequencing differs between self-administered instrument and interviews. In the self-administered questionnaire, it is usually proper to start with interesting but relatively easy questions so that respondents may be motivated to answer them. Routine questions such as background questions are usually placed at the end. In interviews, however, background questions such as those related to demographics, are usually asked in the beginning after a general introduction about the nature of the study. The purpose is to gain rapport so that answers to later questions can be facilitated.

Both self-administered questionnaires and interviews require certain logic in the order of questions. Subheadings may be used to divide the questionnaire into logical sections. Early questions should be easy and interesting and subsequent questions should flow naturally and logically from earlier questions. Difficult, sensitive, or potentially embarrassing questions should be placed near the end when respondents have already committed time and effort and are more likely to complete them. However, if the questionnaire is lengthy, they should be placed at a position where respondents have not become too tired. In general, knowledge, experience, and behavior questions are easier to answer than questions related to feeling, opinion, attitude, or value. As a rule of thumb, qualitative open-ended questions should be placed at or near the end of a questionnaire so that even if respondents do not answer them they would have completed earlier close-ended portions.

The sequencing of questions should also consider the possibility of reactivity, when earlier questions affect responses to later ones. For example, in interviews, earlier questions about the relationship between smoking and lung cancer as well as other diseases may affect later questions relating to respondents' smoking behavior. In general, to reduce reactivity, interviews should ask behavior- and experience-related questions before attitude and value questions. In self-administered questionnaire, since respondents may go back and change previous responses, one should avoid including questions that may cause a particular response set.

Instructions

Questionnaires, whether self-administered or administered by interviewers, must include clear instructions that facilitate their completion. A cover letter often accompanies a self-administered questionnaire. It specifies the purpose, significance, and sponsor of the research; the benefits of completing the instrument; and the length and return method of the questionnaire. In interviews, the contents of the cover letter are read to the respondent by the interviewer.

The purpose of the research gives potential respondents a sense of what type of research they are participating in. People are generally more willing to complete the questionnaire if the study purpose is of interest to them. Likewise, a person's likelihood of responding hinges on how important the research is. The significance section should be carefully worded to make a connection between the targeted respondents and the study objective. The research sponsor refers to the funder or person or organization who has supported the research. When the sponsor is familiar and influential to the research population, the response rate can be improved.

The benefits of completing the questionnaire may be financial or nonfinancial. Financial benefit means respondents receive monetary compensation upon completing and returning the questionnaire. In most situations, nonfinancial benefits are promised. Examples include improvement of social programs, medical practices, productivity, efficiency, effectiveness, or advancement in theories. Respondents may also receive a summary results upon the completion of the study.

The approximate time in completing the questionnaire is suggested so that respondents can plan this activity accordingly. In general, a shorter length is preferred, and respondents are prompted to complete it as soon as possible. Delay in completing a questionnaire often means not responding at all. Finally, the method of returning the completed instrument needs to be specified. Generally, a postage-paid envelope with the return address is provided to the respondent who is encouraged to put the completed questionnaire in the envelope and send it to the mail as soon as possible.

Within the questionnaire, instructions and explanatory statements are provided where appropriate. The beginning of each section may include a short statement ("In this section, we would like to . . .") indicating the objective and major content of the section to create a proper frame of reference for the respondents. At the end of the section, a transitional statement may be placed to smoothly direct the respondents to the next section.

For each question, basic instructions should be given in terms of how to complete it. Instructions are particularly important when there are variations in response formats. For close-ended questions, respondents can be asked to indicate their answers by placing a check mark or an *X* in the box beside the appropriate response category or by writing answers when called for. For open-ended questions, guidance needs to be provided as to the length of the response. If researchers are interested in elaboration to close-ended questions, they should clearly state so and leave sufficient space for written-in answers.

If a single answer is desired, this should be made perfectly clear in the question: "From the list below, please check the *primary* reason that explains why you do not have any health insurance." Or the question may be followed by a parenthetical note: "Please check the *one* best answer." If multiple answers are expected from the respondent, this should also be made clear in the questions or instructions: "Please check as many answers as apply."

When questions are difficult to respond to, examples can be given as guidance in addition to general instructions. For example, ranking questions should illustrate how ranking is to be performed besides indicating whether single or multiple answers are desired: "Please write *1* beside the most important factor, *2* beside the next most important factor, and so forth until you finish ranking all the listed factors."

For interviews, instructions not only provide logic to the respondents but also serve the purpose of standardizing the administration of the instrument, thus reducing interviewer biases. For this reason, separate sheets of instructions are provided to interviewers that detail the background and purpose of study, administrative matters, rules on what to say and how to say it, when to call, how to set appearance, and how to handle different situations. Further, more transitional statements and probing are included in questionnaires to be administered by interviewers so that ad-libbing becomes unnecessary. Transitional statements are included to make the interviewing proceed in a smooth and logical fashion. Examples include: "Hello, my name is . . ."; "That completes our interview. Thank you for . . . ." Probes are necessary when responses are incomplete or vague or when respondents ask for further clarification. Examples are: "What do you mean by . . . "; "Can you explain that a little more?" In writing instructions for interviews, one should differentiate the formats between those to be read out loud and those not to be read. For example, parenthesis or capital letters may be used for words not to be read out ("IF THE RESPONDENT IS HOSTILE IN ANSWERING THIS QUESTION, THEN . . .").

Pretesting

After the questionnaire has been assembled satisfactorily, the next step is to conduct a pretest of the questionnaire. Pretesting is usually conducted among a relatively small number of respondents (say, 10–20) who closely resemble the research population. Purposive sampling method is used to select as heterogeneous a sample of respondents as the research population.

The purpose of pretesting is to find out whether additional revisions of the questionnaire are necessary. Specifically, researchers are interested in knowing the actual time it takes to complete the questionnaire; whether the level of language matches respondents' knowledge; which words, terms, phrases, or sentences are still confusing, ambiguous, and misunderstood; whether response categories are truly mutually exclusive and all inclusive; which questions generate relatively high nonresponse; whether current instructions are understood or additional instructions are needed; and whether responses to open-ended questions are given in the way intended. Those who participate in pretesting may be contacted to talk about their general feelings, interpretations, and comments about the questionnaire items.

SUMMARY

Measurement is the process of specifying and operationalizing a given concept. Various procedures can be used to operationalize a given concept, including relying on existing measures, observation, and self-report. The four levels of measurement into which concepts may be operationalized are nominal, ordinal, interval, and ratio. To ensure that a measurement is valid and reliable, researchers examine a particular measure in terms of its construct, content, concurrent, and predictive validity and its test–retest, split-half, and interrater reliability. In designing a research instrument, researchers take into account the appropriate frame of reference, time span covered, questionnaire response format, composition of questions, assembling of instrument, and pretesting of the completed instrument.

Key Terms

measurement	nominal measures
reliability	validity
ordinal measures	interval measures
ratio measures	measurement errors

measurement validity   measurement reliability
construct validity   concurrent validity
predictive validity   test–retest reliability
split-half reliability   interrater reliability
loaded questions   leading questions
double-barreled questions

Review Questions

1. What are the levels of measurement? What are their characteristics?

2. What are the differences between systematic errors and random errors in measurement?

3. What measures can be taken to ensure measurement validity and reliability?

4. In designing a research instrument for data collection, what considerations must be taken prior to writing the questions?

5. Design a questionnaire on a topic of interest to you using as many of the response formats illustrated in this chapter as possible.

REFERENCES

Babbie, E. (1992). *The Practice of Social Research.* Belmont, CA: Wadsworth Publishing Co.

Singleton, R. A., Straits, B. C., and Straits, M. M. (1993). *Approaches to Social Research.* 2nd ed. New York: Oxford University Press.

Spector, P. E. (1992). *Summated Rating Scale Construction: An Introduction.* Newbury Park, CA: Sage.

Sudman, S., and Bradburn, N. S. (1986). *Asking Questions: A Practical Guide to Questionnaire Design.* San Francisco: Jossey-Bass.

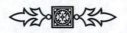

CHAPTER

13

Data Collection and Processing in Health Services Research

LEARNING OBJECTIVES

- To describe the various data collection methods used in health services research.
- To identify situations where some methods are more appropriate than others.
- To specify the measures that can be taken to improve response rate.
- To know how to construct a code book for a research instrument.

Data collection in health services research takes place only after many other research stages have been satisfactorily completed, including conceptualizing the research topic, preparing for research, determining research method and design, sampling, and constructing measurement. This chapter describes various methods of data collection, placing emphasis on the most commonly used methods in health services research: mail questionnaire surveys and personal and telephone interviews. The chapter compares their relative strengths and weaknesses and discuss choices among various methods. It further examines ways to improve both the quantity and quality of responses. Since a data collection instrument may be precoded (i.e., before data are collected), this chapter also introduces concepts related to coding and the components of a code book. Finally, it presents the concepts and procedures of data processing.

DEFINITIONS

Figure 13–1 displays various data collection methods that can be used in health services research. Research data may be collected either empirically or from existing sources. As presented in Chapter 5, studies using existing data are called secondary analysis. Existing data come from both published and nonpublished sources.

Published data may be ordered directly from the publisher, or obtained from university libraries, mostly in the documents section. The federal, state, and local governments regularly publish various kinds of data. Those of particular interest to health services research include official vital statistics abstracted from birth, death, marriage, and divorce certificates (National Center for Health Statistics, 1994c), data on population demographics prepared from census data (U.S. Bureau of the Census, 1994), health statistics (National Center for Health Statistics, 1994b; Centers for Disease Control and Prevention, 1994), health survey results (National Center for Health Statistics, 1994a), and mental health statistics (Center for Mental Health Services and National Institute of Mental Health, 1992). The American Medical Association and the American Hospital Association also periodically publish data on physicians and health services institutions, respectively.

Nonpublished data may be directly obtained from institutions or investigators. The national-level health surveys described in Chapter 3 may be purchased from the federal agencies sponsoring the surveys. Hospitals, insurance companies, and other health services institutions routinely collect data on their patients and clients. Many private foundations, research institutes, and individual researchers have conducted research on many health-related topics. Researchers may negotiate with institutions or individuals to gain access to their data.

Empirical data originate with the research and may be collected either with a data collection instrument (e.g., questionnaire) or through observational methods. As is presented in Chapter 6, the purpose of observational methods is to learn about things first-

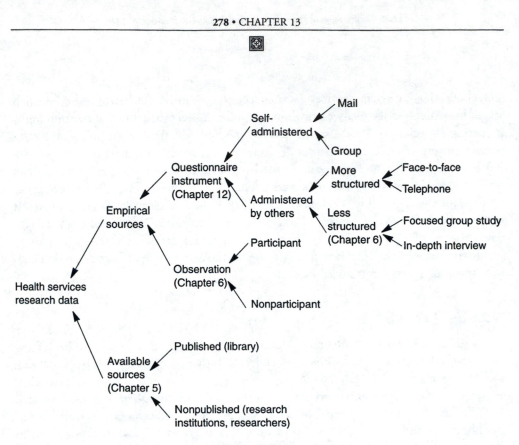

FIGURE 13–1   Health services research data collection methods.

hand. Observation can occur in many settings: homes, community, organizations, programs, and so on. Observational data help describe the research setting, the activities that took place in that setting, the people who participated in these activities, and the meaning of what was observed from the perspective of those observed (Patton, 1990, p. 202). Observation may be conducted either as a participant or nonparticipant. A participant-observer is one who is immersed in the research setting, learning to think, see, feel, and sometimes act as an insider (Powdermaker, 1966, p. 9). A participant-observer describes the program to outsiders as an insider. A nonparticipant-observer is an onlooker who sees what is happening but does not become involved. There are, however, many variations along the continuum between participation and nonparticipation.

   Collecting data with a prepared instrument is the most common method of data collection in health services research. The issues regarding the construction of research instruments were covered in Chapter 12. Data collection instrument may be self-administered by subjects filling out the instrument by themselves, or administered by researchers to the subjects. The mail questionnaire survey is the most common self-administered data collection method. The questionnaire that contains a list of questions for information or opinion is mailed to potential respondents representative of the research population. The respondents are asked to complete the questionnaire and return it by mail. Questionnaires may also be self-administered in group settings where the questionnaire is distributed to group members who are asked to complete and return the instrument either right away or sometime later. Examples of group include classroom students, workplace employees, and association and club members.

When researchers or trained staff administer questionnaires to respondents, they may do so in a more structured or less structured manner. The more structured methods include face-to-face interviews and telephone interviews. In the face-to-face interview, the interviewer administers a highly structured questionnaire with a planned series of questions to a respondent and records the respondent's answers by checking off relevant categories in close-ended questions and taking notes in open-ended questions. In the telephone interview, researchers first locate potential respondents by telephone before administering the prepared research instrument. Almost all residences in the United States now have telephones. The probability of social class bias due to telephone availability has greatly diminished (Groves, 1980). With the increasing availability of telephones, the telephone survey is fast becoming a popular data collection method. However, an increasing number of people, particularly those from upper income households, choose not to list their numbers. Researchers may use random digit dialing, which selects telephone numbers based on tables of random numbers. With random digit dialing, even unlisted numbers have an equal probability of being selected.

The less structured data collection methods include focused group study and in-depth interview. As described in Chapter 6, both are common qualitative research methods. While the in-depth interview refers to a one-on-one interview, the focused group study involves several respondents at a time. In both methods, rather than strictly following the predetermined questions from a questionnaire instrument, interviewers encourage respondents to freely discuss their thoughts, asking questions spontaneously based on the flow of conversation. Often researchers come into the interview with a topic in mind and an interview guide, which may be modified in the course of the interview.

COMPARISONS

Each data collection method has its own strengths and weaknesses. This section compares data collected using the various sources presented earlier. Tables 13–1 and 13–2 summarize the comparisons.

Available versus Empirical Sources

Using available sources generally saves money and time spent in data collection. When the research budget is limited, using available data may be the only viable choice. Data collected empirically, however, tend to be more relevant to the research topic.

TABLE 13–1 Comparison of data collection methods

	(1) Available Sources	Empirical Sources	(2) Available Sources Published	Nonpublished	(3) Empirical Sources Instrument	Observation
Data collection costs	+	−	+	−	=	=
Data collection time	+	−	+	−	+	−
Data collection effort	=	=	+	−	−	+
Sample size for a given budget	+	−	−	+	+	−
Data quality	−	+	−	+	+	−

Note. "+" indicates a relative strength; "−" indicates a relative weakness; "=" indicates the criterion does not distinguish between the methods.

Access can be a problem for both available and empirical sources and is an important consideration in determining data sources. Table 13–1 summarizes these differences in column 1.

Published versus Nonpublished Sources

Among available sources, using published sources saves time, money, and is relatively easy to access. A fundamental weakness of published sources is that often only aggregate summaries are presented, making secondary analysis difficult and, sometimes, impossible. Nonpublished sources are generally more helpful to the researcher, with raw data and large sample sizes. Gaining access to them may be difficult, particularly when the data set contains sensitive questions or is considered confidential. Table 13–1 summarizes these differences under column 2.

Instrument versus Observation Sources

Research based on a prepared instrument generally saves time in data collection, thus increasing the sample size for a given budget. Data collected tend to be more uniform, thus facilitating analysis. However, gaining access to respondents is a potential challenge. Observational methods, on the other hand, have relatively less access difficulty but involve greater time commitment. They are most appropriate for finding out how people behave in public, but not appropriate to learn how people behave in private or what people think. Since not everything may be observed directly, data collected may be incomplete. Table 13–1 summarizes these differences under column 3.

Instrument-Based Data Collection Methods

Table 13–2 compares the data collection methods using research instruments, including self-administered mail or group survey, face-to-face or telephone interview, focused group study, and in-depth interview. The following paragraphs summarize the principal strengths and weaknesses concerning their impact on research project, respondents, interviewer, and instrument.

Impact on Research Project

Data Collection Cost

Self-administered data collection methods such as mail and group questionnaires have the lowest overall costs. Most of the costs are incurred in such categories as postage, printing, and supplies. The significant saving is in labor. Interview methods have relatively higher costs in all phases of the interview operation: staff recruiting, training, supervision, travel, the interview itself, and, sometimes, lodging and meals. Focused group studies and in-depth interviews are potentially most costly due to their labor intensive nature. Face-to-face interviews, although using interviewers as well, are less costly because the interview is more structured and takes considerably less time. Telephone interviews are even less costly due to saving in traveling and related expenses, including personnel and gasoline (Groves and Kahn, 1979; Lavrakas, 1987). The telephone interview also saves money spent in staff supervision. Rather than sending numerous supervisors to the field to monitor face-to-face interviews, telephone interviews allow one supervisor to oversee several interviewers calling from the same office. In addition, call-backs are made more easily and economically than with the face-to-face interview.

Data Collection Time

The group self-administered questionnaire has the greatest saving in time spent on data collection. The mail questionnaire tends to be most time-consuming mainly due to time spent in mailings. The telephone interview saves traveling time compared to the face-to-face interview. Additional time is saved with the use of a **CATI** (computer-assisted telephone interview) system in which survey questionnaires are displayed on computer terminals for interviewers, who type respondents' answers directly into the computer. The focused group method, although involving travels, interviews a number of people at the same time, thus saving time on a per-respondent basis when compared with in-depth interview.

Data Collection Effort

While all data collection methods require researchers to devote a lot of energy, focused group and in-depth interview methods demand the greatest effort on the part of interviewers. Face-to-face and telephone interview methods require less though still significant effort from interviewers. Self-administered methods, on the other hand, require the least effort. The group method requires greater effort than mailing due to the researcher's presence to respond to potential questions.

Sample Size

For a given budget, self-administered methods can achieve the greatest sample size, mainly due to labor savings. Focused group and in-depth interview methods yield the smallest sample size due to labor intensity and lengthy interviews. Telephone interviews yield a larger sample size than face-to-face interviews due to savings in traveling costs.

Data Quality

If data quality is measured by the validity of respondents' statements, then focused group and in-depth interview methods have the highest quality. Both methods afford researchers the opportunity to explore important issues with intensity. The mail survey has the lowest quality, because response validity depends on the ability and willingness of respondents to provide information. Respondents who have trouble understanding and interpreting questions cannot receive any help from researchers. Researchers cannot observe which respondents are reluctant or evasive toward answering what types of questions.

If data quality is measured by the reliability of responses, then focused group and in-depth interview may present the greatest problem because they are not readily susceptible to codification and comparability. Rather, open-ended questions need to be coded, and careful independent observers should establish the validity and reliability of the coding. Other methods have greater uniformity in the manner in which questions are posed.

Impact on Respondents

Dispersed Sample

When potential respondents are geographically dispersed, the mail survey and telephone interview methods are the preferred methods, because they afford a wider geographic contact by reaching people who are difficult to locate and interview. Indeed, it

TABLE 13–2 Comparison of data collection methods using research instruments

	Self-administered		Administered by others			
	Mail	Group	Face-to-face interview	Telephone interview	Focused group	In-depth interview
Research project						
Data collection costs	5	5	2	3	1	1
Data collection time	1	5	3	4	4	2
Data collection effort	5	4	2	2	1	1
Sample size for a given budget	5	5	2	3	1	1
Data quality	1	2	4	3	5	5
Respondents						
Dispersed sample	5	1	1	4	1	1
Low literacy level	1	2	4	3	5	5
Degree of privacy	5	4	2	2	1	2
Rate of nonresponse	1	4	4	3	5	5
Interviewer						
Need interaction with respondents	1	2	4	3	5	5
Presentation of visual aid	2	4	5	1	5	5

TABLE 13–2 *continued*

	Self-administered		Administered by others			
	Mail	Group	Face-to-face interview	Telephone interview	Focused group	In-depth interview
Degree of interview bias	5	4	2	2	1	1
Degree of fieldwork training	5	1	2	2	1	1
Instrument						
Length of survey	2	1	4	2	5	5
Sensitive questions	2	1	4	2	2	5
Check other sources for information	5	1	1	1	4	2
Independent work	1	4	5	4	2	5
Uniformity of questions	5	5	4	4	1	1
Sequencing of questions	1	2	5	5	5	5
Completion rate	1	2	4	3	5	5

Note. 5 indicates most appropriate choice when measured with this criterion; 4 indicates appropriate choice when measured with this criterion; 3 indicates indifferent choice when measured with this criterion; 2 indicates not appropriate choice when measured with this criterion; 1 indicates least appropriate choice when measured with this criterion.

costs no more to conduct a national mail survey than a local one. Group and other interview methods are difficult because either respondents have to travel a long distance to the researcher or vice versa. The cost of a national interview survey would be far more expensive than one conducted at the local level.

Literacy Level

When potential respondents cannot read and write, self-administered methods are automatically excluded from consideration. Among the remaining methods, the telephone interview has greater difficulty than personal interview methods due to distance communication and lack of facial contact.

Privacy

Mail surveys afford the greatest privacy to respondents. Questionnaires administered in group settings also enjoys significant privacy because responses can be given anonymously. The focused group interview has the least privacy because each participant is heard by other participants in addition to the interviewer. Other interview methods have comparatively more privacy: only the interviewer knows who the respondents are and what they say.

Response Rate

High nonresponse rate is perhaps the greatest problem of the mail survey method. Furthermore, it is difficult to separate bad addresses from nonresponses. In contrast, personal interviews generally have higher response rates. Since respondents of the group method are generally a captured audience (i.e., students, employees, members, patients, conference participants, etc.), its response rate is expected to be high. Telephone interviews yield higher responses than mail surveys but lower responses than personal interview methods. The telephone interview requires greater efforts in training interviewers, introducing the study to respondents, and monitoring the interview procedures (Groves and Kahn, 1979, p. 217). A higher nonresponse rate in telephone versus personal interviews reflects the difficulty in establishing rapport between respondents and interviewers in the telephone survey and suggests that respondents find telephone interviews to be a less rewarding experience and more of a chore than personal interviews. The proliferation of bogus telephone surveys, often telemarketing, the use of answering machines as screening devices, and the ease with which people can hang up the phone also contribute to the low response rate.

Low response rate is not a problem in itself. Questionnaires can be sent to more people to achieve the desired sample size. What is problematic is that respondents and nonrespondents are generally significantly different with respect to the research interest.

Typically, responses are bimodal, with those for and against the issue responding and those who are indifferent not responding. Such an unrepresentative sample will likely produce biased results.

Impact on Interviewer

Interaction with Respondents

Mail surveys do not allow any interactions between researchers and respondents. Group surveys allow some interaction when researchers help clarify a particular statement. Telephone interviewers may also clarify misinterpretations, but the interview affords limited interaction due to lack of facial contact. Personal interviews, particularly focused group studies and in-depth interviews that are not constrained by predominantly close-ended questions, afford significantly greater interactions.

The opportunity to interact with respondents have many advantages. In addition to clearing up seemingly inaccurate answers by restating or explaining the questions to the respondents, interviewers can control which person or persons answer the questions, secure more spontaneous reactions, help ensure that every relevant item is answered, and collect supplementary information about the respondent's personal characteristics and environment, which can be valuable in interpreting results. Interaction also improves responses to open-ended questions, because interviewers can elicit a fuller, more complete response than a questionnaire requiring respondents to write out answers. This is particularly true with respondents whose writing skills are weak or who are less motivated to make the effort to respond fully.

Visual Aid

Telephone interviews cannot use visual aids to help explain questions. With all other methods of data collection, visual material can be presented to various extent. Mail surveys can use pictures in the questionnaire, whereas personal interviewers can show various kinds of visual aids, including videos, photos, drawings, cards, objects, and so on. Cards showing response options are useful when they are difficult to remember or when respondents may feel embarrassed to say the options aloud.

Bias

Unfortunately, interviews may also introduce biases related to interactions with respondents. Biases may originate from the interview or respondent. Interviewers may fail to follow the interview schedule in the prescribed manner or may suggest answers to respondents. Bias also may be introduced through a respondent's reaction to the interviewer's gender, race, manner of dress, or personality. Common sources of respondent-originated bias include **social desirability, acquiescence, auspices, prestige,** and

mental set. Social desirability refers to responses based on what is perceived as being socially acceptable or respectable, positive or negative. Acquiescence refers to responses based on the respondent's perception of what would be desirable to the interviewer. Auspices refers to responses dictated by the opinion or image of the sponsor, rather than the actual question. Prestige refers to responses intended to improve the image of the respondent in the eyes of the interviewer. Mental set refers to responses to later items influenced by perceptions based on previous items.

Biases are more likely to be introduced in focused group studies and in-depth interviews. Interviewers with certain biases may unconsciously ask questions so as to secure confirmation of their own views. In face-to-face and telephone interviews, interviewer effect is lessened because the instrument is more structured and there is less opportunity for interviewers to ad lib.

Training

To reduce interviewer biases, interview methods, whether personal or telephone, require substantial efforts in personnel training. Interviewers need to be trained to build rapport with the respondents and to not reveal personal values or let them affect the interview process. Building rapport over the telephone is particularly challenging, because the respondents are called to the telephone unexpectedly and asked to do something they do not anticipate or fully understand. They may be in the middle of other activities (preparing meals, looking after children, watching television, etc.). They may not be in the mood to talk to strangers. Interviewers may have to prove their legitimacy and worth of the time granted to them by reluctant respondents. It is even harder to train interviewers for focused group studies and in-depth interviews. Interviewers not only need to know the proper way of conducting interviews so as not to introduce biases, but also to be very familiar with the research topic so that they can ask the right questions.

Potential interviewers should have a good command of both the spoken and written language. They must understand and believe in the purpose of the study. They need to be familiar with the specific questionnaire items. Desirable qualities of good interviewers include being tactful, careful, sensitive, polite, accurate, adaptable, consistent, interested, honest, assertive (but sensitive enough to know when to be less assertive), persevering, and able to withstand tiring and sometimes boring work. Evening and weekend work is often necessary. Part-time work may be preferable due to the repetitive nature of the interview work.

Interviewer training includes instructions on how to contact a respondent to obtain an interview, how questions must be asked (e.g., order, meaning, probing), and the kinds of behavior to avoid that tend to inhibit respondents (e.g., interrupting, disagreeing, frowning). Before fieldwork, trainees should observe trained interviewers and practice interviews. Role-playing simulations may be set up in which prospective interviewers interview each other with the instructor commenting on proper procedures and mistakes. An interview manual should be prepared that covers techniques specific to the study, including neutral probes and instructions on how to handle problems. For example, in dealing with reluctant respondents, interviewers should be patient and explicit about the interview, explaining what it will demand of the respondent and giving some sample questions. The following summarizes the common dos and don'ts for interviewers (Bailey, 1994; Miller, 1991).

Dos
- Dress formally, to legitimize your role as an interviewer, and unobtrusively, to avoid that attention being diverted to your appearance.
- Introduce yourself and your sponsor to the respondent.
- Explain the purpose of the study, its significance, and the expected length of the interview.
- Tell how the respondent was chosen, assure confidentiality, and ask for permission to be interviewed.
- Follow the interview guide closely by asking questions as worded, following the same sequence and using similar inflection and intonation.
- Use neutral probes, when respondents ask for clarification or indicate misinterpretation, by restating the question, repeating the answer, and explaining the meaning of certain words and phrases in the same manner to all respondents.
- Record respondents' answers exactly as given.
- Thank the respondent for his or her time and leave the name and telephone number of the contact person in case there are questions.

Don'ts
- Do not provide false information concerning the purpose of the study, its expected length, and its benefits to respondents.
- Do not alter the questionnaire by omitting certain questions or changing question wording.
- Do not use biased probing by asking leading questions or offering suggestive answers.
- Do not interpret or modify respondents' answers.
- Do not assume respondents' answers before asking.
- If you made any promise to respondents such as sending them the study results, do not forget to follow it through.

During fieldwork, interviewers should be monitored from time to time to maintain quality control. Regular meetings should be held to collect questionnaires, answer questions, review completed questionnaires, share problems and solutions, and improve morale.

Impact on Instrument

Length

Compared with interviews, self-administered methods generally have a greater preference for shorter questionnaires. Among interview methods, telephone interviews, where interviewers have least control over respondents' behavior, requires a relatively shorter instrument. In personal interviews, the length of interview usually does not affect refusal rate once respondents agree to be interviewed. Focused group studies and in-depth interviews are usually much longer than structured face-to-face interviews.

Sensitive Questions

When sensitive questions are posed, the in-depth interview is most likely to obtain truthful responses. Group-based methods have great difficulty in obtaining frank responses due to concern for confidentiality. Methods that have problem establishing rapport with respondents, including mail surveys and telephone interviews, also are less appropriate for sensitive questions unless complete confidentiality is assured.

Checking Other Sources

When research intends to collect specialized information, the mail survey is the most appropriate choice because it provides the opportunity for more considered answers and for respondents to check and secure information or consult with others. Methods that require respondents to provide answers spontaneously are less suitable for questions that demand more specialized knowledge. The focused group method is relatively less problematic because presumably someone within the focused group knows the answers.

Independent Work

When research intends to find out whether the respondent possesses a particular piece of knowledge or information, methods requiring respondents to provide answers spontaneously are more suitable than mail surveys, where the intended respondent may not be the actual respondent. The focused group method is also not appropriate for knowledge questions because the person responding to a question may or may not be the only person who knows the answer.

Uniformity

Highly structured data collection methods yield more uniform answers than less structured methods, such as focused group studies and in-depth interviews. Among structured methods, interviews, whether face-to-face or by telephone, yield less uniform results than mail or group surveys due to the potential for interviewer effect.

Sequencing

When sequencing of questions is important, interview methods are more appropriate than mail or group surveys because interviewers can control the order in which questions are asked. Mail or group surveys cannot prevent respondents from reading ahead or changing earlier answers based on later information. In addition, interviewers may use a question skip format in which certain questions are skipped when they do not apply to a particular respondent, whereas such a format may be confusing for respondents completing a questionnaire.

Completion Rate

Completion rate is highest among personal interview methods where interviewers have greater control and can be trained to elicit responses to every question. In mail or group survey methods, respondents have greater control and can skip questions without being noticed. Tedious or sensitive items can be passed over easily. Thus, there are usually more missing values in self-administered methods than interviews. The problem of missing items may be alleviated somewhat by instructions stressing the need to answer every item, assuring confidentiality, and making items easy to understand.

Choices among Methods

In deciding which data collection method(s) to use, researchers compare the strengths and weaknesses of these methods with their unique research situation and select the method(s) that optimally matches their situation. Sometimes it is obvious which method should be used. If many respondents are illiterate, then interview methods have to be used instead of self-administered questionnaires. When research funding is limited, a cheaper method, such as the mail survey, may be the only viable choice. The nature of the questions also dictates which method should be chosen. If many questions are sensitive, then more honest and valid responses may be obtained by self-administered methods than through interviews, as the former is more assuring in terms of anonymity and confidentiality. Many research situations, however, are not so clear-cut. Researchers have to weigh the pros and cons of various methods and select the most appropriate method(s). To facilitate choosing the right method(s), researchers should be familiar with conditions most appropriate to each data collection method.

The conditions a self-administered mail questionnaire has to satisfy include: (1) respondents must be literate, (2) survey questions and instructions are relatively simple and straightforward, (3) questionnaire order is not important, and (4) consultation by respondents with other sources for information will not affect the validity of the response. In addition, the self-administered mail questionnaire is most appropriate when research budget is limited, when a large sample size is desired, when a sampling list representative of the study population is readily available, when the sample is more dispersed, when privacy is important, and when respondents have to check other sources to give appropriate responses.

A self-administered group survey has to satisfy the following conditions: (1) respondents can be gathered in the same setting, (2) the gathered respondents are representative of the research population, and (3) questionnaire order is not important. The self-administered group survey can be used for respondents who are less educated than in a mail survey situation. With the assistance of the researcher, survey questions and instructions can be relatively more difficult. The method is appropriate when research budget and time are both limited, and consultation with other sources for information is not allowed.

The conditions for a face-to-face interview include: (1) researchers have access to respondents or organizations in which respondents are located, (2) interviewers are adequately trained to perform the interview in an unbiased manner, and (3) a sufficient budget exists to perform an adequate number of interviews. The face-to-face interview is preferred when (1) respondents are illiterate or have little education and interviewers have to do the recording, (2) interaction with the respondents is required, (3) the sample size can be relatively small, (4) respondents are concentrated in a confined geographic area, (5) question order is important, (6) questions are relatively complex and difficult, (7) questions are not so sensitive that respondents feel threatened or embarrassed to talk to someone, (8) visual aids have to be used, (9) the research instrument is relatively lengthy because better rapport and cooperation can be achieved with personal presence, and (10) checking other sources for information is not allowed.

A telephone interview requires that a telephone directory or other lists serve a representative sample frame and interviewers are properly trained to establish rapport with respondents within a short time. The telephone interview is preferred when (1) respondents are spread throughout a broad geographic area, (2) rapid data collection is needed, (3) the questionnaire is relatively short and easy, (4) question sequence is important, (5) questions are somewhat sensitive and anonymity of response is desired, (6) no visual aid is required, (7) respondents should not receive help in answering questions, (8) respondents are illiterate or have little education, and (9) the research setting is not important to observe.

Both the focused group method and the in-depth interview may be used either at the initial stage of research, to identify issues and measures to be used in the survey instrument, or after the survey research, to collect additional information that explores the factors and details associated with survey findings. Both methods are time-consuming and require a small sample size. They are the most valid ways to collect qualitative data and sensitive information. Both demand greater interviewer skill with the language and techniques that encourage respondents to speak frankly and at length. Interviewers should also have considerable knowledge about the research topic. However, quantitative analysis of the collected information is difficult. The data elements obtained can vary significantly among subjects depending on their interests and the approach adopted by the interviewer. It is difficult to code and use these data in a quantitative way. While the in-depth interview can better ensure privacy and confidentiality, the focused group study is more suitable to find out the impact of group interactions.

In many situations, researchers may combine different data collection methods in the same research. For example, the focused group study or the in-depth interview may be used first to explore important issues related to the topic that may be incorporated in the research instrument. Mail surveys may be used in combination with telephone and personal interviews to improve the response rate. Telephone interviews may be used as a screening method to determine study eligibility before face-to-face interviews. On the other hand, respondents may be notified via mail and followed up with a telephone interview.

IMPROVING RESPONSE RATE

High response rate is critical for research results to be valid. Many researchers believe an adequate response rate should be at least over 50 percent (Babbie, 1973, p. 165). The importance of a high response rate is that those who answer the questionnaire may differ significantly from nonrespondents, thereby biasing the sample. In most situations, nonrespondents tend to be less educated, less wealthy, or less interested in the research topic. Research thus has an inherent bias toward overrepresenting the better-educated population and underrepresenting the poor and minorities. As a minimum effort, researchers should make special efforts to assess how nonrespondents compare with respondents. Examples include using registered letters, telephone calls, personal interviews, and so on (Wallace, 1954).

More importantly, researchers should incorporate various means to improve response rate in the data collection process. The following, as summarized in Table 13–3, presents these measures as well as their relative need for different data collection methods.

Follow-up Efforts

Intensive follow-up efforts are the best means to increase returns. When completed questionnaires are returned, they should be assigned serial identification numbers to keep track on returns and facilitate follow-up. Follow-up is particularly important for mail surveys and telephone interviews. Often, more than one follow-up may be needed. In their comprehensive reviews of published studies, Herberlein and Baumgartner (1978) found that the average response rate for the initial mailing was 48 percent (based on 183 studies). Response rate increased by an additional 20 percent with a second mailing (based on 58 studies), 12 percent with a third mailing (based on 40 studies), and 10 percent with a fourth mailing (based on 25 studies).

TABLE 13–3   Methods of data collection and means to improve response rate

	Self-administered		Administered by others			
	Mail	Group	Face-to-face interview	Telephone interview	Focused group	In-depth interview
Follow-up	5	3	2	4	1	1
Sponsor	5	5	4	5	4	4
Length	5	4	2	4	1	1
Introductory letter	5	2	3	4	1	1
Type of questions	5	3	1	4	1	1
Inducement	3	3	4	4	5	5
Type of population	5	3	3	4	2	1
Anonymity/confidentiality	5	3	5	4	1	5
Time of contact	4	4	3	5	2	1
Method of return	5	1	1	1	1	1

Note. A Likert-type scale ranging from 1 to 5 is used with 5 indicating the item to be the most needed measure to improve response rate and 1 the least needed measure.

Telephones can often be used effectively for follow-up. Researchers can find out if respondent needs another copy of the questionnaire to replace the original one, which may have been destroyed or misplaced. The telephone may be used to collect information directly from respondents, especially when the questionnaire is relatively short and the respondent has lost the questionnaire form. Waves of mailed questionnaires and a final telephone interview can generate a very high response rate. Research experience with Community and Migrant Health Center administrators indicates that a second mailing after a three-week interval improved the response rate from 50 to 70 percent (Shi, Samuels, and Glover, 1994). A third contact by telephone improved response rate by an additional 15 percent.

Sponsor

The appeal of the sponsor is an important factor in improving the response rate. Preferably, the sponsor should be a person or agency that the respondents know and respect. Examples of legitimate sponsors are scientific, governmental, university, professional associations, and well-known nonprofit agencies. A cover letter by the prestigious and respected sponsor making an appeal to respondents can significantly influence returns. The sponsor factor is important for all data collection methods, particularly those where little or no direct personal contact is involved and establishing rapport with respondents is difficult.

Length

The length of a questionnaire is a critical factor for a high response rate, particularly for mail surveys and other methods where researchers have no or limited personal contact with respondents. For these methods, the shorter the questionnaire, the higher the response rate (Berdie, 1973). For personal methods such as face-to-face and in-depth interviews, the length of the interview is less critical. Respondents giving permission to be interviewed generally do not mind if the interview is somewhat lengthy.

Introductory Letter

An introductory or a cover letter explains the nature and purpose of the research and stresses its importance. A good cover letter is short and concise. It should not exceed one page in length. The letter ends with a solicitation to participate. Use of an actual signature on the cover letter is more appealing than using copies of a signed cover letter. The personalization of large numbers of letters can be accomplished with word processing software using the "replace" command so that respondent's name and address can be inserted in the body of the text.

An introductory letter is particularly important for survey methods where researchers have the least control over respondents' behavior and respondents have the greatest need for motivation. An introductory letter may be sent by mail prior to telephone interviews to explain the study and inform that a study representative will call soon so that respondents are not caught by surprise.

Type of Questions

The type of questions in a questionnaire is most critical for mail surveys than for other methods to affect response rate. In general, respondents are more likely to complete questions that are interesting, relevant, or judged as salient to them. Questionnaires asking for objective information receive a better response rate than those asking for subjective information. Those containing simpler questions receive better returns than those with difficult questions or ones that require consultation with additional sources. Response rate drops substantially if questions probe areas regarded by respondents as private, sensitive, and/or a threat to them or their immediate groups. Examples of sensitive questions include sexual behavior, deviant behavior (e.g., drug use, smoking), income, and education level. Questionnaires using a complex format also receive lower responses. A questionnaire with many contingency questions is too confusing for the average respondent. Complex questionnaire may be used in an interview because interviewers have been given extensive training in understanding the format and skip pattern. Finally, clean, neat, less cluttered, and straightforward questionnaires improve response rate.

Inducement

Researchers may offer certain inducements to enhance response rate. Inducements can be both financial and nonfinancial. Financial incentives are provided particularly when the questionnaire or interview is lengthy and research results are important (Armstrong, 1975). The problem with offering financial inducement, besides its costliness, is that some respondents will be offended that the researcher considers their time to be worth so little.

Nonfinancial inducement includes sending reports of study results to respondents, enclosing a souvenir such as a ball-point pen, emphasizing study significance, or making an altruistic appeal. Nonfinancial means are preferred if monetary inducement is insignificant. Using a deadline is another nonfinancial inducement. Its advantage is that respondents can plan completing the questionnaire based on the deadline. Its disadvantage is that once the deadline is passed, respondents may decide it is too late to return the questionnaire and throw it away instead.

Type of Population

Response rate varies significantly with the type of population surveyed or interviewed. Response generally varies with education, income, and occupation. Better-educated people are more likely to return questionnaires, and among them, professionals and those who are more wealthy are more likely to return questionnaires (Herberlein and Baumgartner, 1978). Minority populations have a lower response rate than the white population.

Anonymity/Confidentiality

Among data collection methods, only self-administered methods and telephone interviews are capable of maintaining anonymity. The anonymous nature of surveys enhances response rate, particularly when questions are sensitive. The downside of anonymity is the inability to use follow-up. An alternative is to send everyone a second questionnaire with the instruction to disregard the questionnaire if they have already completed and returned the first one. However, this method will be expensive, particularly when the sample size is large. Questionnaires using identification codes to track responses are not truly anonymous because they can be traced to individual respondents. Another method for identifying nonrespondents while maintaining anonymity involves mailing a postcard with the questionnaire to the respondents. The postcard contains the respondent's name and address. Respondents are asked to return the postcard when they complete the questionnaire. The questionnaire is mailed back separately with no name or identification code (Babbie, 1973, p. 169; Bailey, 1994). Because of the difficulty and deficiency of anonymity, most researchers promise complete confidentiality rather than anonymity to improve response rate.

Time of Contact

The time to contact respondents for interviews or to send questionnaires in mail surveys can play a significant role in returns. When respondents are working, they are best located at the end of the day or during weekends. The questionnaire, if sent home, should arrive near the end of the week. When sending questionnaires to administrators in organizations, summer or near a holiday season is the worst time to pick because many people take time off for vacation and holidays.

Method of Return

The method of returning completed questionnaires may be psychologically important to respondents. Including a regularly stamped (preferably with a new commemorative stamp), self-addressed envelope has a personal touch and produces better results than business reply or metered envelopes. If the questionnaire is short and simple, double postcards may be used as a convenient way to secure returns. A double postcard contains the questionnaire as well as the return address so that respondents, upon receiving the postcard, can easily fill out the questionnaire, fold it up, and mail it back to the researcher.

QUESTIONNAIRE CODING

Coding consists of assigning numbers to questionnaire answer categories and specifying column locations for these numbers in the computer data file. Such standardization and quantification of data is necessary in order to permit computer storage, retrieval, manipulation, and statistical analysis. Coding is a critical part of data preparation.

In general, data should be coded into relatively more categories to maintain details. Code categories can always be combined during data analysis if it is deemed that less detailed categories are more desirable. Conversely, if too few categories are used, it is impossible to capture the original detail. Code categories should be both exhaustive and mutually exclusive. Every data element should fit into one and only one category. Code categories may be determined before data collection (i.e., precode) or after data collection (i.e., postcode, recode). A code book is usually prepared after data collection.

Precoding

Precoding assigns numbers to data categories and indicates their column locations prior to data collection. Assigning columns may be unnecessary if data are directly entered into a statistical program or spreadsheet that assigns a field instead of columns to each variable. Precoding can be prepared when the questionnaire is being written so that coding categories and column locations appear in the questionnaire instrument itself. Because data collected by questionnaires are typically transformed into some type of computer format, it is usually appropriate to include data-processing instructions on the questionnaire itself. These instructions indicate where specific pieces of information will be stored in the machine-readable data files.

Figure 13–2 presents a precoded questionnaire studying respondents' attitude toward a single-payer health care system. Precoding appearing in the margin of a questionnaire is also called *edge-coding*. Note the numerical codes in the right-hand margin of the questionnaire, which indicate the column location for the questions. For example, Question 6 requires respondents to check only one answer. The number in the right-hand margin, 20, indicates the column of the computer data file in which the code for Question 6 is to be entered.

When a code for a particular variable is greater than nine, then two columns must be used to code one variable. Question 1, for example, requires respondents to record their age. Unless we expect a respondent to be 100 years old or more, two columns will be sufficient to capture all variations in respondents' age. Question 4 asks about respondents' annual income and uses six columns. More columns may be used if you suspect higher income levels.

When multiple answers to a single question are needed, as in Question 5, they cannot be coded into a single column. Rather, separate columns should be allotted for every

RECORD 1

1. Your current age _____   5–6/

2. Your sex: male (1)   female (2)   7/

3. Your race: White (1)   Black (2)   Asian (3)   Other (4) _____   8/

4. What was your annual income last year? $ _____   9–14/

5. Which of the following health insurance plans do you currently have?
   (Check all that apply)

   Medicare   ___ (1)   15/

   Medicaid   ___ (2)   16/

   Blue Cross/Blue Shield   ___ (3)   17/

   Other (specify _____)   ___ (4)   18/

   No insurance   ___ (5)   19/

6. Indicate your agreement with a single-payer health care system.   20/
   (Check one only)

   Strongly agree   ___ (1)

   Agree   ___ (2)

   Unsure   ___ (3)

   Disagree   ___ (4)

   Strongly disagree   ___ (5)

FIGURE 13–2   Mini survey: Opinion toward single-payer system.

potential answer. Such coding is equivalent to transforming one variable containing five different response categories into five variables. Each of the variables now becomes binary, coded either as present (when respondent checks off the response) or absent (when respondent leaves the response blank). For example, suppose a respondent checks off Medicare and Blue Cross/Blue Shield, then the researcher will enter one in column 15, zero in column 16, three in column 17, and zero in columns 18 and 19.

Using precoding has two time-saving advantages. In face-to-face interviews, respondents can tell the interviewer the numerical codes for response categories rather than remembering the complete categories and repeating the appropriate one to the interviewer. In self-administered questionnaire surveys, respondents can jot down the numerical codes in the appropriate spaces rather than writing out the answers. The second advantage is with data entry. There is no need to code respondents' answers again. The actual questionnaire can also serve as a code book that defines the meaning of each numerical code and specifies its column location. Data entry can be accomplished by reading directly from respondents' questionnaire and entering their responses into the computer according to the column locations specified in the right-hand margins. In addition to time saved from compiling a new code book and transferring data from the questionnaire to a transfer sheet, using precoded questionnaires also reduces the number of errors made in data transferring.

However, precoding can only be used when questions are close-ended. When researchers cannot predict what answer categories or how many additional "other" categories exist for a given question, open-ended questions will have to be used. Postcoding will become necessary.

Postcoding

Postcoding assigns numbers to data categories and indicates their column locations after data collection, that is, after respondents have answered the questions in the questionnaire. Postcoding is necessary mainly for open-ended questions for which researchers cannot anticipate response categories. For example, the following open-ended question may be added to the single-payer survey as Question 7.

7. Why are you in favor, unsure, or opposed to the "single-payer" system?

Since we are not certain about all the possible answers to this question, we have to leave it as open-ended. After reviewing the actual responses from respondents, we can decide the number of categories to use and assign numerical codes accordingly.

Questions with "other" as a response category may also need to be postcoded if many people have chosen it as their choice. For example, the "other" category in Question 3 may encounter many responses from Hispanics. Similarly, Question 5's "other" category may generate many answers such as HMO, PPO, or other managed care arrangements. New response categories may be needed to better represent the research population. A rule of thumb is to add new categories when the "other" response accounts for 10 percent or more of the total responses.

Since open-ended questions are the principal reason for postcoding and postcoding is more labor intensive and time-consuming, researchers often use open-ended questions in small-scale exploratory research or qualitative research where the sample size is small. These preliminary studies help identify not only the right questions to ask but also the most common categories for a given question. These findings pave the way for the design of a close-ended and precoded questionnaire instrument to be used for large scale survey research.

Recoding

Recoding changes earlier coding assignments of the attributes of a variable. Similar to postcoding, recoding is done after data have been collected. However, rather than assigning numerical codes to attributes before data analysis as is the case with postcoding, recoding is generally done after some preliminary data analysis so that researchers have some feel of the nature of the data. Data recoding may be known as process editing, using a computer to edit the data so that they can be analyzed in the most meaningful manner.

For example, the variable "age" in our single-payer survey may be recoded from a continuous variable into a categorical one (e.g., over 65: old age, 45–64: middle age, under 45: young age) to compare people within different age groups and their attitude toward a single-payer system. In addition to collapsing categories, other forms of recode include adding together the responses to several items to form an index, and creating new variables based on combinations or mathematical transformations of existing variables (for example, creating a dummy variable by assigning one to all those with any form of insurance and zero to those without). The number of variables to be recoded is limited only by the need of data analysis and the knowledge of researchers.

Code Book

A **code book** is a document that describes the locations allocated to different variables and lists the numerical codes assigned to represent different attributes of the variables (Babbie, 1992). Its primary purpose is to assist in the coding process. Like a dictionary, a code book guides researchers to find the right code for each answer category and record the code either on a coding sheet or directly into the computer. It may also contain instructions on how to code missing values or when two answers are circled to a single-response question. Another purpose of a code book is to guide in locating variables and interpreting results in data analysis.

Table 13–4 is a **code sheet** for the single-payer survey questionnaire. The code sheet may be called a *data transfer sheet* because responses from the instrument are recorded or transferred on to the code sheet before they are entered into the computer. A code sheet is usually necessary for a questionnaire with open-ended questions for which it is impossible to precode. Reading responses from the questionnaire and checking the correct code from the code book could lead to numerous errors in data entry. Transfer sheets are used to reduce the number of errors. For a precoded questionnaire, such as our example, a code sheet is usually not necessary because data recorded on the questionnaire can be directly entered into the computer following the column location instructions.

Note the word *record* indicates the row of the responses. Since our survey example has only six questions, only one record will be needed for each respondent. Lengthier questionnaires require more records per respondent because the number of columns per record is limited.

Table 13–5 presents the code book for the single-payer survey questionnaire. The code book is required primarily for open-ended questions. If a questionnaire can be completely precoded, as with our example, then a separate code book is not necessary because the questionnaire itself can be precoded and used as a code book. Or, if a questionnaire contains predominantly close-ended questions with only one or two open-ended questions near the end, a partial code book can be prepared separately for the open-ended, postcoded questions, and data from close-ended questions can still be entered directly from the questionnaire.

TABLE 13–4 Code sheet for mini survey: Opinion toward single-payer system

	RECORD 1 **Column Location**
Q. 1. __ __	5–6/
Q. 2. __	7/
Q. 3. __	8/
Q. 4. __ __ __ __ __ __	9–14/
Q. 5.1. __	15/
Q. 5.2. __	16/
Q. 5.3. __	17/
Q. 5.4. __	18/
Q. 5.5. __	19/
Q. 6. __	20/

Note a code book usually contains the following information: questions or statements, column location, variable name, and codes. Questions or statements are exactly the same as appeared in the questionnaire, serving as a linkage between the questionnaire and the code book. Column location specifies the exact place in a data file that responses to a particular question or statement are to be placed. The process of storing information, in the computer data file, for each variable in the same column for all respondents is termed **fixed-column format.** Variable name is the abbreviated name of the question or statement and usually contains less than eight characters. To facilitate data analysis at a later stage, researchers can assign names that easily remind them of the particular questions or statements. Codes refer to the numerical assignments of the attributes of the question or statement.

While missing data are usually unavoidable in research, too many missing data reflect deficiency in the choice of the data collection method and threaten the validity of research findings. Missing data are particularly common with mail surveys where researchers have the least control. Other sources include respondents refusing to be interviewed or not answering all the questions in an interview, and participants dropping out of an experiment or program, particularly from the control group where they

❖

TABLE 13–5 Code book of mini survey: Opinion toward single-payer system

Question/Statement	Column location	Variable name	Codes
	RECORD 1		
Respondent ID	1–3	RESPID	001–200
Coder ID	4	CODERID	1—John 2—Mary 3—David
1. Your current age.	5–6	AGE	Precoded 99—Missing
2. Your sex.	7	SEX	1—male 2—female 9—missing
3. Your race.	8	RACE	1—White 2—Black 3—Asian 4—Other 8—Don't know 9—Missing
4. What was your annual income last year?	9–14	INCOME	Precoded. 888888—Don't know 999999—Missing
5. Which of the following health insurance plans do you currently have?			
5.1. Medicare	15	MEDICARE	1—Yes 0—No
5.2. Medicaid	16	MEDICAID	2—Yes 0—No
5.3. Blue Cross/ Blue Shield	17	BLUES	3—Yes 0—No
5.4. Other	18	OTHER	4—Yes 0—No
5.5. No insurance	19	NONE	5—Yes 0—No

TABLE 13–5   *continued*

Question/Statement	Column location	Variable name	Codes
6. Indicate your agreement with a single-payer health care system.	20	SINGLPAY	1—Strongly agree 2—Agree 3—Unsure 4—Disagree 5—Strongly disagree 9—Missing

derive few or no benefits. Attrition rate is likely to be higher in longitudinal than cross-sectional studies.

When nonresponses are received, researchers should devise a consistent scheme to code them so that they can be easily singled out in data analysis. Avoid leaving missing values blank because some computer programs may treat blanks as zeros or change the original format of the data file. A conventional way is to represent missing values with nines so long as nine is not a legitimate response. For example, if one of the respondents is 99 years old, it would be necessary to use three columns for the variable age in order to represent missing values (i.e., 999). Similarly, eights are used to indicate "don't know" responses and sevens are used to indicate "not applicable" responses.

DATA ENTRY

Because health services research typically uses large sets of data, computers, ranging from mainframe computers to personal microcomputers, are becoming indispensable to data analysis. The development of portable computers, or laptops, has revolutionized the data collection process. Direct data entry is no longer limited to telephone interviews. The interviewer can easily carry a laptop to the respondent's residence or workplace, read questions off the screen, and record the answers directly into the computer. In addition, computers may be used for self-administered questionnaires where respondents can be asked to sit at computer terminals and enter their own answers to the questions that appear on the screen. Data may be stored on computer disks or tapes. At least one back-up copy should be made of the data set.

There are many computer statistical software packages that data can be directly entered into. These include SAS, SPSS, SYSTAT, Minitab, Statview, Microstat, StatPro, JUMP, to name just a few. An easier alternative is to enter the data into a spreadsheet package (e.g., Excel for Apple computers or Windows, and Lotus for IBM computers or its compatibles). A more cumbersome way is to enter the data into a mainframe computer via a terminal using X-edit, for example. Direct data entry not only saves time incurred in transferring data from the questionnaire to the computer data file (a computer file that contains only raw data) but also reduces the chance for data-transferring errors. In addition, data entry in the field, either by interviewers or respondents, is less boring compared to data entry after their collection.

Indeed, data entry is often considered the least glamorous aspect of research. However, "probably at no other stage is there a greater chance of a really horrible error being made" (Davis and Smith, 1992, p. 60). Sources for error include incorrect reading of written codes, incorrect coding of responses, incorrect column location assignment, missed entry, repeated entry, and so forth. Unlike nonresponses or missing values, data entry errors are largely avoidable. Since a mail questionnaire survey still relies on data entry after collection, great efforts should be made to reduce the chances for errors. These efforts include screening personnel so that careless people are given other work or are not hired at all. Those assigned to transfer or enter the data must be trained so that they carry out their tasks correctly and simple clerical errors are reduced if not avoided. Incentives should be built into data entry to promote accurate work.

Data entered must be checked for accuracy. The process of checking for, and correcting errors related to data coding, transferring, and entering is often called **data cleaning.** One method is to reenter the data by another person or use a verifier to check for errors. When noncompatible entries are noted, the source document, the respondent's questionnaire, is consulted with and the errors are then corrected.

Another method is to visually examine the data file to see if all records have the same pattern and whether blank entries can be found. Since a fixed-column format is used, any aberration in pattern by a record indicates the presence of coding errors due to misassignment of column locations. Data from the case containing the record should be reentered to correct the errors. Blank entries also indicate errors in entry since even missing values have codes.

A further method is to use the computer to do the cleaning. Since for every variable there is a specified range of legitimate numerical codes assigned to the variable's attributes, the computer can be used to check for possible code violations. Many computer data entry or text editor packages (e.g., EPI-INFO) can be programmed to accept only legitimate codes for each variable. They check for errors automatically as the data are being entered and will beep when wrong codes are being entered. Even if one does not have such a program, a frequency distribution analysis can be easily performed to examine if the categories are legitimate for each variable. When errors are discovered, the researcher can perform a cross tabulation between the variable "respondent ID" and the variable with the coding error. This will help identify the case(s) where coding errors occur. Next, the researcher should go to the source document and correct the errors accordingly.

Finally, more complicated surveys may use a process called *consistency checking* to examine whether responses to certain questions are logically related to responses to other questions (Sonquist and Dunkelberg, 1977, p. 215). For example, coding errors are suspected if one finds a respondent who is 25 years old and has Medicare insurance. Consistency checking is usually accomplished through computer programs using a set of if–then statements (e.g., "if MEDICARE, then AGE ≥ 65").

SUMMARY

Data used for health services research may be collected either from existing sources or empirically. Existing data come from both published and nonpublished sources. Empirical data may be collected by the researcher either with a data collection instrument (e.g., questionnaire) or through observational methods. More structured data collection methods include face-to-face interviews and telephone interviews. Less structured methods include focused group studies and in-depth interviews. Each data collection method has its own strengths and weaknesses. In choosing the most appropriate method, researchers compare each method's impact on the research project (e.g., cost, time, effort, sample size, quality), respondents (e.g., nature of the sample, literacy, privacy, response rate), interviewer (e.g., interaction, visual aids, biases, training), and instrument (e.g., length, sensitive questions, checking for information, knowledge questions, uniformity, sequencing, completion rate). They then select the method(s) that optimally matches their situation. A number of measures have proven effective in improving response rate. These include intensive follow-up, sponsorship, shorter length, introductory letter, questionnaire design, inducement, maintaining anonymity, time of contact, and method of return. Once data have been collected, they need to be coded before analysis. A code book may be prepared that assists in data coding and analysis.

Key Terms

CATI	social desirability
acquiescence	auspices
prestige	mental set
coding	code book
code sheet	fixed-column format
data cleaning	

Review Questions

1. What are the methods of data collection used in health services research? Describe their characteristics.

2. What do researchers take into account in selecting a data collection method?

3. Compare the strengths and weaknesses of mail questionnaire surveys and personal and telephone interviews. What situations are most suitable for each of these methods?

4. What measures can be used to improve both the quantity and quality of responses?

5. Find an existing questionnaire either constructed by yourself or others. Design a code book for that questionnaire.

6. What are the components in data processing?

REFERENCES

Armstrong, J. S. (1975). Monetary incentives in mail surveys. *Public Opinion Quarterly,* 39, 111-116.

Babbie, E. R. (1973). *Survey Research Methods.* Belmont, CA: Wadsworth Publishing Co.

Babbie, E. (1992). *The Practice of Social Research.* Belmont, CA: Wadsworth Publishing Co.

Bailey, K. D. (1994). *Methods of Social Research.* New York: The Free Press.

Berdie, D. R. (1973). Questionnaire length and response rate. *Journal of Applied Psychology,* 58, 278-280.

Center for Mental Health Services and National Institute of Mental Health. (1992). *Mental Health, United States, 1992.* Washington, DC: Government Printing Office.

Centers for Disease Control and Prevention. (1994). *Morbidity and Mortality Weekly Report.* Washington, DC: Government Printing Office.

Davis, J. A., and Smith, T. W. (1992). *The NORC General Social Survey: A User's Guide.* Newbury Park, CA: Sage.

Groves, R. M. (1980). Telephone helps solve survey problems. *Newsletter of the Institute of Social Research* (University of Michigan), 6(1), 3.

Groves, R. M., and Kahn, R. L. (1979). *Surveys by Telephone: A National Comparison with Personal Interviews.* New York: Academic Press.

Herberlein, T. A., and Baumgartner, R. (1978). Factors affecting response rate to mailed questionnaires. *American Sociological Review,* 43, 451.

Lavrakas, P. J. (1987). *Telephone Survey Methods: Sampling, Selection, and Supervision.* Newbury Park, CA: Sage.

Miller, D. C. (1991). *Handbook of Research Design and Social Measurement.* Newbury Park, CA: Sage.

National Center for Health Statistics. (1994a). *Catalog of Publications 1993.* Hyattsville, MD: Public Health Service.

National Center for Health Statistics. (1994b). *Health, United States.* (since 1975, annual). Hyattsville, MD: Public Health Service.

National Center for Health Statistics. (1994c). *Vital Statistics of the United States, Vol. I, Natality; Vol. II, Mortality; Vol. III, Marriage and Divorce.* Washington, DC: Government Printing Office.

Patton, M. Q. (1990). *Qualitative Evaluation and Research Methods.* Newbury Park, CA: Sage.

Powdermaker, H. (1966). *Stranger and Friend.* New York, NY: Norton.

Shi, L., Samuels, M. E., and Glover, S. (1994). *Educational Preparation and Attributes of Community and Migrant Health Center Administrators.* Columbia, SC: University of South Carolina.

Sonquist, J. A., and Dunkelberg, W. C. (1977). *Survey and Opinion Research: Procedures for Processing and Analysis.* Englewood Cliffs, NJ: Prentice-Hall.

U.S. Bureau of the Census. (1994). *Statistical Abstract of the United States.* (since 1878, annual). Washington, DC: Government Printing Office.

Wallace, D. (1954). A case for—and against—mail questionnaires. *Public Opinion Quarterly,* 18, 40-52.

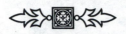

CHAPTER

14

Statistical Analysis in Health Services Research

LEARNING OBJECTIVES

- To explore and prepare data for analysis.
- To become aware of the common statistical methods used in research analysis.
- To identify appropriate statistical methods for the analysis of nominal-, ordinal-, and interval-ratio-level data.

Although data analysis follows data collection, planning for analysis comes before data collection. Analysis decisions are related to the research question or hypothesis, level of measurement, sampling method and size, and computer programs used. If there are more than one research questions or hypotheses, several statistical procedures may be performed. If the relationship between two variables is explored, some statistical measure of association is needed. If the differences between two groups are examined, the significance of the difference between the groups would be tested. If the impact of certain predictors on dependent variables is assessed, a multivariate measure is usually appropriate.

The choice of statistics is also determined by the level of measurement of the variables used. Different statistics exist for nominal, ordinal, and interval-ratio measures. Sampling consideration is important because many statistics are founded on the randomized, probability sampling method. Indeed, inferential statistics, which deals with the kinds of inferences that can be made when generalizing from sample data to the entire population, are based on samples being randomly selected. Sample size influences analysis because the more the variables that are to be analyzed simultaneously, the larger the sample size would be required.

One way that facilitates making analysis decisions well before data collection is to construct dummy statistical tables, which represent the actual tables to be used for analysis when data are collected and frequencies or values are inserted within them (Miller, 1991). These dummy statistical tables become the statistical plan. By setting them in advance, researchers can make a careful appraisal of the relevant statistics to be used, design the most appropriate research instrument, and select sampling and data collection methods pertinent to the analysis to be undertaken. Constructing dummy statistical tables means data analysis is projected in advance for appraisal and evaluation. Improvement of the study design can be made with minimum waste of time and money, and risks of failure are also reduced.

Data analysis can seldom be performed without computer software. Among the more commonly used statistical computer software packages by health services researchers include SAS (Statistical Analysis System), SPSS (Statistical Package for the Social Sciences), BMD (biomedical computer programs), and LISREL (Analysis of Linear Structural Relationships by the Method of Maximum Likelihood). These programs generally have both mainframe and PC (personal computer), versions, and technical support is usually available from both the manufacturers and researchers' institutional computer centers.

This chapter describes the process of conducting data analysis and illustrates the most commonly used statistical measures. Specifically, this process involves data exploration, **univariate analysis, bivariate analysis,** and **multivariate analysis** (Singleton, Straits, and Straits, 1993). Statistical measures can be based on one or more variables. Univariate analyses examine the characteristics of one variable at a time. Univariate analyses often produce descriptive statistics. Bivariate analyses examine the relationship between two variables at a time. Multivariate analyses examine the relationship among three or more variables at a time. Throughout the chapter, the emphasis is placed on choosing the appropriate methods based on the nature of the variables and the level of measurement. The chapter is not a substitute for statistics textbooks. Readers who want in-depth description and illustration of statistics described in this chapter are encouraged to consult current biostatistics and econometrics textbooks.

DATA EXPLORATION

After the collected data have been entered into the computer and the process editing completed, researchers often spend a considerable amount of time exploring the data before launching a formal analysis. One of the purposes of data exploration is to make sure all data elements are included in one data file. If a research project uses several data sources, the separate data files have to be combined and merged. The files can be merged based on shared variables but different cases, or similar cases but different variables. Data can also be sorted in a different order based on the value of one or more variables. On the other hand, if the data file is too large for the research purpose, a subset of cases may be selected to restrict the analysis to that subset. The unit of analysis can also be altered by grouping cases together.

Another purpose of examining data carefully before analysis is to prepare it for hypothesis testing and model building. Researchers may display the data in tabular (e.g., frequency table) or graphic (e.g., scatterplots, histograms, stem-and-leaf plots, box plots) forms. Inspecting the distribution of values is important for evaluating the appropriateness of the statistical techniques to be used for hypothesis testing or model building. Since normal distribution is important to statistical inference, a normal probability plot may be used to pair each observed value with its expected value from a normal distribution. If the sample is drawn from a normal distribution, the points will fall more or less on a straight line. In such a case, a simple linear regression model may be needed. If the distribution does not appear to be normally distributed, data transformation might be necessary, or some nonparametric techniques can be used. If the plot resembles a mathematical function, that function may be used to fit the data. For example, when the data do not cluster around a straight line, the researcher can take the log of the independent variables. If this does not coax the data to linearity, a more complicated model of data transformation may have to be used. Some commonly used transformations include cube (3), square (2), square root (½), natural logarithm (0), reciprocal of the square root (−½), and reciprocal (−1).

UNIVARIATE ANALYSIS

Univariate analysis, which examines one variable at a time, may be conducted as part of data exploration, as a major component of descriptive analysis, or as a prelude to bivariate and multivariate analysis. As part of data exploration, univariate analysis is performed to help assess whether assumptions of statistical tests have been met, for example, whether the data are normally distributed. Very large standard deviations often imply outliers, that is, extreme values that may disproportionally affect the statistics (Grady and Wallston, 1988, p. 152). Examination of variable distribution may reflect departures from normality and require transformation of variables. Lack of variation in responses makes it more difficult to determine how differences in one variable are related to differences in another variable. Univariate analysis also helps decide collapsing categories of a variable.

When information on a group of individuals or other units has been systematically gathered, it needs to be organized and summarized in an intelligible way. As a major component of descriptive analysis, univariate analysis helps describe a sample in terms of the variables measured so that a profile of the sample can be delineated. Research often goes beyond descriptive analysis, and univariate analysis serves as a prelude to more complex analysis by providing readers a complete picture of the bases of the conclusions.

Commonly used univariate statistics include frequency and percentage distributions, measures of central tendency (e.g., mean, median, and mode), variability or dispersion (e.g., range, standard deviation, variance), shape (e.g., frequency or percentage polygon, skewness, kurtosis, leptokurtic, platykurtic), and standard scores (z score, rate, ratio). The choice of these statistics typically depends on the level of measurement of the variables (see Table 14–1).

TABLE 14–1   Level of measurement and statistics for analyzing one variable a time

Level of Measurement	Statistics				
	Distributions	*Averages*	*Dispersion*	*Shape*	*Standardized Scores*
Nominal	Frequency Percentage	Mode			Ratio Rate
Ordinal	Frequency Percentage	Mode Median	Range Maximum Minimum		Ratio Rate
Interval-Ratio		Mode Median Mean	Range Maximum Minimum Variance Standard Deviation	Skewness Kurtosis	z Score

Distributions

A **distribution** organizes the values of a variable into categories. A frequency distribution, also known as a marginal distribution, shows the number of cases that fall into each category. Data measured at the nominal- or ordinal-level can be organized in terms of the categories of responses given. Interval-ratio-level data usually have to be grouped into a distribution in terms of categories that are convenient and substantively meaningful.

Another way of summarizing a variable is to report its percentage distribution, obtained by dividing the number or frequency of cases in the category by the total N, or corrected total if missing data are to be excluded, and then multiplying by 100 to convert to a percent. Thus frequency distribution can easily be converted into percentage distribution. The advantage of percentage distribution is to facilitate comparisons across distributions based on different sample sizes since all numbers are converted to a base 100. The distribution of a variable can also be shown graphically to highlight certain aspects of a distribution. Examples are bar charts, histograms, polygons, and pie charts.

Table 14–2 displays a frequency and percentage distribution of the insurance status of emergency room patients in a large urban county teaching hospital. When tables are used, it is necessary to present the data clearly so that readers can easily understand it. Each table should stand by itself. It ought to be possible for the reader to understand a table without referring to the text that surrounds it. Each table should have a unique and detailed title describing what the variables are and what the cell entries are. Columns and rows should be clearly labeled. A table should also show the relevant sample size. If a percentage table is used, marginals are typically reported as well. Marginals refer to the frequency counts and percentages for the row and column variables taken separately. Foot-

TABLE 14–2 Frequency and percentage distribution of emergency room patients' insurance status

Insurance	Frequency	Percentage
Medicaid	16,130	29.4%
Medicare	4,660	8.5%
Private	16,882	30.8%
No Insurance	17,161	31.3%
TOTAL	54,833	100.0%

notes may be used to indicate sources, explain symbols and missing values, or summarize procedures used.

Measures of Central Tendency

Measures of central tendency summarize information about the average value of a variable, some typical value around which all the values cluster. The three commonly used measures are **mode, median,** and **mean.** The mode is the value (or category) of a distribution that occurs most frequently. Although the mode can be reported for any level of measurement, it is most often used for nominal-level data. For grouped data, the mode may be affected by the way in which values are grouped into categories. Therefore, it is necessary to verify that the categories are of the same width, or else adjustments have to be made.

The median is the middle position, or midpoint, of a distribution. It is computed by first ordering the values of a distribution and then dividing the distribution in half, that is, half the cases fall below the median and the other half are above it. In general, researchers may find the observation that has the median value for an ordered distribution simply by computing $(N + 1)/2$.

The median is used for both ordinal and interval-ratio levels of measurement. It is a meaningless statistic for nominal data. Since the median is a stable measure of central tendency and is not affected by extreme values, it is typically used when the distribution is skewed, that is, when there are extreme values in one of its ends (e.g., income data).

The most commonly used measure of central tendency is the mean, the arithmetic average computed by adding up all the values and dividing by the total number of cases. Where X_i equal the "raw" or observed values of a variable and N equal total number of cases or observations, then mean is calculated with the following formula:

$$\frac{\sum x_i,}{N} \quad \text{or} \quad \frac{(x_1 + x_2 + x_3 + \ldots + x_N)}{N} \tag{14.1}$$

Mean is only used for the interval-ratio level of measurement. It is the preferred measure of central tendency because it has important arithmetic and other properties useful in inferential statistics. It is also a good summary measure because its computation utilizes every value of a distribution. However, extreme values do affect the mean. Therefore, for skewed distributions, it is best to report both the mean and the median to avoid misleading interpretations.

Measures of Variability

While measures of central tendency identify a single, most representative value of the distribution, **measures of variability** or **dispersion** refer to the spread or variation of the distribution. A simple measure of variability or dispersion is the **range,** the difference between the highest (maximum) and lowest (minimum) values in a distribution. Range can be used for both ordinal and interval-ratio levels of measurement. Since range only takes into account those minimum and maximum values in a distribution, it does not reflect the rest of the distribution.

Other distance-based measures of dispersion have been developed that are more informative about the middle of a distribution. One such measure is the interquartile range, which is the range of values in the middle half (50 percent) of a distribution. Such a measure is more sensitive to the way values are concentrated around the midpoint of the distribution, but it still only provides the difference between two values of the distribution and tells little about the aggregate dispersion of a distribution.

A more informative characterization of dispersion is the extent to which each of the values of a distribution differs from the mean. The **variance** is such a measure and is defined as the average squared deviation from the mean.

$$\text{variance} = S^2 = \frac{\sum (x_i - \text{mean})^2}{N - 1} \tag{14.2}$$

However, variance does not have a direct interpretation for descriptive purposes. A more intuitive measure of variability is the **standard deviation,** defined as the square root of the variance. The standard deviation is expressed in the original unit of measurement of the distribution. Both the variance and standard deviation can be used only for the interval-ratio level of measurement.

Measures of Shape

When a distribution of observations is not symmetric, that is, when more observations are found at one end of the distribution than the other, such a distribution is called **skewed.** If the tail is skewed toward larger values, the distribution is positively skewed, or skewed to the right. Conversely, if the tail is skewed toward smaller values, the distribution is negatively skewed, or skewed to the left. *Kurtosis* refers to the extent cases or observations cluster around a central point. When cases cluster around the central point more than in a normal distribution, the distribution is called *leptokurtic*. When cases cluster around the central point less than in a normal distribution, the distribution is called *platykurtic.*

Statistics measuring skewness and kurtosis are generally automatically generated by computer statistical software in univariate analysis. If the observed distribution is normal, skewness and kurtosis measures will fluctuate around zero. A researcher may get some sense of possible skewness and kurtosis by examining a histogram. Both skewness and kurtosis measures can only be validly used in interval-ratio level of measurement.

Standard Scores

Standard scores describe the relative position of an observation within a distribution. One standard score, the z score, uses both the mean and standard deviation to indicate the number of standard deviations above or below the mean an observation falls. A positive z score indicates that a particular score is above the mean, whereas a negative z score indicates that a particular score is below the mean. The distribution of z scores has two important properties: the mean of z scores is always zero, and the standard deviation is always one. The z score is calculated by obtaining the difference between the value of a particular case x_i and the mean of the distribution, and dividing this difference by the standard deviation.

$$z_i = \frac{(x_i - \text{mean})}{SD} \tag{14.3}$$

Suppose a student wants to see how the performance in two exams (90 in the first and 80 in the second) compared with that of the class. The distribution of the first exam scores had a mean of 75 and standard deviation of five. The second exam scores had a distribution with a mean of 60 and standard deviation of four. (Note that the second exam was harder, and there was less variation around the mean than for the first exam). The z scores for the two exams are 3 [(90 − 75)/5] and 5 [(80 − 60)/4] respectively, indicating that the person performed better in the second exam than the first one relative to the average score and variation in each of the class distributions. In other words, 90 is equivalent to three standard deviation units higher than the mean, but 80 is equivalent to five standard deviation units higher than the mean. The z score is used only with interval-ratio level of measurement.

In addition to the z score, ratios and rates may be used to standardize and make meaningful comparisons across different numbers. Computing ratios and rates are called *norming* or *standardizing operations*. Both involve dividing one number (or a set of numbers) by another. A **ratio** is simply one number divided by another: the frequency of observations in one category is divided by the frequency in another category of a distribution. A **rate** is similar to a percentage since it is computed by dividing the number of cases or events in a given category by the total number of observations. The resulting proportion is then expressed as any multiple of 10 that clears the decimal, usually 100 or 1,000. The formula is:

$$\text{rate} = \frac{\text{number of events during a time period}}{\text{total } N \text{ (or number of possible events)}} \times 100 \text{ (or 1,000)} \tag{14.4}$$

For example, natality or birth rate is usually expressed as the number of births in a population per 1,000: if there are 10,000 births during a year, and the population at the middle of the year is 500,000, the crude birth rate is 50 births per 1,000 (10,000 ÷ 500,000 × 1,000).

A rate of change is useful in comparing the distribution of a variable through time, say before (Time 1) and after (Time 2) an intervention program. A positive result indicates rate of gain whereas a negative result indicates rate of loss. The result can be multiplied by 100 to remove the decimal and reflect percentage change. The formula is:

$$\text{rate of change} = \frac{\text{value at Time 2} - \text{value at Time 1}}{\text{value at Time 1}} \qquad (14.5)$$

BIVARIATE ANALYSIS

Bivariate analysis that examines two variables at a time may be conducted to determine whether there exists a relationship between two variables (i.e., association), and if a relationship exists, how much influence one variable has on the other (i.e., magnitude). Bivariate analysis is commonly used in subgroup comparisons and as a preparation for multivariate analysis. In subgroup comparisons the researcher can choose any stratification variable and describes each subgroup of that variable in terms of any other variable. The examination of the relationship between pairs of variables helps select appropriate variables in multivariate analysis.

The bivariate measure of association is a correlation usually ranging from −1 to +1 and assesses the strength and direction of the relation between two variables. A negative sign means that higher values of one variable are associated with lower values of another, and vice versa. When the statistic is close to zero, the variables are considered to be uncorrelated. Statistical tables are used to assess the probability that a correlation is significantly different from zero. The closer the number is to one (perfect correlation), the greater the magnitude of correlation or association.

Commonly used bivariate procedures include cross-tabulation, **Chi-square** (χ^2), phi coefficient (ϕ), coefficient of contingency (C), Cramér's V, Goodman-Kruskal's lambda (λ), relative risk ratio, Kendall's tau (τ), Goodman-Kruskal's gamma (γ), ANOVA, Pearson correlation coefficient (r), and paired t test. The choice of these statistics depends on the level of measurement of the variables (see Table 14–3 for these and other statistics that may be used for bivariate analysis).

Cross-tabulation

The first step in determining the existence of a relationship between two variables is to cross-tabulate them, or to examine their joint distribution. In general, we study the influence of an independent variable on a dependent variable, or how the distribution of the dependent variable varies within the categories of the independent variable. The

TABLE 14–3 Level of measurement and statistics for analyzing two variables a time

Level of Measurement	*Statistics*		
	Nominal	*Ordinal*	*Interval-Ratio*

Nominal	Cross-tabulation
	Chi-square (χ^2)
	Phi coefficient (ϕ)
	Coefficient of
	  contingency (C)
	Cramér's V
	Goodman-Kruskal's
	  lambda (λ)
	Relative risk ratio
	Fisher's exact test		

Ordinal	Cross-tabulation
	Chi-square (χ^2)
	Goodman-Kruskal's
	  lambda (λ)
	Kruskal-Wallis test
	Median test
	Sign test
	Wilcoxon signed-rank test
	Somers' d
	Kolmogorov-Smirnov
	  two sample test
	Runs test
		Cross-tabulation
		Chi-square (χ^2)
		Goodman-Kruskal's
		  gamma (γ)
		Kendall's tau (τ)
		Spearman's coefficient
		  of rank order
		  correlation (r)
		
		Somers' d	

Interval-Ratio	Paired t test
	ANOVA
	F test
	Multiple comparison
	  procedures (Bonferroni
	  test, Duncan's multiple
	  range test, Tukey's b,
	  Scheffé test)
		Simple regression	Pearson correlation
			  coefficient (r)
			Simple regression
			F test

contingency table where cross-tabulation is presented is set up so that the categories of the independent variable are in the columns (i.e., across the top of the table) and the categories of the dependent variable are in the rows of the table. Three different percentages can be computed for each cell, each conveying a different meaning. Specifically, the

◙

TABLE 14-4 Hospital setting and patient sex

Hospital Setting	Sex		
	Male	Female	Total
Emergency Room	25,427 (46.37%)	29,406 (53.63%)	54,833
Inpatient	10,383 (41.77%)	14,475 (58.23%)	24,858
Outpatient	26,518 (33.86%)	51,808 (66.14%)	78,326
Clinics	19,060 (26.14%)	3,850 (73.86%)	72,910
Dental	2,523 (36.63%)	4,365 (63.37%)	6,888
TOTAL	83,911 (35.28%)	153,904 (64.72%)	237,815

column percent divides the cell entry by the total for its column. The row percent divides the cell entry by the total for its row. The total percent divides the cell entry by the total in the sample. Table 14–4 is a contingency table about hospital setting and patient sex. The row percent is displayed.

Chi-Square Test for Independence

For cross-tabulation, chi-square (χ^2) is a very common test for independence. It is based on a comparison between an observed frequency table with an expected frequency table, or the table one would expect to find if the two variables were statistically independent, that is, unrelated to one another. An expected frequency table is computed from the marginal frequency totals only and represents a frequency table showing no relationship between the variables. Table 14–5a shows the expected cell frequencies (derived from Table 14–4), assuming no relationship between sex and hospital setting, and Table 14–5b shows the derived bivariate percentage distribution with cell percentages the same as the marginals. The chi-square statistic may be calculated using the following formula:

$$\chi^2 = \sum \frac{(O_{ij} - E_{ij})^2}{E_{ij}}$$

$$= \frac{(25427 - 19347)^2}{19347} + \frac{(10383 - 8771)^2}{8771} + \ldots + \frac{(4365 - 6888)^2}{6888} \tag{14.6}$$

$$= 45011$$

The calculated chi-square value is compared against the critical points of the theoretical chi-square distribution corresponding to the preestablished level of significance and de-

TABLE 14–5 Hospital setting and patient sex

Hospital Setting	a. Frequencies			b. Percentages		
	Sex			Sex		
	Male	Female	Total	Male	Female	Total
Emergency Room	19,347	35,486	54,833	23%	23%	23%
Inpatient	8,771	16,087	24,858	11%	11%	11%
Outpatient	27,637	50,689	78,326	33%	33%	33%
Clinics	25,726	47,184	72,910	30%	30%	30%
Dental	2,430	4,458	6,888	3%	3%	3%
TOTAL	83,911	153,904	237,815	100%	100%	100%
				(83,911)	(153,904)	(237,815)

grees of freedom. The degrees of freedom are $(r - 1)(c - 1)$ where r is the number of rows and c the number of columns. In this example, the degrees of freedom are $(5 - 1)(2 - 1)$ or 4 and the p value (i.e., significance level) is less than .001, indicating that sex and hospital setting are not independent. This should be obvious from the observed frequencies. For example, while males and females are relatively similar in emergency room visits (46.37% vs. 53.63%), there is a much large difference in clinic visits (26.14% vs. 73.86%).

However, chi-square is a test of independence and provides little information about the strength of the association. Chi-square statistics also depend on sample size and will increase as the sample size becomes larger. Conversely, when the expected cell frequencies are very small, the chi-square test statistic is not distributed exactly as the chi-square distribution. Thus, the rule of thumb is not to use the chi-square test for independence when the expected frequency (f_e) of the smallest cell is five or less.

Chi-Square-Based Measures of Association

Once the researcher has found a significant relationship, the next step is to examine the nature and magnitude of such a relationship. Measures of association refer to statistics that quantify the relationship between variables in cross-tabulation and indicate the magnitude or strength of that relationship. For nominal-level variables, several **chi-square-based measures** can be used to assess the extent of the relationship. These measures modify the chi-square statistics to reduce the influence of sample size and degrees of freedom and restrict the values between zero and one.

The phi coefficient (ϕ) divides chi-square by the sample size and takes the square root of the result:

$$\phi = \sqrt{\chi^2 / N} \tag{14.7}$$

In our example, the phi coefficient is 0.44 (or $\sqrt{45011/237815}$). When the chi-square value is greater than the sample size, the phi coefficient lies beyond zero and one.

Pearson's coefficient of contingency (C) and Cramér's V are always between zero and one:

$$C = \sqrt{\chi^2/(\chi^2 + N)} \tag{14.8}$$

$$V = \sqrt{\chi^2/[N(k - 1)]} \tag{14.9}$$

In our example, C and V are respectively 0.40 [or $\sqrt{45011/(45011 + 237815)}$] and 0.25 [or $\sqrt{45011/(237815 \times 3)}$]. Although chi-square-based measures of association can be used to compare magnitude or strength of association across different contingency tables, they are difficult to interpret due to the nominal nature of the variables.

PRE-Based Measures of Association

PRE, or **proportional reduction in error,** is a broad framework that helps organize a large number of measures for nominal-, ordinal-, and even interval-ratio-level data. PRE-based measures are typically ratios of a measure of error in predicting the values of one variable based on that variable alone and the same measure of error based on knowledge of an additional variable (Goodman and Kruskal, 1954). The logic behind this framework is that if prior knowledge about another variable improves the knowledge of this variable, then these two variables are related. PRE may be summarized below:

$$PRE = \frac{\text{error using dependent variable only} - \text{error using independent variable}}{\text{error using dependent variable only}} \tag{14.10}$$

For example Table 14–6 presents the one-day frequency distribution of patient race and their insurance status. If we only use the distribution about insurance, we would predict private insurance (the mode) and be correct 52.5 percent of the time (105/200) and wrong 47.5 percent of the time [(55 + 40)/200].

However, if we also use the distribution of insurance within each racial category, we would predict Medicare/Medicaid when the sampled individual was black and be correct in 35 of 70 guesses (i.e., 35 errors). We would predict private insurance when the sampled individual was white and be right in 90 of 110 guesses (i.e., 20 errors). We would predict Medicare/Medicaid when the sampled individual was Hispanic and be right in 10 of 20 guesses (i.e., 10 errors). When we do not know the person's race, we make 95 errors in 200 guesses. When we do know the person's race, we make only 65 errors in 200 guesses. That our predictions improve when we know ethnicity over the predictions we make when we do not indicates that race and insurance status are related. Applying the PRE formula, our predictions may be computed as follows:

TABLE 14–6 Patient race and insurance status

INSURANCE	RACE			
	White	Black	Hispanic	Total
Medicare/Medicaid	10	35	10	55
Private	90	10	5	105
No Insurance	10	25	5	40
Total	110	70	20	200

$$PRE = \frac{95 - (35 + 20 + 10)}{95} = .32$$

Goodman and Kruskal's lambda (λ) is a measure of association for nominal-level data based on PRE method. The computing formula for lambda is:

$$\lambda = \frac{\text{Sum of modal frequency for each category of } x - \text{modal frequency of } y}{N - \text{modal frequency of } y} \quad (14.11)$$

where x is the independent variable, y is the dependent variable, and N is the sample size. Applying this formula to the data in Table 14–6, we can calculate lambda as:

$$\lambda = \frac{(90 + 35 + 10) - 105}{200 - 105} = \frac{135 - 105}{95} = \frac{30}{95} = .32$$

This is the same as the proportional reduction in our guessing errors. Lambda ranges between zero and one. A value close to one indicates the independent variable closely specifies the categories of the dependent variable. When the two variables are independent, lambda is close to zero.

For measures of association for ordinal-level data based on PRE method, we may use either Goodman-Kruskal's gamma (γ) or Kendall's tau (τ). For ordinal-level data, we can make our predictions not only based on the mode of a distribution, but also the rank-ordering of the categories. The computation of gamma is as follows:

$$\text{gamma} = \frac{s - d}{s + d} \quad (14.12)$$

where s is the number of same-ordered pairs, d is the number of different-ordered pairs. To compute gamma, the table must be consistently ordered: both the column and row must be ordered either from low to high or from high to low. To find s, or the number of same-ordered pairs, we start with the upper left-hand cell and multiply the cell frequency by the sum of the frequencies of all the cells that are both to the right and below the reference cell. This procedure is repeated for each cell until all the cells to the right and below that cell have been included. We then sum up all those pairs to obtain s. To find d, or the number of different-ordered pairs, we start with the lower left-hand cell and multiply the cell frequency by the sum of the frequencies that are both to the right and above the reference cell. This procedure is repeated for each cell until all the cells to the right and above that cell have been included. We then sum up all those pairs to obtain d.

For example, Table 14–7 presents the distribution of patient education and income level. The values s and d may be obtained by summing up all same-ordered or different-ordered pairs, respectively:

$$60(30 + 10 + 10 + 45) = 5700 \qquad 5(15 + 5 + 30 + 10) = 300$$
$$15(10 + 45) = 825 \qquad 10(5 + 10) = 150$$
$$20(10 + 45) = 1100 \qquad 20(15 + 5) = 400$$
$$30(45) = 1350 \qquad 30(5) = 150$$
$$s = 8975 \qquad d = 1000$$

Gamma may then be calculated as:

$$\text{gamma} = \frac{8975 - 1000}{8975 + 1000} = .80$$

This means there is a 80 percent reduction in error if we predict ranking on income based on ranking on education, as opposed to predicting randomly.

TABLE 14–7 Patient education and income level

INCOME	EDUCATION			
	Elementary	Secondary	College	Total
Low	60	15	5	80
Medium	20	30	10	60
High	5	10	45	60
Total	85	55	60	200

Since gamma ignores all the tied pairs, it tends to overestimate the strength of association. Kendall's tau (τ) does take into account tied pairs and is:

$$\tau = \frac{s - d}{\sqrt{(s + d + t_x)(s + d + t_y)}} \tag{14.13}$$

where s = number of same-ordered pairs, d = number of different-ordered pairs, t_x = number of pairs tied on the independent variable, and t_y = number of pairs tied on the dependent variable. To compute t_x and when the categories of the independent variable are in the columns, we look for cells that are in the same column and below the referent cell. To compute t_y and when the categories of the dependent variable are in the rows, we look for cells that are in the same row and to the right of the referent cell. Using the same example in Table 14–7, t_x may be calculated as: $60(20 + 5) + 15(30 + 10) + 5(10 + 45) + 20(5) + 30(10) + 10(45) = 1500 + 600 + 275 + 100 + 300 + 450 = 3225$. t_y may be calculated as: $60(15 + 5) + 20(30 + 10) + 5(10 + 45) + 15(5) + 30(10) + 10(45) = 1200 + 800 + 275 + 75 + 300 + 450 = 3100$. Kendall's tau ($\tau$) may then be calculated as:

$$\tau = \frac{8975 - 1000}{\sqrt{(8975 + 1000 + 3225)(8975 + 1000 + 3100)}} = .61$$

By adjusting for tied pairs, the measure of association is reduced from .80 to .61.

Another ordinal measure of association is **Spearman's coefficient** of rank correlation (r_s). To compute r_s, the two variables are rank-ordered, with each person having two ranks, one on each variable. The values of the two variables are ranked from the smallest to the largest for all cases. The difference between the pairs of ranks for each person is denoted by d. For example, if a person ranks first on one variable and fifth on another, the d score would be 4 (5 − 1). The values of r_s range from 1 (when $\sum d_i^2 = 0$ or all pairs of ranks are identical) to −1 (when no pairs of ranks are identical). The formula for r_s is:

$$r_s = 1 - \frac{6 \sum d_i^2}{N(N^2 - 1)} \tag{14.14}$$

When data are collected with interval-ratio-level measurement, researchers have the choice to convert interval-level data to ordinal and categorical variables and then use measures of association appropriate to these levels. For example, income, if obtained as a dollar amount, can be converted into ordinal- (e.g., < \$10,000, \$10,000–\$20,000, etc.) or nominal- (e.g., above poverty line vs. below poverty line) level measure, depending on the purpose of the research.

Alternatively, researchers may use measures appropriate only for interval-ratio measures. A commonly used measure of association is the **Pearson product–moment cor-**

relation coefficient (r). As with most other measures, r ranges from 1 (perfect positive relationship) to -1 (perfect negative relationship). Zero indicates no relationship or independence between the two variables. The computation formula for r is:

$$r = \frac{N\sum xy - (\sum x)(\sum y)}{[N\sum x^2 - (\sum x)^2][N\sum y^2 - (\sum y)^2]} \tag{14.15}$$

The correlation coefficient may be tested for statistical significance based on sample size. In general, a correlation coefficient may be interpreted as follows (Miller, 1991; Herman, Morris, and Fitz-Gibbon, 1987):

.00–.20: little or no positive correlation
.20–.40: some slight positive correlation
.40–.60: substantial positive correlation
.60–.80: strong positive correlation
.80–1.00: very strong positive correlation
−.80– −1.00: very strong negative correlation
−.60– −.80: strong negative correlation
−.40– −.60: substantial negative correlation
−.20– −.40: some slight negative correlation
.00– −.20: little or no negative correlation

However, statistical significance does not mean substantive importance. Suppose that we find that two groups are significantly different at the .05 level. Our finding only means that there is a 5 percent chance that we would make a mistake in concluding that the two groups are not exactly equal, that is, the difference is zero. Thus, two groups can be significantly different in a statistical sense, even though the difference between them is very close to zero.

From a practical sense, statistical significance tests are highly sensitive to sample size. With a large enough sample size, even a trivial difference will likely be statistically significant. Thus, statistical significance only expresses the degree of confidence in the conclusion. Being confident that there is a difference does not imply that the difference is either large or important. Substantive and theoretical considerations must be involved when decisions are based on statistical tests, particularly in applied health services research.

Other Bivariate Measures

Other commonly used measures of association include **relative risk ratio** or **odds ratio,** testing hypotheses about differences in sample means or proportions, and **simple regression** procedure.

Relative Risk Ratio

The relative risk ratio can be used for two nominal-level measures. Specifically, it measures the strength of association between the presence of a factor (x) and the occurrence of an event (y). For example, data have been collected on lung cancer (y) between those who smoke and those who don't (x). A two-by-two table may be created as Table 14–8. The relative risk ratio is the ratio of the incidence of disease (i.e., lung cancer) among the exposed (i.e., those who smoke) to the incidence of disease among the unexposed (i.e., those who don't smoke):

$$\text{relative risk} = \frac{\text{Incidence rate of disease in exposed group}}{\text{Incidence rate of disease in nonexposed group}} = \frac{ad}{bc} \tag{14.16}$$

Although incidence rates are not determined in a retrospective study, the relative risk can be estimated by the cross product of the entries in a two-by-two table. However, two assumptions are necessary to make such an estimate: (a) the frequency of the disease in the population must be small and (b) the study cases should be representative of the cases in the population and the controls representative of the noncases in the population (Lilienfeld and Lilienfeld, 1980). The relative risk ratio for our example is 2.11. If the 95 percent confidence interval does not include one, then this ratio is significant. For retrospective or case-control studies, the term *odds ratio* is often used in lieu of relative risk. Odds ratio may be defined as the ratio of two odds, that is, the ratio of the probability of occurrence of an event to that of nonoccurrence (Last, 1983).

Measures of Differences

When there is a single independent variable with only two categories (i.e., nominal level, e.g., sex) and a single continuous dependent variable (i.e., interval-ratio, e.g., income), *t test* may be used. The *t* value may be calculated as follows:

$$t = \frac{x_1 - x_2}{\sqrt{(S_1^2/N_1) + (S_2^2/N_2)}} \tag{14.17}$$

TABLE 14–8 Smoking and lung cancer

Lung Cancer	*Smoking*		
	Yes	No	Total
Yes	100 (*a*)	900 (*b*)	1000
No	50 (*c*)	950 (*d*)	1000
Total	150	1850	2000

where x_1 is the mean of one category, x_2 is the mean of another category, S_1^2, S_2^2 are the variances, and N_1, N_2 are the sample sizes for the two categories respectively. The t value can be checked for its observed significance level from a statistics table (e.g., critical values for a student's t). If the observed p level is sufficiently small (e.g., less than .05, or .01), we can then reject the hypothesis that the means of the two categories are equal.

When there are more than two categories within a single nominal variable (e.g., race), the analysis of variance (ANOVA) method is used to test the differences among these categories in terms of the continuous dependent variable. The null hypothesis in ANOVA states that the means for the different categories or groups are equal in the population ($\mu_A = \mu_B = \mu_C$). The test statistic is the F ratio, which compares the variations in the scores due to different sources: variation between categories or groups (or treatment variation) and variation within categories or groups (or error variation). The variation between groups reflects the treatment and random error; the variation within groups reflects random error only. Thus, the F ratio can be conceptualized as follows:

$$F = \frac{\text{Treatment} + \text{Error}}{\text{Error}} = \frac{\text{Mean square between groups}}{\text{Mean square within groups}} \qquad (14.18)$$

The larger the F ratio, the more likely there is a true difference in means among various categories or groups. However, a significant F value only indicates that the means are not all equal. It does not identify which pairs of categories or groups appear to have different means. A post hoc or multiple comparison procedures can be used to test which means are significantly different from one another. Examples of multiple comparison procedures include the Bonferroni test, Duncan's multiple range test, Tukey's b, and the Scheffé test (Norusis, 1994).

A test for significant difference between two proportions can be performed with the same logic as a test for significant difference between means. The computation formula is as follows:

$$z = \frac{p_1 - p_2}{\sqrt{(p_1 q_1 / n_1) + (p_2 q_2 / n_2)}} \qquad (14.19)$$

where p_1 is the proportion of one group (e.g., male) with a particular characteristic (e.g., those who smoke), p_2 is the proportion of another group (e.g., female) with the same characteristic, $q = 1 - p$, and n is the sample size. If the z statistic is significantly large, then we reject the hypothesis that the proportion of one group with a particular characteristic is the same as that of another group.

Simple Regression Procedure

Another way to examine the relationship between two interval-ratio-level variables is to perform a simple regression procedure:

$$y = \alpha + \beta_x + \text{random error} \qquad (14.20)$$

where y equals the variable to be predicted (or the dependent variable), x equals the variable to be used as a predictor of y (or the independent variable), α (alpha) equals the y-intercept of the line, and β (beta) equals the slope of the line.

The intercept (α) gives the predicted value of y when x is zero. In general, it is technically incorrect to extend the regression line beyond the range of values of x for which it was estimated, because the procedure produces the best-fitting (ordinary least squares) line through the observed data points. Other data points beyond the ones used as the basis of the calculations might change the nature and extent of the relationship drastically. For example, the relationship may be nonlinear if additional observations are included.

The regression coefficient (β) is interpreted as the change in y for a unit change in x. The procedure is referred to as the regression of y on x. If the coefficient is positive, a unit change in x produces an increase in y (i.e., the line slopes upward). If the coefficient is negative, a unit change in x produces a decrease in y (i.e., the line slopes down).

The estimated regression equation allows researchers to calculate a predicted value of y for every observed value of x by simple substitution into the prediction equation. For example, if x equals the mother's years of education, and y equals the child's birthweight, an estimated regression line might look like this: $y = 5.75 + (.15)(x)$. For a mother with six years of education ($x = 6$) the predicted birthweight of the child is 6.65 pounds.

When the Pearson correlation coefficient (r) is squared, the resulting number (r^2) can be interpreted as the proportion of variance in y explained by x. For example, if $r^2 = .45$, we would say that mother's education accounts for or explains 45 percent of the variance in child's birthweight. Another way to calculate r^2 would be as follows:

$$r^2 = \frac{\text{total sum of squares} - \text{error sum of squares}}{\text{total sum of squares}} = \frac{\text{explained variation}}{\text{total variation}} \qquad (14.21)$$

MULTIVARIATE ANALYSIS

Multivariate analysis examines three or more variables at a time. In health services research as in social research, two-variable relationships seldom suffice. Often, instead of one independent variable and one dependent variable, researchers usually need to sort out the effects of several variables on a dependent variable. The inclusion of additional variables is based on both theoretical and practical knowledge, which helps specify the direction of influence and test for spuriousness. A model is properly specified when it correctly reflects the underlying or real world phenomena. Specification error occurs when the model is not properly stated, that is, when important explanatory variables have been excluded from the model, when unimportant variables have been included, or when the wrong form of the relationship has been assumed. A researcher could introduce many additional variables as control variables, but such analyses are potentially mindless unless guided by theoretical and practical considerations. Moreover, unless the sample size is very large, the investigator rapidly runs out of observations in each cell when many control variables are used simultaneously.

In reporting statistical results, the researcher should not only describe the techniques or models used but also examine the assumptions of the models and how they are consistent with the nature of the data. Otherwise, the techniques may not be appropriate for the analysis of the dataset. In addition to reporting significance level of the test results (e.g., p values), researchers may also report the confidence intervals of the estimates and the power of statistical tests.

Table 14–9 summarizes some statistical techniques used to analyze three or more variables based on nominal (categorical), or interval levels of measurement. Ordinal measures may be treated as nominal or interval measures (if equal distance among intervals can be assumed) and the appropriate techniques for those levels may then be used. It should be emphasized that the table is by no means exhaustive. In addition, many multivariate procedures investigate relationships among variables without designating some as independent and others as dependent. For example, principal component and factor analyses examine relationships within a single set of variables. Canonical correlation analysis examines the relationship between two sets of variables. Interested readers should consult with a multivariate textbook and an econometric textbook for detailed discus-

TABLE 14–9 Level of measurement and analysis involving three or more variables

Dependent Variable	Independent Variable	
	Nominal/Categorical	Interval-Ratio
Nominal/Categorical	Logistic regression (Dummy variables)	Logistic regression
	Binary segmentation techniques	Logit and Probit analysis
	Multidimensional contingency table analysis	Discriminant analysis
Interval-Ratio	Multiple regression (Dummy variables)	Multiple correlation
	ANOVA	Multiple regression
	Multivariate analysis of variance (MANOVA)	Multiple curvilinear regression
	Covariance analysis	Path analysis
	Multivariate binary segmentation techniques	Factor analysis
		Principal component
		Time-series analysis
		Survival analysis
		Cox regression
		Canonical correlation
		Structural models with latent variables

sions of those and many other multivariate techniques (Andrews, Klem, Davidson, Malley, and Rodgers, 1981; Kshirsagar, 1972; Mardia, Kent, and Bibby, 1979; Mu-laik, 1972; Nishisato, 1980; Mansfield, 1994; Poirer, 1995). This section discusses some of the more commonly used statistical analysis techniques: **multiple regression, logistic regression,** and **path analysis.**

Multiple Regression

Multiple regression is among the most versatile and powerful statistical techniques for analyzing the relationships among variables (Duncan, Knapp, and Miller, 1983). Multiple regression may be used simply to examine the relationships among variables or as an inferential method, to test hypotheses about population parameters.

The general formula for a multiple regression equation may be stated as follows:

$$y = \beta_0 + \beta_1 x_1 + \beta_2 x_2 + \beta_3 x_3 + \ldots + \beta_i x_i + e \tag{14.22}$$

where y is the dependent variable, each x_i represents an independent variable, β_0 is the y-intercept or the predicted value of y when all x's are equal to zero, β's are the regression coefficients of the associated independent variables or partial regression coefficients, and e is the error term, or the prediction error.

For example, in addition to mother's education, empirical evidence indicates that a mother's smoking habit may also affect the child's birthweight. A multiple regression model of child's birthweight on mother's education and smoking habit is: $y = 5.37 + .17x_1 - .21x_2$, where y equals weight (pounds), x_1 equals education (years of education), and x_2 equals the mother's smoking habit (packs of cigarettes/day).

β_0 is the predicted birthweight (5.37 pounds) for infants from mothers who have no education and do not smoke. β_1 is the predicted change in weight (0.17 pound) for every additional year of mother's education, holding constant the effect of smoking. β_2 is the predicted change in weight (−0.21 pound) for every additional pack of cigarettes smoked per day, holding constant the effect of education. For a woman with six years of education who smokes two packs of cigarettes a day, then, the predicted birthweight of her child would be 5.97 pounds [(5.37 + .17(6) − .21(2)].

In multiple regression, the multiple correlation coefficient R, which reflects the correlation between the observed values of y and the predicted values y, is a measure of how well the model fits the data. The square of the multiple correlation coefficient, R^2, is a measure of the proportion of the variance in y explained by all the independent variables in the model. For example, $R^2 = .70$, indicating that 70 percent of the variance in child's birthweight is explained by mother's education and smoking habit.

In addition to R^2, analysis of variance test can be performed for the whole equation. The null hypothesis amounts to all the regression coefficients being zero. The test statistic is an F ratio of the variance explained by the regression equation to the residual or error variance.

In multiple regression, it is sometimes useful to report the standardized coefficients when a researcher is interested in examining the relative effects of the independent variables on the dependent variable. The raw (unstandardized) regression coefficients give the predicted change in y for a unit change in x, but the unit that attaches to each coefficient depends on the metric underlying each variable. Therefore, the magnitudes of the raw coefficients are not directly comparable. The standardized coefficients, on the other hand, are expressed in the standard deviation units and the variables are comparable within a single equation.

So far, the multiple regression model presented assumes an additive effects, that is, y is determined by x_1 plus x_2. However, this is not a necessary assumption for a regression model. If the presence of an interaction effect (i.e., the impact of one independent variable depends on the value of another independent variable) is suspected, the interaction term of these two variables may be introduced. The model with interaction term may be specified as follows (Lewis-Beck, 1980):

$$y = \beta_0 + \beta_1 x_1 + \beta_2 x_1 x_2 + e \tag{14.23}$$

For example, in examining the impact of education on income, if one wants to test if the impact of education (x_1) on income (y) varies by sex (x_2, i.e., sexual discrimination in income determination) an interaction term of sex and education ($x_1 x_2$) may be included in the regression model. If the regression coefficient of the interaction term (β_2) is significant, there is evidence that sexual discrimination might exist in income determination.

Assuming the following is the result of the regression estimate: $y = 8050 + 630 \, x_1 + 250 \, x_1 x_2$, where y equals annual income (dollars), x_1 equals education (years), and x_2 equals sex (1 = male, 0 = female). The regression equation for women is thus: $y = 8050 + 630 x_1 + 250 x_1 (0)$, or $y = 8050 + 630 x_1$. The regression equation for men is: $y = 8050 + 630 x_1 + 250 x_1 (1)$, or $y = 8050 + (630 + 250) x_1$, or $y = 8050 + 880 \, x_1$. According to the model, a woman with 10 years of education will make \$14,350 a year [$y = 8050 + 630(10)$], but a man with 10 years of education will make \$16,850 a year [$y = 8050 + 880(10)$].

When a multiple regression model includes two or more independent variables that are highly intercorrelated, the results become difficult to interpret. This problem is known as multicollinearity. The problem with collinear variables is that they provide very similar information, and it is difficult to separate the effects of the individual variables. The tolerance of a variable is one common measure of collinearity. It is defined as $1 - R_i^2$, where R_i is the multiple correlation coefficient when the ith independent variable is predicted from the other independent variables. A small tolerance score indicates the presence of collinearity.

The multiple regression model presented so far is a technique for estimating linear relationships in the data. In many cases, it is necessary to convert the data to forms amenable to analysis by the general linear model by means of mathematical transformations. If researchers are convinced, based on theoretical or empirical evidence, that relationships among variables are nonlinear, a mathematical specification may be found that is consistent with the type of nonlinearity expected or observed. For example, the researcher can take the logarithm of y. Other arithmetic manipulations include taking a square function (e.g., $y = \beta_0 + \beta_1 x_1 + \beta_2 x_2 + \beta_3 x_2^2 + e$), a cube function ($y = \beta_0 + \beta_1 x_1 + \beta_2 x_2 + \beta_3 x_2^2 + \beta_4 x_2^3 + e$), and so on.

Examples of mathematical transformations include the polynomial model, the exponential model, and the hyperbolic model. The polynomial model may be specified as:

$$y = \beta_0 + \beta_1 x_1 + \beta_2 x_1^2 + \beta_3 x_1^3 + \ldots + \beta_m x_1^m + e \qquad (14.24)$$

This model is appropriate when the slope of the relationship between an independent variable x_1 and dependent variable y is expected to change sign as the value of x_1 increases. The exponential model may be specified as:

$$y = \beta_0 x^{\beta_e} \qquad (14.25)$$

This model is appropriate when the slope of the curve representing the relationship between x and y does not change sign, but increases or decreases in magnitude as the value of x changes. For example, the relationship between health care expenditure and health status in the United States indicates a declining rate of return.

To estimate the coefficients of the exponential model, the researchers could take the logarithm of both sides so that the equation is in linear form and can be estimated by the general linear model:

$$\log y = \log \beta_0 + \beta (\log x) + \log e \qquad (14.26)$$

The hyperbolic model may be specified as:

$$y = \beta_0 + \beta (1/x) + e \qquad (14.27)$$

This model may also be called the reciprocal model. It is used when as the value of x gets infinitely large, the value of y approaches β_0. For example, the relationship between marketing expenditure and sales may look like this model. As marketing expenditure is increased indefinitely, sales first increase accordingly but later remain constant when the market is close to saturation.

When independent variables are nominal (e.g., race, sex), the investigator may choose to include these variables in a multiple regression model by creating a set of dummy variables or binary indicators that uniquely code a case into a category of the nominal variable. Dummy variables are typically indexed by the numerical values zero and one. An ordinal-level variable can also be transformed into a set of dummy variables and entered into a regression equation, for example, a variable whose categories are high, medium, and low. Alternatively, ordinal variables may be used as continuous variables if the investigator is willing to assume that the categories are separated by equal intervals.

Table 14–10 reports the raw data about the number of patients' emergency room visits and their insurance status for a county general hospital. The variable insurance may be recoded into three dummy variables, d_1, d_2, and d_3, as shown. Since any one of the three dummies is a perfect linear function of the other two, (i.e., if we know that a patient has neither public nor private insurance, we also know the patient must have no insurance), including all three dummies in the regression model will cause perfect multicollinearity so that the regression coefficients cannot be calculated. Therefore, we have to omit one of the dummy variables from the regression model. Thus, given a variable with k categories, $k-1$ dummy variables may be created and entered into the regression model.

Estimating the model, that number of emergency room visits is a function of insurance status, requires that the dummy variable representing insurance be used. The results calculated for this model are: $y = 6.25 - 1.22d_1 - 4.95d_2$ and $R^2 = .48$. Specifically, β_0 (the intercept) is the predicted value of y when all independent variables equal zero. The independent variables in this model both equal zero when the patient has neither public ($d_1 = 0$) nor private insurance ($d_2 = 0$), or in other words, when the patient has no insurance. The intercept (6.25) is therefore interpreted as the predicted number of emergency room visits for a patient with no health insurance and is exactly equal to the mean

TABLE 14–10   Raw data on number of emergency room visits, and insurance status

Observation	y = Number of E.R. visits	x = Insurance	d_1 = Public	d_2 = Private	d_3 = None
1	13	1	1	0	0
2	4	1	1	0	0
3	3	1	1	0	0
4	2	2	0	1	0
5	1	2	0	1	0
6	2	2	0	1	0
7	1	2	0	1	0
8	6	3	0	0	1
9	9	3	0	0	1
10	19	3	0	0	1
...					
N					

Note. For insurance, the codes are: 1 = public (Medicare or Medicaid), 2 = private, and 3 = no insurance or self-pay.

number of emergency room visits for a patient with no health insurance in the sample. Thus, in dummy variable regression involving a single set of dummies, the intercept value is equal to the mean of the dependent variable for the omitted category.

The coefficient β_1 for the dummy variable corresponding to patients with public health insurance represents the change (over the intercept value) in number of emergency room visits for those in the d_2 category. In dummy variable regression involving a single set of dummies, the regression coefficients are interpreted as the difference in means between any one category and the omitted category. The β_1 coefficient, −1.22, therefore infers that the mean number of emergency room visits by patients with public health insurance is 1.22 times less than the mean number of emergency room visits by patients with no insurance. The predicted number of emergency room visits by patients with public health insurance is 5.03 [or 6.25 − 1.22(1) − 4.95(0)]. Similarly, the predicted number of emergency room visits by patients with private insurance is 1.30 [or 6.25 − 1.22(0) − 4.95(1)], the mean for patients with private insurance. Finally, the R^2 for this model (.48) means that 48 percent of the variance in number of emergency room visits are explained by patients' insurance status.

Logistic Regression

The distinction between a logistic regression model and a linear regression model is that the dependent variable is binary or dichotomous in logistic regression (e.g., whether one smokes or not, has health insurance or not) but continuous in linear regression (Hosmer and Lemeshow, 1989; Draper and Smith, 1981; Kleinbaum and Kupper, 1978; Cox, 1970; Yarandi and Simpson, 1991). Logistic regression is based on the assumption that the logarithm of the odds of belonging to one population is a linear function of several predictors (independent variables) in the model. The multiple logistic regression model may be presented as follows:

$$\ln \left(\frac{p}{1 - p} \right) = \beta_0 + \beta_1 x_1 + \beta_2 x_2 + \ldots + \beta_k x_k + e \tag{14.28}$$

When we solve for probability, p, the model can be represented as:

$$p = \frac{e^{\beta_0 + \beta_1 x_1 + \beta_2 x_2 + \ldots + \beta_k x_k}}{1 + e^{\beta_0 + \beta_1 x_1 + \beta_2 x_2 + \ldots + \beta_k x_k}} \tag{14.29}$$

For the multiple logistic regression model in 14.29, the odds ratio relating to a dichotomous independent variable x_i, which is coded as one if present and zero if absent, may be estimated by:

$$\text{Odds ratio} = e^{\beta_i} \tag{14.30}$$

As an example, the impact of financial characteristics of rural primary care programs (PCPs) on the chance of program survival was examined (Shi et al., 1994). A randomly selected national cohort of rural PCPs (n = 162) was used to compare financial measures of programs that were continuing and those that were noncontinuing. Financial data were obtained from 1978–1987 BCRR (Bureau Common Reporting Requirements) forms submitted to the Bureau of Health Care Delivery and Assistance of the U.S. Department of Health and Human Services as part of the requirement to receive federal grant support for the programs. A stepwise logistic regression procedure was used to calculate the significant predictors of program survival (see Table 14–11).

The dependent variable is the status of program survival (1 = continuing, 0 = noncontinuing). Independent variables include self-sufficiency (Payments for Services ÷ Total Costs × 100), grant revenue (the percentage of total revenues that come from federal, state, local, or private grants), average personnel costs (Costs of Total Salaried Personnel ÷ Total Number of Salaried Personnel), and patients (the annual number of patients of all ages who have received treatment at the community health centers). Knowing the estimated logistic coefficients (Table 14–11) and using Equation 14.29, we can compute the probability of program survival under different conditions. For example, a program that is 20 percent self-sufficient, receives 20 percent grant revenue, has $15,000 average personnel cost, and an annual patient load of 5,000 has a 29 percent chance of surviving. This probability is obtained by plugging the estimated coefficients from Table 14–11 into Equation 14.29 as follows:

TABLE 14–11   Logistic regression of predictors of primary care programs' continuation

Independent Variables	Dependent Variable		
	(Continuing programs = 1 Noncontinuing programs = 0)		
(x_i)	Regression Coefficient (β_i)	Standard Error (S_{β_i})	P Value (x^2)
Intercept	−.306	.275	0.27
Self Sufficiency	.629	.251	0.01
Grant Revenue	.438	.221	0.05
Average Personnel Costs	.00001	.00000	0.02
Patients	.00001	.00000	0.06

Note. N = 162. Adapted from the author's study.

$$p = \frac{e^{[-1\ 306\ +\ 629(\ 20)\ +\ 438(.20)\ +\ 00001(15000)\ +\ 00001(5000)]}}{1\ +\ e^{[-1.306\ +\ 629(\ 20)\ +\ 438(.20)\ +\ 00001(15000)\ +\ 00001(5000)]}}$$

$$p = \frac{e^{-.8926}}{1\ +\ e^{\ 8926}}$$

Since $e = 2.71828$, then,

$$p = \frac{(2.71828)^{-\ 8926}}{1\ +\ (2.71828)^{-\ 8926}} = \frac{.40958968}{1.40958968} = 0.29057369, \text{ or } 29\%$$

The odds ratio (relative risk) of a program noncontinuing given the extent of a specific condition can be computed using the estimated regression coefficients (Table 14–11) and Equation 14.30. For example, the odds ratio of grant revenue is 1.55 ($e^{\beta_i} = 2.7182^{438}$) indicating that for a 1 percent increase in grant revenue, the chance of program survival improves by 1.55 times. Similarly, improvement in the self-sufficiency ratio by 1 percent increases the chance of program survival by 1.88 times (2.71828^{629}). Thus, the use of logistic regression provides an efficient way to estimate the probability of the occurrence of an event or condition and the odds ratio (relative risk) of having that event or condition.

Path Analysis

Path analysis is a popular form of multivariate analysis which provides the possibility for causal determination among a set of measured variables (Miller, 1991). It is a procedure that gives a quantitative interpretation of an assumed causal system. Path analysis may consist of a series of regression equations, with many variables in the model taking their places respectively as dependent and independent variables (Duncan, 1975). In other words, most of the variables in the model will be a dependent variable in one equation and an independent variable in one or more different equations. A four-variable path model may be delineated as follows:

(1) $x_2 = p_{21}\ x_1 + p_{2u} R_u$

(2) $x_3 = p_{31}\ x_1 + p_{32}\ x_2 + p_{3v} R_v$

(3) $x_4 = p_{41}\ x_1 + p_{42}\ x_2 + p_{43} x_3 + p_{4w} R_w$ (14.31)

where p represents the path coefficient, x is the variable, and R is the residual or unexplained variance. The path coefficients (p's) can be derived from the standardized regression coefficients, computed by multiplying an unstandardized coefficient by the ratio of the standard deviation of the independent variable to the standard deviation of the dependent variable (Pindyck and Rubinfeld, 1981). Specifically, path coefficients are identical to partial regression coefficients (the betas) when the variables are measured in standard form. With path analysis, both direct and indirect effects of one variable may be computed.

Developing **causal modeling** is the first step in path analysis (Wang, Eddy, and Westerfield, 1992). Causal modeling requires the researcher to think causally about the research question and construct an arrow diagram that reflects causal processes. Such a process identifies variables for analysis based on a theoretical framework, literature review, and observations; and the ensuring models are likely to be theory driven.

Examples of causal structures are provided in Figure 14–1. Panel A depicts a situation where X is causally related to Z but not to Y, and Y is causally related to Z but not to X. Panel B indicates that X is a direct cause of Y and an indirect cause of Z, mediated by Y. Panel C shows X has a co-causal relationship between Y and Z. Finally, panel D demonstrates that Z is causally dependent on both X and Y, plus an indirect cause of X via X's impact on Y. The result of causal modeling is the completion of a path diagram that indicates the theoretical or expected relationships among the measured variables in the model.

The second step in path analysis is to compute the path coefficients. Path coefficients reflect the amount of direct contribution of a given variable on another variable when the effects of other related variables are taken into account. Path coefficients may be calculated either through regression programs or zero order correlations among variables (Loether and McTavish, 1974). The results of the path coefficients may then be entered in the path diagram.

The third step in path analysis is to conduct a "goodness of fit" test. Land (1969) suggests three approaches: (1) examine the amount of variation in the dependent variables that is explained by variables specified in the model; (2) examine the size of path coefficients to see whether they are large enough to warrant the inclusion of a variable or path in the model; and (3) evaluate the ability of the model to predict correlation coefficients that were not used in computation of the path coefficients themselves. The first approach may be used by examining the R^2's of the various equations. The second approach entails examining whether the path coefficients are significant. In applying the third approach, the researcher could test an alternative model by substituting factors in the basic model believed to be more important and by adding new factors to the basic model.

The fourth and final step in path analysis is to interpret the results. Both direct and indirect effects of the variables in the causal model may be studied. It should be understood that path analysis does not discover causal relationships but rather gives a quantitative estimate of an assumed causal system based on both theoretical and empirical evidence.

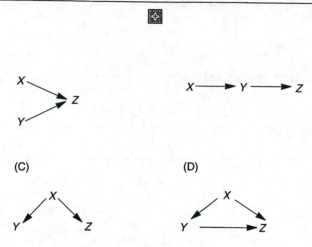

FIGURE 14–1 Examples of causal structure diagrams.

As an example, the relationship between family planning, socioeconomic conditions, and fertility was investigated in six rural villages of China, based on a 1989 random household survey (Shi, 1992). The theoretical model (see Figure 14–2) guiding the analysis concerns the extent to which family planning programs and socioeconomic conditions affect fertility among rural inhabitants. Both family planning programs and socioeconomic conditions are hypothesized to have negative direct effects on fertility. The indirect effects of socioeconomic conditions on fertility through family planning and proximate fertility variables are hypothesized to be positive. The indirect effects of family planning programs on fertility through proximate fertility variables are hypothesized to be positive. Finally, the proximate fertility variables are hypothesized to inversely affect fertility.

Table 14–12 displays the path coefficients estimated from regression procedures. All family planning measures and all but one (income level) socioeconomic measures are significantly related to fertility. Further, the family planning measures and female educa-

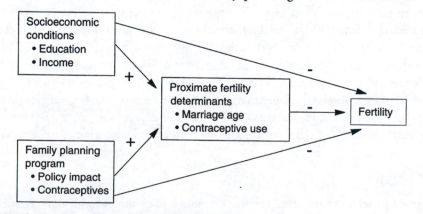

FIGURE 14–2 Theoretical model specifying the relationships of family planning and socioeconomic conditions with fertility.
Source: Adapted from the author's study.

TABLE 14–12 Direct, indirect, and total effects of predictor variables on fertility

Predictor	Direct Effects	Indirect Effects			Total Effects
	(1)	Marriage age (2)	Contraception (3)	Total indirect (4)	(5)
Policy impact	−.096	−.006	−.017	−.023	−.119
Male education	.018	−.006	.004	−.002	.016
Female education	−.077	−.007	−.015	−.022	−.099
Per capita income	.0004	.00009	−.00008	.00001	.00005
Income level	−.183	−.026	.020	−.006	−.189
Marriage age	−.043	–	–	–	−.043
Contraception	−.017	–	–	–	−.017
Free contraceptives	−.256	−.021	.020	−.001	−.257

Source: Adapted from the author's study.

tion are significantly related to both proximate fertility measures that are related to fertility. Male education and per capita income are both related to contraceptive use. Consistent with the temporally ordered structural model, it is possible for the predictor variables to have sizable effects on fertility decline through indirect paths. These are described in columns 2 through 4 of Table 14–12. When the indirect effects of each variable are added to its direct effects (column 1), we obtain the total effect of that variable on fertility (column 5). Examination of all total effects shows that policy impact, female and male education, free contraceptive provision, and income level assume somewhat greater importance than was implied by consideration of their direct effects alone.

SUMMARY

Before formal analysis, data are first explored to make sure all data elements are included in one data file and prepared for hypothesis testing and model building. The choice of appropriate statistics is determined by the level of measurement and the number of variables analyzed. Commonly used descriptive statistics for analyzing one variable a time include frequency and percentage distributions, measures of central tendency (e.g., mean, median, and mode), variability or dispersion (e.g., range, standard deviation, variance), shape (e.g., frequency or percentage polygon, skewedness, kurtosis, leptokurtic, platykurtic), and standard scores (z score, rate, ratio). Commonly used bivariate procedures include cross-tabulation, chi-square (χ^2), phi coefficient (ϕ), coefficient of contingency (C), Cramér's V, Goodman-Kruskal's lambda (λ), relative risk ratio, Kendall's tau (τ), Goodman-Kruskal's gamma (γ), ANOVA, Pearson correlation coefficient (r), and paired t test. Commonly used multivariate statistical procedures include multiple regression, logistic regression, and path analysis.

Key Terms

univariate analysis	bivariate analysis
multivariate analysis	distribution
measures of central tendency	mode
median	mean
measures of variability	measures of dispersion
range	variance
standard deviation	skewedness
standard scores	ratio
rate	chi-square
chi-square-based measures	Spearman's coefficient
proportional reduction in error (PRE)	
Pearson product–moment correlation coefficient	
relative risk ratio	odds ratio
simple regression	multiple regression
logistic regression	path analysis
causal modeling	

Review Questions

1. Why do researchers explore and examine data prior to formal analysis?

2. What descriptive statistics have you learned from the chapter? How can they be used (i.e., what level of measurement are they suitable for)?

3. What bivariate statistics have you learned from the chapter? How can they be used (i.e., what level of measurement are they suitable for)?

4. What multivariate analysis procedures have you learned from the chapter? How can they be used (i.e., what level of measurement are they suitable for)?

◼

REFERENCES

Andrews, F. M., Klem, L., Davidson, T. N., Malley, P. M., and Rodgers, W. L. (1981). *A Guide for Selecting Statistical Techniques for Analyzing Social Science Data.* 2nd ed. Ann Arbor, MI: Institute for Social Research, the University of Michigan.

Cox, D. R. (1970). *The Analysis of Binary Data.* London: Metheum.

Draper, N. R., and Smith, H. (1981). *Applied Regression Analysis.* New York: John Wiley.

Duncan, O. D. (1975). *Introduction to Structural Equation Models.* New York: Academic Press.

Duncan, R. C., Knapp, R. G., and Miller, M. C. (1983). *Introductory Biostatistics for the Health Sciences.* Albany, NY: Delmar.

Goodman, L. A., and Kruskal, W. H. (1954). Measures of association for cross-classification. *Journal of the American Statistical Association, 49,* 732–764.

Grady, K. E., and Wallston, B. S. (1988). *Research in Health Care Settings.* Newbury Park, CA: Sage.

Herman, J. L., Morris, L. L., and Fitz-Gibbon, C. T. (1987). *Evaluator's Handbook.* Newbury Park, CA: Sage.

Hosmer, D. W., and Lemeshow, S. (1989). *Applied Logistic Regression.* New York: John Wiley.

Kleinbaum, D. G., and Kupper, L. L. (1978). *Applied Regression Analysis and Other Multivariate Methods.* Belmont, CA: Wadsworth Publishing Co.

Kshirsagar, A. M. (1972). *Multivariate Analysis.* New York: Marcel Dekker.

Land, K. C. (1969). Principles of path analysis. In E. F. Borgatta (Ed.), *Sociological Methodology 1969.* San Francisco: Jossey-Bass.

Last, J. M. (1983). *A Dictionary of Epidemiology.* New York: Oxford University Press.

Lewis-Beck, M. S. (1980). *Applied Regression.* Beverly Hills, CA: Sage.

Lilienfeld, A. M., and Lilienfeld, D. E. (1980). *Foundation of Epidemiology.* New York: Oxford University Press.

Loether, H. J., and McTavish, D. C. (1974). *Descriptive Statistics for Sociologists.* Boston: Allyn and Bacon.

Mansfield, E. (1994). *Statistics for Business and Economics: Methods and Applications.* 5th ed. New York: Norton.

Mardia, K. V., Kent, J. T., and Bibby, J. M. (1979). *Multivariate Analysis.* London: Marcel Dekker.

Miller, D. C. (1991). *Handbook of Research Design and Social Measurement.* Newbury Park, CA: Sage.

Mulaik, S. A. (1972). *The Foundation of Factor Analysis.* New York: McGraw-Hill.

Nishisato, S. (1980). *Analysis of Categorical Data: Dual Scaling and Its Applications.* Toronto: University of Toronto Press.

Norusis, M. J. (1994). *SPSS Advanced Statistics.* Chicago, IL: SPSS.

Pindyck, R. S., and Rubinfeld, D. L. (1981). *Econometric Models and Economic Forecasts.* New York: McGraw-Hill.

Poirer, D. J. (1995). *Intermediate Statistics and Econometrics: A Comparative Approach*. Cambridge, MA: MIT Press.

Shi, L. (1992). Determinants of fertility: Results from a 1989 rural household survey. *The Social Science Journal*, 29(4), 457–477.

Shi, L., Samuels, M. E., Konard R., Porter, C., Stoskopf, C. H., and Richtor, D. (1994). Rural primary care program survival: An analysis of financial variables. *Journal of Rural Health*, 10(3), 173–182.

Singleton, E. A., Straits, B. C., and Straits, M. M. (1993). *Approaches to Social Research*. Oxford: Oxford University Press.

Wang, M., Eddy, J. M., and Westerfield, R. C. (1992). Causal modeling in health survey studies. *Health Values*, 16(4), 55–57.

Yarandi, H. N., and Simpson, S. H. (1991). The logistic regression model and the odds of testing HIV positive. *Nursing Research*, 40(6), 372–373.

CHAPTER

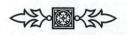

15

Applying Health Services Research

LEARNING OBJECTIVES

- To become aware of the channels of communicating the results of health services research.
- To understand the general format of research report for refereed journals.
- To appreciate the training needs for a successful health services researcher.

Scientific research is cumulative. Without communicating research findings to other health services researchers, researchers cannot contribute to the cumulative body of knowledge that defines scientific disciplines. Thus, one purpose for researchers to publicize their findings is to add to the stock of scientific knowledge so that the research is connected with past research and future research can build upon the present.

In addition to the advancement of knowledge, health services researchers are eager to communicate their findings due to the applied nature of their inquiry. Chapter 1 stated that the priorities of health services research are largely established by societal questions and problems about health services for population groups. Much of health services research is conducted to solve health-related problems. Indeed, the products of health services research are often assessed primarily in terms of their usefulness to people with decision-making responsibilities, whether they be clinicians, administrators of health services organizations or government agencies, or politicians and elected officials charged with formulating national health care policy.

This chapter delineates specific communication channels through which research findings can be publicized. The format of writing a scientific report for publication will be described. The potential and constrains of implementing research findings will be discussed. The chapter completes with a review of the 10 major stages in health services research as covered throughout the book, and examines the skills needed to become an effective health services researcher.

COMMUNICATING HEALTH SERVICES RESEARCH

Before communicating research findings, researchers must know who their intended audiences are, because the types of communication channels vary depending on who the audiences are. Potential audiences may be divided into three groups: the research community, the stakeholders, and the public. The research community includes scientists or would-be scientists who share similar research interests. Stakeholders are those who provide funding for research or have a key role to play in implementing research findings. The public are those who are neither researchers nor stakeholders. Often, the same research can have several different types of audiences, and researchers should adapt their communication style to specific audiences to maximize comprehension and acceptance. Table 15–1 summarizes the commonly used channels of communication for the different audiences.

Research Community

When the intended audiences are members of the research community, certain assumptions may be made as to their existing knowledge. Research findings may be summarized rather than explained in great detail. Similarly, more technical terms can be used than would be the case for other audiences.

TABLE 15–1 Health services research communication and audience

Audience	Research Community	Stakeholders	Public
	journal articles	research proposals	newspapers
	conference presentations	reports	magazines
	working papers	symposiums	television
	monographs	testimonies	radio
	books	research notes	brochures

The most popular means of communicating research results to the scientific community is to write an article to be published in a refereed scientific journal. Appendix 1 lists journals commonly used by health services researchers as well as other social scientists. The length and style of the articles may vary among journals. Before submitting articles for publication, researchers should examine manuscript preparation guidelines of the journal and samples of articles previously published by the journal in question.

Another popular means of communicating research findings is through professional conferences. Researchers typically join a number of professional associations related to their research interest. These associations generally organize periodic (e.g., annual) conferences or meetings to allow members an opportunity to present their research. Since it is usually more difficult to have a paper accepted by a journal than a conference, professional conferences provide an excellent opportunity for a larger number of researchers to communicate their research. Another advantage of conferences over journals is that it is also more timely to publicize the research. Refereed journals, particularly those more sought-after ones, usually have a backlog of articles to be published. Researchers may wait many months between submission and request for revision, and formal acceptance and final publication. A further advantage of conferences is that they can be used to invite comments, suggestions, and criticisms for the research. Thus, many researchers use conference presentations as a means of gathering suggestions for revising their paper before formal submission to an academic journal. Since each presentation session has limited time allotment, to achieve maximum feedback, researchers may distribute the draft manuscript and leave their addresses to the audience.

Working papers and monographs are another form of reporting to the research community. A working paper implies the article is still in progress and not fully polished. It is circulated among colleagues or those who share the same research interest with an implicit request for comments and suggestions. Working papers can vary in length and may present only a portion of the research findings. Since researchers' professional reputations are not at stake in a working paper, they can present rather tentative analysis and interpretations and invite comments on them. While working papers are often the prelude to journal articles, monographs are preparations for books. Monographs are usually written for large and complex projects. Similar to working papers, monographs may be circulated among peers for comments and suggestion. Monographs may also be published internally by some research institutions.

Books generally represent the most comprehensive if not prestigious form of research report. It has all the advantages of a monograph—length, detail—but is more polished. Since the publication of research findings as a book gives the findings an appearance of greater authenticity and worth, the researcher has a special obligation to the audience to maintain truthfulness because many readers may be led to accept the findings uncritically.

Stakeholders

When stakeholders are the intended audiences, researchers cannot assume that the stakeholders are as knowledgeable as they are about the research subject and terminologies. Introductions and explanations are necessary whenever technical terms and concepts are introduced.

A common means of securing funding is the preparation of a research proposal. In a research proposal, the researcher tries to convince a prospective sponsor or funder that she or he is qualified to perform the research activities necessary to answer the questions deemed important to the sponsor or funder. Most funding sources require the same basic information for a research proposal, although the details and required format may vary. See Chapter 3 for a review of writing the research proposal.

Perhaps the most common means of communicating with stakeholders is through the preparation of technical reports, often required by funders or sponsors. In preparing such a report, researchers should bear in mind the audience for the report—scientific or lay—and their initial reasons for sponsoring the project. The report should be focused and consistent with the purposes of the sponsors or funders for this research. It is usually unwise to include research findings that have no interest or value to the sponsors. At the same time, it may be useful to summarize the ways in which the research has advanced basic scientific knowledge, if it has. In finalizing the funding contract and research protocol, researchers and sponsors should work out an agreement in terms of whether permission is granted to the investigator(s) for publishing research findings in academic journals.

Stakeholders, such as sponsors and policymakers, may be invited to symposiums conducted to discuss the research and its implications to decision makers. Symposiums provide an opportunity not only to communicate research findings but also to discuss and debate research issues of interest to the stakeholders.

Expert testimony is another means that researchers may promote awareness and use of their research. Testifying before stakeholders, such as during congressional hearings or state Certificate of Need meetings, requires researchers to be well focused, speak in nontechnical terms, and explain in greater detail.

Finally, research notes can be prepared that summarize the basic research design, major findings, and the policy implications. Research notes may be adapted from the executive summary portion of the research report. Research notes are sent to stakeholders to inform them about a relevant policy issue.

Public

When the intended audiences are the general public, researchers can rely on the mass media to publicize significant research findings. Examples include newspapers (both national and local), popular magazines and journals, television programs, and radio talk shows. In addition, special brochures may be prepared that summarize the research and its significant findings. It is critical that presentations be given in nontechnical language and any key terms and concepts be defined and explained. No assumptions should be made about the audience's existing knowledge on the research topic.

PUBLISHING HEALTH SERVICES RESEARCH

To publish research in a peer-reviewed, academic journal, researchers need to be familiar with the journal requirements, follow these requirements in the preparation of manuscript, and be prepared for rejection and resubmission.

Familiarity with Journal Requirements

Each journal has its own goals, standards of quality, and preferred style. The more accurately these requirements are met, the better is the chance of getting accepted for publication. As a first task, researchers should become thoroughly familiar with the journals in which they wish to publish. The guidelines for manuscript preparation published in the journals should be thoroughly studied. If such a guide cannot be found, the journal office should be contacted to request a copy. The articles that have been published in the journal should be read and attention paid to the content, writing style, structure and organization, use of tables and charts, and length. The manuscript, if published, is likely to be very similar to these. Table 15–2 presents the general format for scholarly papers.

Title

The title of a paper should succinctly and accurately reflect the study contents. Since the title of a paper will be recorded in the researcher's curriculum vitae, preferably it would reflect the area of research the researcher wants to be associated with. Some journals may place a limit on the number of words to be used in a title. If there is such a requirement, it should be adhered to.

TABLE 15–2 General format for scholarly papers

Title	succinct and reflects study contents
Abstract	objectives, methods, results, conclusion
Introduction	problem statement, study purpose, significance
Literature Review	current literature, conceptual framework, research questions or hypotheses
Methods	• design (type of research, implementation procedures) • subjects (research population, sample size, sampling procedure, response rate, sample characteristics, biases) • measures (operational definitions, validity and reliability of measures) • analysis (statistical and modeling techniques, data assumptions)
Results	• findings that answer the research questions or hypotheses • use of subheadings, tables, and figures
Discussion	key research findings and implications, comparisons with previous research, limitations, future research direction
References	cited literature
Appendix (optional)	questionnaire instrument, tables

Abstract

An abstract is a capsule version of the full article and prepared after the article is written. There is usually a word limit imposed by the journal (e.g., 150 to 200 words). The purpose of an abstract is to help readers decide whether the report is consistent with their interest. An abstract can be prepared by using the same words and phrases in the finished article. Typically, a well-prepared abstract includes a statement of purpose, a description of design, a description of setting and research subjects, a statement of intervention (if applicable), a concise summary of major measures used, a clear quantified presentation of results, and a conclusion statement. Some journals require a specific format for the abstract. For example, the *American Journal of Public Health* (1996) requires authors to use the following subheadings for their abstracts: Objectives, Methods, Results, and Conclusions. Since titles and abstracts are often the only things researchers have access to in computerized databases, they often decide whether or not to retrieve a paper based solely on its title and abstract.

Introduction

The introduction section lays the groundwork for the rest of the paper. It contains a clear statement of the problem, the major purpose of the study, and its theoretical as well as practical significance. The problem and its significance play an important role in paper acceptance. Studies that are potentially important often address important questions either from a theoretical or practical perspective. Articles that use a new methodological approach could also be valuable contributions.

Literature review

The literature review section focuses on the current literature that clearly frames the study, describes the conceptual framework of the study, and states the research questions or hypotheses. Key studies are reviewed in terms of theoretical and methodological approaches, as well as major findings that document the evolution of the research problem. Such a review provides the framework for the current research, which builds on previous theories and research. The hypotheses or research questions to be addressed fill a gap in the current knowledge and/or research. The theoretical model used by the study can be presented in a figure, such as an arrow diagram. The hypotheses or research questions should be precisely stated and testable. Some journals require literature review to be incorporated in the introduction section. If this is the case, authors need to prepare a more concise summary of the literature and their conceptual framework.

Methods

The research methods section summarizes how the study was done so that others can replicate the study based on the information given. The following subheadings may be used to assist in the preparation of this section: design, subjects, measurement, and analysis. The design of the study tells what type of research was conducted, whether it be experiment, survey, longitudinal, qualitative field study, or using available data. The procedures of implementing the study should be described in sufficient detail to allow approximate replication. If available data were used, the sources of the data and their completeness, validity, and reliability should be addressed in detail. The design should be appropriate to the research purpose.

The subjects of the study refer to those who participated in the study. The research population, the sample size, the sampling procedure, response rate, sample characteristics, and biases, if any, should all be described. Critical evaluation criteria for submitted manuscripts often include appropriate control or comparison group(s), proper selection or assignment of subjects, sufficient sample size, sufficient response rate, and appropriate handling of missing data and attrition.

Measurement describes the operational definitions of the variables used in the study, specifies the way in which the observations were translated into variables, and assesses the validity and reliability of the measures. If the study is complicated and lengthy, a complete questionnaire may be attached as an appendix.

The analysis specifies the statistical and modeling techniques used and reviews assumptions made concerning the data. The analysis procedures should be appropriate to the research purpose and data. There should be adequate testing and control for violations of data assumptions (e.g., distribution, linearity, collinearity, residuals, etc.).

Results

The results section presents the findings of the study, which answers the research questions or hypotheses that frame the study. Findings should be presented judiciously but completely. The significance, power, and confidence intervals regarding the findings should also be reported. Tables and figures may be constructed to facilitate the presentation of findings and are placed near the text describing the findings. However, authors should consult with the guidelines to see if there is any restriction on the number of tables that can be included in a manuscript. Subheadings may be used to help organize the presentation. They may be phrased to reflect the research questions or hypotheses. A critical concern in presenting the results is to present findings that specifically address the research questions or hypotheses.

Discussion

The discussion section provides a succinct summary of key research findings relevant to the research questions or hypotheses, discusses the implications of the findings in terms of theoretical and practical significance, compares the findings to other relevant studies, points out the various limitations of the study and their impact on the findings, and suggests directions for future research.

References

The reference section generally includes literature cited in the text of the article. The format of the references varies by journals, and authors should consult with the preferred style of the particular journal to which they are submitting before preparing the references.

Appendix

An appendix is usually not required or encouraged by journals. Unless it is a lengthy and complicated study, authors need not use an appendix. An appendix may include such items as the complete research questionnaire, additional tables not already presented in the results section, as well as other items the authors perceive as being relevant to the understanding of the research.

Length

Finally, the length of the paper is usually restricted by journals. Twenty-five typed, double-spaced pages, including references and tables, can be used as a rough guide. However, the investigator should check with the specific instruction of the journal. If a study is complicated and of great significance, many journals make exceptions in terms of restrictions on the length of paper or number of tables included.

Dealing with Rejections

When reports are prepared according to journal guidelines, they have a better chance of being accepted for publication. However, there is no guarantee this will happen. Even experienced researchers receive rejections from time to time. Many factors could influence a rejection decision. The competitiveness of a particular journal is a critical factor. If the acceptance rate is low, say 10 percent of all manuscripts submitted, then, by design, many articles, including those of good quality will be rejected. Authors may target several journals so that once the paper is rejected by one journal, they may proceed to submit elsewhere. Young scholars may be advised to choose among journals where the competition is less intense. After accumulating some experience and confidence, they can then submit to more competitive journals.

Another factor that affects a paper's acceptance is the review process. Usually, a submitted paper is reviewed by two or more professionals with relevant experience or interest. A good reviewer studies the manuscript carefully, prepares a balanced critique, and points out ways to improve the article. The evaluations are subsequently weighed by the editor who makes the final decision with regard to acceptance, revision and resubmission, or rejection. Unfortunately, editors do not always know the qualification of reviewers. Some reviewers could be incompetent themselves. Qualified reviewers may be very busy themselves and turn down the chance to review. Both reviewers and editors could have their own biases with a particular topic or methodology. Most authors usually have no way of finding out these factors prior to the submission of their paper. However, once a rejection letter is received, the concerns of the editor and reviewers should be studied carefully. If they make sense, these concerns should be addressed prior to resubmitting the paper either to the same journal (if allowed) or elsewhere. If the criticism is irrelevant or indicates misunderstanding, authors can write to the editor to state their concern over the review and request that the editor appoint someone else to reevaluate the paper.

However, the most common reason for rejection is that the paper is not good enough. Sometimes the topic is not relevant to the journal, not significant enough, or the design of the study is flawed. Some of the concerns are easier to handle than others. If the article is inappropriate for the journal, more relevant journals may be targeted for submission. Usually, a more specialized journal related to the authors' area is more likely to accept their paper than a more general journal whose interest borders on theirs. If the submitted article misses certain elements, the missing elements should be included. If the wrong analysis was used, the data should be reanalyzed with the proper approach. However, if the design is flawed or the topic is not significant, there is little an investigator can do about it other than accept this as a lesson for future benefit. After all, not all research is published.

IMPLEMENTING HEALTH SERVICES RESEARCH

Perhaps the ultimate challenge for health services researchers is to see their research findings implemented in policy decisions. The applied nature of health services research indicates that one of its major goals is to apply disciplinary knowledge to solve current and emerging health-related problems so that resources can be better utilized to improve the health status of the population. The synthesis and the dissemination of health services research have played and continue to play an important role in health policy formulation and implementation (Ginzberg, 1991). For example, health services research has improved the public's knowledge and understanding of the health care system. It has benefited health policy formulation and implementation and management and clinical practices with respect to HIV/AIDS-related illness and primary care (National Center for Health Services Research and Health Care Technology Assessment, 1985; United States Agency for Health Care Policy and Research, 1990). The analyses made of the effects of alternative RBRVS configurations are a good example of health services research application. Health services research that has identified disturbingly large gaps in access to needed health care has served as an impetus to policies toward health care reform that aims at reducing these gaps. The community snapshots study sponsored by the Robert Wood Johnson Foundation represents a nice integration of research and practice (Ginsburg and Fasciano, 1996). The study represents the first major initiative to provide a portrait of the U.S. changing health system by capturing the process of change in 15 local health systems throughout the country. Major topics studied include developments in managed care, health services organizational change, state and local policies, and activities of purchasers, insurers, providers, and consumers.

However, application of research knowledge is not always smooth sailing, and researchers are often frustrated that their research is not taken seriously or reflected in policies. This section points out some inherent barriers hindering such goal attainment and identifies the requisites to overcoming these barriers (Patton, 1990; Frenk, 1993).

Priorities

There is a potential conflict between policy and research priorities. Decision makers, who make decisions to determine a course of action in response to a given health problem, are generally concerned about the most pressing problems that hinder the progress of their work. One of the limiting factors in the production of useful health services research is the failure by researchers to study problems that are of most concern to decision makers. Similarly, the failure of decision makers to clearly communicate their problems and concerns to health services researchers often impedes the production of useful and relevant research. The concerns of decision makers may be unknown to researchers or do not coincide with the topics that researchers consider to be of greatest scientific merit.

To overcome this barrier, the policy and research community need to have frequent dialogues. Frequent meetings between researchers and decision makers would help in understanding and appreciating the policy priorities, and research may then be planned to address these priorities. Another possible solution involves ensuring the presence of decision makers in the governing or consultative bodies of research institutions or teams, so that they can express their needs and identify opportunities in current projects.

Timetable

A potential conflict between decision makers and researchers is their different timetables expected of research. Decision makers facing a pressing problem expect the research to be completed immediately to help solve the problem. Researchers, on the other hand, are concerned with the validity of the study design and findings. To ensure all phases of the research are accomplished properly, they often demand more time than decision makers envision.

One way to reduce this gap is to involve decision makers in the planning phase of the proposed research so that the two sides may come to an agreement as to the timetable for the project. The benefit of such consultation and negotiation is that there will be few surprises. Another way to shorten the gap is to create a series of useful progress reports and intermediate results from the study. For example, a review of the current literature on related topic may be provided to decision makers shortly after the research project begins. The results of a pilot test can be forwarded. Analysis of secondary data maintained by the agency may also be presented. During data collection, the participation of respondents and their characteristics can be summarized and reported. Shortly after data collection, descriptive summaries can be shared with decision makers before in-depth analyses are conducted. These intermediate reports can be useful for decision making even before the project has been completed.

Communication

Decision makers and researchers often do not share a common set of vocabulary. For decision makers, research results must be expressed in understandable vocabulary and free of technical jargon. For researchers, as required by publication in scientific journals, results must be communicated in precise scientific terms after a detailed description of research design and analysis. Many decision makers have trouble understanding the logic of study design or the various statistics used to analyze the data set.

Both researchers and decision makers can contribute to reducing the communication barrier. For researchers, in addition to technical reports for scientific journals, they can write nontechnical reports for decision makers that summarize the most pertinent results to decision makers. If certain jargon must be used to describe the design or analysis, detailed explanations should be given. In addition, researchers can meet with decision makers to help interpret research findings and answer questions. Decision makers can also improve their knowledge of scientific research by taking research-related courses and seminars and reading scientific journals related to their areas.

Scope

Differences between policy and research scopes is another barrier to the implementation of research findings. Since social problems are inherently complicated, involving multiple factors and interconnections, decision makers require useful and relevant research to provide broad, integrated information that assesses all the dimensions of a problem and reflects all the relevant factors. In contrast, researchers are trained to focus on a well-defined, narrow subject matter in order to yield conclusive results.

To reduce the differences between policy and research scopes, it behooves researchers to be knowledgeable about the institution or problem under investigation, to be fully aware of the dimensions and related issues their research will affect, and to design an integrated project that takes into account all important policy concerns. Effective research should provide information and analysis that take into account the multiplicity of interests that exist in both the political system and the health care system. If there are research constraints, decision makers need to be informed and their expectations directed accordingly.

Values

Researchers and decision makers may place different values on research. For researchers, the value of research may be to receive publication in prestigious scientific journals and contribute to existing literature. For decision makers, the value in a research project is its immediate application to problem solving. While decision makers are concerned with problems at hand, researchers are also concerned with their peers and reputation. In addition, personal values or ideological preferences may influence decision makers' acceptance of research based on scientific evidence.

To narrow the gap in values, decision makers should have a proper and realistic expectation of the value of research. They should be better educated and informed about research. As a minimum, they need to value the type of contribution research has made toward improved decision making, and to understand the criteria for judging the quality of research. For their part, the research community should place a higher premium on efforts toward research applications. Excellence in research should be defined as not only the pursue of scientific knowledge but also the transformation of that knowledge into health policies and problem solving. Researchers should also recognize their personal biases and predilections and guard against their interference with the conduct of research. Only when both sides value each other can research findings be more properly and widely used.

Leadership

Health services research is not a substitute for leadership in implementing research. While researchers can conduct relevant and timely analysis and summarize the research results in understandable reports that can be easily used by decision makers, leadership is required to translate the knowledge derived from health services research into politically acceptable policy. Health services research cannot empower individuals who do not have the necessary authority to implement policies. The development and implementation of health care policy fundamentally depends on the leadership and initiatives of decision makers at various levels and sectors of society.

Rapport

A close rapport needs to be built up between researchers and decision makers. Both sides need each other and are interdependent. Decision makers rely on researchers to assist them in making sound and legitimate decisions that are based on scientific evidence and existing knowledge. Researchers need decision makers to identify, conduct, and implement research, including selecting research problems, obtaining funding, gaining access to research sites and subjects, and implementing research finding. The sooner both sides recognize this interdependency and work towards collaboration, the greater will be the value of health services research to policy formulation and implementation.

TRAINING NEEDS FOR HEALTH SERVICES RESEARCHER

We complete this book by identifying the needed knowledge and skills of competent health services researchers. These skills, summarized in Table 15–3, are related to each of the 10 stages in the conduct of health services research described throughout the book. They include knowledge about subject matter, methodology, statistics, computers, writing, and public relations. Without these skills and knowledge, researchers have to make sure that others in the research team possess the missing elements or that outside consultants are employed. Many of these skills can be acquired in the classroom setting, through the integration of theories and practices. However, the proficiency in research can be achieved only through numerous research projects that integrate the many phases of health services research.

TABLE 15–3 Health services research stages and skills

Research Stage	Subject	Methodology	Knowledge and Skills			
			Statistics	Computers	Writing	Public Relations
1. Conceptualization	x					
2. Groundwork	x				x	x
3. Research method		x				
4. Research design		x	x			
5. Sampling		x	x			
6. Measurement	x		x			
7. Data collection		x				x
8. Data processing				x		
9. Data analysis			x	x		
10. Application					x	x

Subject

The foremost research skill is subject-related knowledge. An in-depth knowledge of the subject matter; available research data, instruments, and funding sources; and the design of survey questionnaires is critical for the conceptualization, groundwork, and measurement stages of health services research. The conceptualization phase requires the researcher to understand the general purpose of the research, determine the specific research topic, identify relevant theories and literature, specify the meaning of concepts and variables, and formulate hypotheses or research questions. A thorough command of the subject matter with respect to literature and theories is crucial to accomplishing these research components. The groundwork phase of research requires the researcher to identify relevant data sources, explore potential funding sources, develop a research plan or proposal, and prepare organizationally and administratively to carry out the research. Knowledge of data and funding sources are fundamental requisites to fulfill these tasks. The measurement, or operationalization, phase is concerned with devising measures linking specific concepts to empirically observable events or variables. Researchers are therefore required to be knowledgeable about the general guidelines and specific techniques in constructing research instruments such as the survey questionnaires.

Methodology

The second research skill is the command of general research methods or methodology. Understanding the general approaches to research is critical in the selection of research method(s), designing studies, sampling, and data collection phases of research. Competent researchers should know the pros and cons of the various types of research approaches, including research review, meta-analysis, secondary analysis, research analysis of administrative records, qualitative research, case study, experiment, survey research, longitudinal study, and evaluation research; and assess their suitability for a given research problem. Researchers should be capable of developing an overall plan or framework for investigation. They must know how to identify the research population, choose the appropriate sampling method, and decide the optimal sample size. They must know the advantages and disadvantages of different data collection methods and select the one that maximizes both response and completion rates.

Statistics

The third important research skill is the command of statistical knowledge, particularly critical in the data analysis, design, sampling, and measurement phases of research. In data analysis, researchers use statistical procedures to analyze collected data and interpret study findings to draw conclusions about hypotheses or research questions. Knowledge about the choice and application of statistical procedures is necessary for the conduct of research independently without having to hire a statistician. Statistical knowledge can also enhance research design and sampling, which are based on statistical principles. Measurement decisions are also related to statistical knowledge because different levels of measures are subject to different types of statistical procedures. The design of a research instrument can benefit greatly from statistical knowledge. In finalizing a questionnaire, researchers should not only think about the hypotheses or research questions to be addressed but also the statistical procedures to be used in analyzing the data. Many projects get delayed when data collection is not integrated with analysis. A bad practice is to hire a statistical consultant well after data collection. The consultant is forced to deal with the existing data format, which may restrict the use of more powerful analyses.

Computers

The fourth research skill particularly critical for large data analyses is computer knowledge, especially relevant during the data processing and analysis phases. In data processing, researchers typically transform the collected raw data to some computer format. In the case of using available data, data sorting and merging are often integral parts of data preparation. In analyzing data, researchers use either mainframe or PC-based statistical software to help apply various statistical and modeling procedures.

Writing

The ability to write is another critical research skill. Whether in writing proposals for funding (the groundwork phase) or reports for publication (the application phase), good writing is a required skill and essential to convey the research to potential funders or users. In many cases, it is a matter of following structured formats (e.g., research proposals, journal articles). However, the ability to write concise and clear sentences and to organize thoughts is also important. Excellent booklets exist that help improve research writing (Becker, 1986; Cuba, 1988; Friedman and Steinberg, 1989; Strunk and White, 1979; University of Chicago Press, 1993; Wilkinson, 1991; Wolcott, 1990).

Public Relations

Last but not least is public relations skills, particularly useful in the groundwork, data collection, and application phases of research, and in project management. In the groundwork phase, seeking funding support for research requires good public relations. In data collection, getting access to research sites or subjects necessitates patience and rapport. Finally, in the application phase, collaboration with decision makers is vital for policy formulation and implementation based on research findings.

The successful completion of a research project, particularly a large one, requires that the researcher is a capable administrator. Administrative skills are reflected in hiring the research staff, supervising and coordinating research activities, managing time to keep on schedule, and responding to changes and crisis. Good human relation is a prerequisite for a good project director.

SUMMARY

The audiences for scientific research include the research community, the stakeholders, and the public. For the research community, the common means of communicating research results consist of publications in refereed scientific journals, reading research results in professional conferences, and writing working papers, monographs, or even books. Familiarity and adherence to journal requirements on content, writing style, structure, organization, use of tables and charts, and length is crucial to publication. When stakeholders are the intended audience, researchers communicate findings through research proposals, technical reports, symposiums, expert testimony, or research notes. To enhance the chance of implementing research findings in policy decisions, both researchers and policymakers should strive to improve communication, mutual understanding, and collaboration and to reduce gaps in research priorities, scope, and timetables. When the intended audience is the general public, researchers may communicate through the mass media or brochures. Health services researchers should continuously improve knowledge in subject matter, methodology, statistics, computer applications, writing, and public relations.

Review Questions

1. What are the channels of communicating research results?

2. What components are commonly shared by scientific journals when publishing scientific research?

3. How can a person develop the skills necessary to become a capable health services researcher?

REFERENCES

American Journal of Public Health. (1996). What AJPH authors should know. *American Journal of Public Health,* 86(4), 470.

Becker, H. S. (1986). *Writing for Social Scientists.* Chicago: University of Chicago Press.

Cuba, L. J. (1988). *A Short Guide to Writing About Social Science.* Glenview, IL: Scott, Foresman.

Frenk, J. (1993). The new public health. *Annual Review of Public Health,* 14, 469-490.

Friedman, S., and Steinberg, S. (1989). *Writing and Thinking in the Social Sciences.* Englewood Cliffs, NJ: Prentice-Hall.

Ginzberg, E. (1991). *Health Services Research: Key to Health Policy.* Cambridge, MA: Harvard University Press.

National Center for Health Services Research and Health Care Technology Assessment. (1985). *Health Services Research on Primary Care.* Rockville, MD: National Center for Health Services Research and Health Care Technology Assessment.

Patton, M. Q. (1990). *Qualitative Evaluation and Research Methods.* 2nd ed. Newbury Park, CA: Sage.

Strunk, W., and White, E. B. (1979). *The Elements of Style.* 3d ed. New York: Macmillan.

United States Agency for Health Care Policy and Research. (1990). *Health Services Research on HIV/AIDS-Related Illness.* Rockville, MD: Agency for Health Care Policy and Research.

University of Chicago Press. (1993). *The Chicago Manual of Style.* 14th ed. Chicago: Author.

Wilkinson, A. M. (1991). *The Scientist's Handbook for Writing Papers and Dissertations.* Englewood Cliffs, NJ: Prentice-Hall.

Wolcott, H. T. (1990). *Writing up Qualitative Research.* Newbury Park, CA: Sage.

APPENDICES

APPENDIX 1

Selected journals publishing health services research papers

- Academic Medicine
- AIDS Care
- American Journal of Nursing
- American Journal of Medicine
- American Journal of Preventive Medicine
- American Journal of Public Health
- American Journal of Medical Quality
- American Journal of Epidemiology
- American Journal of Hospital Care
- Annual Review of Public Health
- Asia-Pacific Journal of Public Health
- Australian Journal of Public Health
- British Journal of Preventive and Social Medicine
- Bulletin of the World Health Organization
- Business and Health
- Canadian Journal of Public Health
- Cancer Research
- Carolina Health Services Review
- Community Health
- Community Health Education
- Contemporary Longterm Care
- Demography
- Ethnicity and Health
- Evaluation and the Health Professions
- Family and Community Health
- Frontiers in Health Services Management
- Geriatrics
- Gerontologist
- Hastings Center Report
- Health Administration Education
- Health Affairs
- Health and Place
- Health and Social Work
- Health Care Financing Review
- Health Care for Women International
- Health Care Management Review
- Health Care Strategic Management
- Health Economics
- Health Education
- Health Education Quarterly
- Health Education Research
- Health Legislation and Regulation
- Health Management Quarterly
- Health Planning and Management
- Health Policy, Politics and Law
- Health Progress
- Health Promotion
- Health Reports
- Health Services Manager
- Health Services Research and Policy
- Health Services Research
- Health Technology Assessment Reports
- Health United States
- Health Values
- Healthcare Financial Management
- Home Health Care Services Quarterly
- Hospital and Health Services Administration
- Hospital Ethics
- Hospital Physician
- Hospital Practice
- Hospital Progress
- Hospital Statistics

- Hospital Topics
- Hospitals
- Human Services in the Rural Environment
- Inquiry
- International Journal of Health Services
- International Journal of Health Education
- International Quarterly of Community Health Education
- Issues in Law and Medicine
- Journal of Aging and Social Policy
- Journal of Allied Health
- Journal of Ambulatory Care Management
- Journal of Community Health
- Journal of Epidemiology and Community Health
- Journal of Family Practice
- Journal of Gerontology
- Journal of Health Administration Education
- Journal of Health and Human Resources Administration
- Journal of Health and Social Behavior
- Journal of Health Care for the Poor and Undeserved
- Journal of Health Care Management
- Journal of Health Care Marketing
- Journal of Health Economics
- Journal of Health Politics, Policy, and Law
- Journal of Hospital Marketing
- Journal of Human Resources
- Journal of Law and Medicine
- Journal of Long-term Care Administration
- Journal of Medicine and Philosophy
- Journal of Medical Ethics
- Journal of Medical Practice Management
- Journal of Nurse Midwifery
- Journal of Nursing Administration
- Journal of Occupational Medicine
- Journal of Perinatal and Neonatal Nursing
- Journal of Professional Nursing
- Journal of Public Health Dentistry
- Journal of Public Health Policy
- Journal of Rural Health
- Journal of Social Issues
- Journal of the American Medical Association
- Journal of the Foundation of the American Association College of Healthcare Executives
- Journal of the National Medical Association
- Journal of the Society for Health Systems
- Journal of the Society of Public Health
- Journal of Women's Health
- Lancet
- Law, Medicine and Health Care
- Managed Health Care Today
- Maternal Child Nursing Journal
- Medical Care
- Medical Care Research and Review
- Medical Decision Making
- Medical Economics
- Medical Group Management Journal
- Milbank Quarterly
- Modern Healthcare
- Monthly Vital Statistics Report
- Morbidity and Mortality Weekly Report
- Nation's Health
- New England Journal of Human Services
- New England Journal of Medicine
- Nurse Management
- Nursing Administration Quarterly
- Nursing and Health Care
- Nursing Economics
- Nursing Outlook
- Occupational Health
- Patient Care
- Perspectives in Healthcare Risk Management
- Prevention
- Preventive Medicine
- Provider

- Psychology Health and Medicine
- Public Health
- Public Health Reports
- Public Health Review
- Qualitative Health Research
- Quality Assurance in Health Care
- Quality Review Bulletin
- Reports on Health and Social Subjects
- Research in Community and Mental Health
- Research in Nursing and Health
- Scandinavian Journal of Primary Health Care
- Sciences
- Social Policy
- Social Science and Medicine
- Social Work in Health Care
- Sociology of Health and Illness
- Southern Medical Journal

- Topics in Health Care Financing
- Vital and Health Statistics. Series 1: Programs and Collection Procedures
- Vital and Health Statistics. Series 2: Data Evaluation and Methods Research
- Vital and Health Statistics. Series 3: Analytical and Epidemiological Studies
- Vital and Health Statistics. Series 4: Documents and Committee Reports
- Vital and Health Statistics. Series 5: Comparative International Vital and Health Statistics Report
- Vital and Health Statistics. Series 10–14: Data from National Health Survey.
- Vital and Health Statistics. Series 21: Data on Natality, Marriage, and Divorce
- Western Journal of Medicine
- Western Journal of Nursing Research

APPENDIX 2
Selected health services-related professional associations

Academic health science centers
Association of Academic Health Science Centers (AAHC)

Administrators
American College of Health Care Executive (ACHCE)
American College of Health Care Administrators (ACHCA)
Association of Group Medical Administrators (AGMA)
Medical Group Management Association (MGMA)
American Society of Hospital Personnel Administration
Association of Mental Health Administrators

Allied health personnel
American Society of Allied Health Professions (ASAHP)

Dentistry
American Association of Dental Schools (AADS)

Dentists
American Dental Association (ADA)

Group health organizations
American Group Practice Association (AGPA)

Health professionals and schools of public health
American Public Health Association (APHA)

Hospitals
American Hospital Association (AHA)

Medical schools
Association of American Medical Colleges (AAMC)

Nurses
American Nurses Association (ANA)

Nursing
National League of Nursing (NLN)

Pharmacy
American Association of colleges of Pharmacy (AACP)

Physicians
American Medical Association (AMA)
American College of Physician Executive (ACPE)
American Academy of Medical Directors (AAMD)

Programs/departments of health services policy and administration
Association of University Programs in Health Administration (AUPHA)
Association for Health Services Research

Rural health
American Rural Health Association

APPENDIX 3
A list of funding sources

Annual Register of Grant Support

A definitive reference book that is published annually. The volume for 1995 has 3,155 entries representing billions of dollars to potential grant seekers. It is published by National Register Publishing Co., Wilmette, IL 60091.

Aris

Monthly newsletter for biomedical sciences, social and natural sciences, creative arts, and humanities that lists program guidelines, deadlines, and contacts for government and private funding sources.

Broad Agency Announcements

Funding information from specific federal agencies.

Catalog of Federal Domestic Assistance

A comprehensive catalog of federal programs, guidelines, funding amounts, and contact persons.

Commerce Business Daily

Carries announcements of sponsored program opportunities through federal contracts.

Contracts and Grants Weekly

A weekly publication that lists the most current deadlines for funding agencies that support a variety of programs.

Directory of Research Grants

A well-indexed source of private and federal programs.

Federal Register

A daily publication for making federal agency regulations, proposed regulations, and official deadline notices available to the public.

The Foundation Directory

A listing and brief description of all major national and state foundations.

The Foundation Directory and Supplements

The national collections of source materials on the foundations and their grant-making activities. Includes basic records filed by every private foundation with the Internal Revenue Service, annual reports, and the Foundation Center's standard reference works. Information has been compiled on about 26,000 American foundations. National collections are located at the following addresses: The Foundation Center, 888 Seventh Ave., New York, NY 10019; The Foundation Center, 1001 Connecticut Ave., NW Washington, DC 20036; and Donors' Forum, 208 South Lasalle St., Chicago, IL 60604.

National Institute of Health

Offers research and research-training grants and awards in the biomedical and health-related sciences.

National Institute of Mental Health

Supports programs designed to increase knowledge and improve research methods on mental and behavioral disorders.

Source Book Profiles

Lists activities, purposes, and funding ranges of most foundations.

Taft Corporate Giving Directory

Comprehensive profiles of America's major corporate foundations and charitable giving programs.

APPENDIX 4
Public Health Service Grant Application Forms

Form Pages Only

Application for a

Public Health Service Grant
PHS 398

Includes Research Career Awards

and Institutional National

Research Service Awards

The following form pages are a *part* of the complete PHS 398 application packet. The packet also includes a booklet with instructions for preparing and submitting your application, as well as definitions, assurances, and other relevant information. Please retain the instructional booklet for future submission of applications.

AA

Form Approved Through 9/30/97
OMB No. 0925-0001

Department of Health and Human Services
Public Health Service

Grant Application

Follow instructions carefully.
Do not exceed character length restrictions indicated on sample.

LEAVE BLANK—FOR PHS USE ONLY.		
Type	Activity	Number
Review Group	Formerly	
Council/Board *(Month, Year)*		Date Received

1. TITLE OF PROJECT *(Do not exceed 56 characters, including spaces and punctuation.)*

2 RESPONSE TO SPECIFIC REQUEST FOR APPLICATIONS OR PROGRAM ANNOUNCEMENT ☐ NO ☐ YES *(If "Yes," state number and title)*
Number: Title:

3. PRINCIPAL INVESTIGATOR/PROGRAM DIRECTOR

3a. NAME *(Last, first, middle)*	3b. DEGREE(S)	3c. SOCIAL SECURITY NO.

3d POSITION TITLE

3e MAILING ADDRESS *(Street, city, state, zip code)*

3f. DEPARTMENT, SERVICE, LABORATORY, OR EQUIVALENT

3g. MAJOR SUBDIVISION

3h. TELEPHONE AND FAX *(Area code, number and extension)*
TEL:
FAX:

E-MAIL ADDRESS:

4 HUMAN SUBJECTS	4a If "Yes," Exemption no or		4b Assurance of compliance no	5 VERTEBRATE ANIMALS	5a If "Yes," IACUC approval date	5b Animal welfare assurance no
☐ No ☐ Yes	IRB approval date	☐ Full IRB or ☐ Expedited Review		☐ No ☐ Yes		

6 DATES OF PROPOSED PERIOD OF SUPPORT *(month, day, year—MM/DD/YY)*		7 COSTS REQUESTED FOR INITIAL BUDGET PERIOD		8 COSTS REQUESTED FOR PROPOSED PERIOD OF SUPPORT	
From	Through	7a Direct Costs ($)	7b Total Costs ($)	8a Direct Costs ($)	8b Total Costs ($)

9 APPLICANT ORGANIZATION	10 TYPE OF ORGANIZATION
Name	Public: → ☐ Federal ☐ State ☐ Local
Address	Private: → ☐ Private Nonprofit
	Forprofit:→ ☐ General ☐ Small Business

	11. ORGANIZATIONAL COMPONENT CODE
	12 ENTITY IDENTIFICATION NUMBER Congressional District

13. ADMINISTRATIVE OFFICIAL TO BE NOTIFIED IF AWARD IS MADE	14 OFFICIAL SIGNING FOR APPLICANT ORGANIZATION
Name	Name
Title	Title
Address	Address
Telephone	Phone
FAX	FAX
E-Mail Address	E-Mail Address

15. PRINCIPAL INVESTIGATOR/PROGRAM DIRECTOR ASSURANCE: I certify that the statements herein are true, complete and accurate to the best of my knowledge. I am aware that any false, fictitious, or fraudulent statements or claims may subject me to criminal, civil, or administrative penalties. I agree to accept responsibility for the scientific conduct of the project and to provide the required progress reports if a grant is awarded as a result of this application.	SIGNATURE OF PI / PD NAMED IN 3a *(In ink "Per" signature not acceptable.)*	DATE
16. APPLICANT ORGANIZATION CERTIFICATION AND ACCEPTANCE: I certify that the statements herein are true, complete and accurate to the best of my knowledge, and accept the obligation to comply with Public Health Service terms and conditions if a grant is awarded as a result of this application. I am aware that any false, fictitious, or fraudulent statements or claims may subject me to criminal, civil, or administrative penalties.	SIGNATURE OF OFFICIAL NAMED IN 14 *(In ink "Per" signature not acceptable)*	DATE

PHS 398 (Rev. 5/95)   Face Page   AA

BB   Principal Investigator/Program Director *(Last, first, middle):* _____

DESCRIPTION. State the application's broad, long-term objectives and specific aims, making reference to the health relatedness of the project. Describe concisely the research design and methods for achieving these goals. Avoid summaries of past accomplishments and the use of the first person This description is meant to serve as a succinct and accurate description of the proposed work when separated from the application. If the application is funded, this description, as is, will become public information. Therefore, do not include proprietary/confidential information. **DO NOT EXCEED THE SPACE PROVIDED.**

PERFORMANCE SITE(S) *(organization, city, state)*

KEY PERSONNEL. See instructions on Page 11 *Use continuation pages as needed* to provide the required information in the format shown below.

Name	Organization	Role on Project

⬙

CC   Principal Investigator/Program Director *(Last, first, middle):* _____

Type the name of the principal investigator/program director at the top of each printed page and each continuation page. (For type specifications, see instructions on page 6.)

RESEARCH GRANT

TABLE OF CONTENTS

Page Numbers

Research Plan

*Type density and type size of the entire application must conform to limits provided in instructions on page 6

Appendix *(Five collated sets No page numbering necessary for Appendix)*

    Number of publications and manuscripts accepted or submitted for publication *(not to exceed 10)* _____

    Other items *(list):*

☐ Check if Appendix is included

DD   Principal Investigator/Program Director *(Last, first, middle):* _____

DETAILED BUDGET FOR INITIAL BUDGET PERIOD
DIRECT COSTS ONLY

FROM	THROUGH

PERSONNEL *(Applicant organization only)*					DOLLAR AMOUNT REQUESTED *(omit cents)*		
NAME	ROLE ON PROJECT	TYPE APPT. *(months)*	% EFFORT ON PROJ.	INST. BASE SALARY	SALARY REQUESTED	FRINGE BENEFITS	TOTALS
	Principal Investigator						
SUBTOTALS ⟶							

CONSULTANT COSTS

EQUIPMENT *(Itemize)*

SUPPLIES *(Itemize by category)*

TRAVEL

| **PATIENT CARE COSTS** | INPATIENT |
| | OUTPATIENT |

ALTERATIONS AND RENOVATIONS *(Itemize by category)*

OTHER EXPENSES *(Itemize by category)*

SUBTOTAL DIRECT COSTS FOR INITIAL BUDGET PERIOD	$

| **CONSORTIUM/CONTRACTUAL COSTS** | DIRECT COSTS |
| | INDIRECT COSTS |

TOTAL DIRECT COSTS FOR INITIAL BUDGET PERIOD *(Item 7a, Face Page)* ⟶	$

EE   Principal Investigator/Program Director *(Last, first, middle)*: _____

BUDGET FOR ENTIRE PROPOSED PERIOD OF SUPPORT
DIRECT COSTS ONLY

BUDGET CATEGORY TOTALS		INITIAL BUDGET PERIOD *(from Form Page 4)*	ADDITIONAL YEARS OF SUPPORT REQUESTED			
			2nd	3rd	4th	5th
PERSONNEL: *Salary and fringe benefits* *Applicant organization only*						
CONSULTANT COSTS						
EQUIPMENT						
SUPPLIES						
TRAVEL						
PATIENT CARE COSTS	INPATIENT					
	OUTPATIENT					
ALTERATIONS AND RENOVATIONS						
OTHER EXPENSES						
SUBTOTAL DIRECT COSTS						
CONSORTIUM/ CONTRACTUAL COSTS	DIRECT					
	INDIRECT					
TOTAL DIRECT COSTS						

TOTAL DIRECT COSTS FOR ENTIRE PROPOSED PERIOD OF SUPPORT *(Item 8a, Face Page)* → | $ |

JUSTIFICATION. Follow the budget justification instructions exactly. Use continuation pages as needed

FF   Principal Investigator/Program Director *(Last, first, middle):* _____

BIOGRAPHICAL SKETCH

Provide the following information for the key personnel in the order listed on Form Page 2.
Photocopy this page or follow this format for each person.

NAME	POSITION TITLE

EDUCATION/TRAINING *(Begin with baccalaureate or other initial professional education, such as nursing, and include postdoctoral training.)*

INSTITUTION AND LOCATION	DEGREE *(if applicable)*	YEAR(s)	FIELD OF STUDY

RESEARCH AND PROFESSIONAL EXPERIENCE: Concluding with present position, list, in chronological order, previous employment, experience, and honors. Include present membership on any Federal Government public advisory committee. List, in chronological order, the titles, all authors, and complete references to all publications during the past three years and to representative earlier publications pertinent to this application. If the list of publications in the last three years exceeds two pages, select the most pertinent publications **DO NOT EXCEED TWO PAGES.**

GG

Other Support

There is no form page for other support. Information on other support should be provided in the *format* shown below, using Continuation Pages. *Include the Principal Investigator's name at the top and number consecutively with the rest of the application.* The sample is intended to provide guidance regarding the type and extent of information requested. For the instructions and explanation of the sample below, see page 14. For information pertaining to the use of and policy for other support, see page 25.

Format

NAME OF INDIVIDUAL		
ACTIVE/PENDING		
Project Number (Principal Investigator) Source Title of Project *(or Subproject)*	Dates of Approved/Proposed Project Annual Direct Costs	Percent Effort
The major goals of this project are…		
OVERLAP *(summarized for each individual)*		

Samples

ANDERSON, R.R.

ACTIVE

2 R01 HL 00000-13 (Anderson) NIH/NHLBI Chloride and Sodium Transport in Airway Epithelial Cells	3/1/94 – 2/28/97 $186,529	30%

The major goals of this project are to define the biochemistry of chloride and sodium transport in airway epithelial cells and clone the gene(s) involved in transport.

5 R01 HL 00000-07 (Baker) NIH/NHLBI Ion Transport in Fetal Lung	4/1/91 – 3/31/96 $122,717	10%

The major goal of this project is to study chloride and sodium transport in normal and cystic fibrosis fetal lung.

R000 (Anderson) Cystic Fibrosis Foundation Gene Transfer of CFTR to the Airway Epithelium	9/1/93 – 8/31/95 $43,123	10%

The major goals of this project are to identify and isolate airway epithelium progenitor cells and express human CFTR in airway epithelial cells.

PENDING

DCB 950000 (Anderson) National Science Foundation Liposome Membrane Composition and Function	12/01/95 – 11/30/97 $82,163	20%

The major goals of this project are to define biochemical properties of liposome membrane components and maximize liposome uptake into cells.

OVERLAP

There is scientific overlap between aim 2 of NSF DCB 950000 and aim 4 of the application under consideration. If both are funded, the budgets will be adjusted appropriately in conjunction with agency staff.

RICHARDS, L.

NONE

(Format Page 7)   GG

GG

Other Support *(Continued)*

HERNANDEZ, M.

ACTIVE

5 R01 CA 00000-07 (Hernandez)	4/1/91 – 3/31/96	40% academic
NIH/NCI		
Gene Therapy for Small Cell Lung Carcinoma		

The major goals of this project are to use viral strategies to express the normal p53 gene in human SCLC cell lines and to study the effect on growth and invasiveness of the lines.

5 P01 CA 00000-03 (Chen)	7/1/92 – 6/30/97	20% academic
NIH/NCI	$104,428 (sub only)	100% summer
Mutations in p53 in Progression of Small Cell Lung Carcinoma		

The major goals of this subproject are to define the p53 mutations in SCLC and their contribution to tumor progression and metastasis.

BE 00000 (Hernandez)	9/1/93 – 8/31/96	20% academic
American Cancer Society	$86,732	
p53 Mutations in Breast Cancer		

The major goals of this project are to define the spectrum of p53 mutations in human breast cancer samples and correlate the results with clinical outcome.

OVERLAP

Potential commitment overlap for Dr. Hernandez between 5 R01 CA 00000-07 and the application under consideration. If the application under consideration is funded with Dr. Hernandez committed at 30 percent effort, Dr. Hernandez will request approval to reduce her effort on the NCI grant.

BENNETT, P.

ACTIVE

Investigator Award (Bennett)	9/1/93 – 8/31/97	70%
Howard Hughes Medical Institute	$581,317	
Gene Cloning and Targeting for Neurological Disease Genes		

This award supports the PI's program to map and clone the gene(s) implicated in the development of Alzheimer's disease and to target expression of the cloned gene(s) to relevant cells.

OVERLAP

None

CHU, H.

ACTIVE

94RD000 (Chu)	5/1/94 – 5/30/96	30%
Univ. Respiratory Diseases Coordinating Committee	$48,000 (no salary)	
Improved Detection of Non-malignant Lung Diseases		

The major goals of this project are to develop and test a sensitive, PCR-based method to discriminate among respiratory fungal infections.

OVERLAP

None

(Format Page 7, continued)

GG

HH   Principal Investigator/Program Director *(Last, first, middle):* _____

RESOURCES

FACILITIES: Specify the facilities to be used for the conduct of the proposed research Indicate the performance sites and describe capacities, pertinent capabilities, relative proximity, and extent of availability to the project. Under "Other," identify support services such as machine shop, electronics shop, and specify the extent to which they will be available to the project. Use continuation pages if necessary

Laboratory:

Clinical:

Animal:

Computer:

Office:

Other:

MAJOR EQUIPMENT: List the most important equipment items already available for this project, noting the location and pertinent capabilities of each.

II

Principal Investigator/Program Director *(Last, first, middle):* _____

CHECKLIST

TYPE OF APPLICATION *(Check all that apply.)*

☐ **NEW** application *(This application is being submitted to the PHS for the first time)*

☐ **REVISION** of application number: _____
(This application replaces a prior unfunded version of a new, competing continuation, or supplemental application)

☐ **COMPETING CONTINUATION** of grant number: _____
(This application is to extend a funded grant beyond its current project period)

INVENTIONS AND PATENTS *(Competing continuation appl.only)*
☐ No
☐ Yes I: "Yes," ☐ Previously reported
☐ Not previously reported

☐ **SUPPLEMENT** to grant number: _____
(This application is for additional funds to supplement a currently funded grant.)

☐ **CHANGE** of principal investigator/program director.
Name of former principal investigator/program director: _____

☐ **FOREIGN** application or significant foreign component

1. ASSURANCES/CERTIFICATIONS

The following assurances/certifications are made and verified by the signature of the Official Signing for Applicant Organization on the Face Page of the application. Descriptions of individual assurances/certifications begin on page 27 of Section III. If unable to certify compliance where applicable, provide an explanation and place it after this page

•Human Subjects; •Vertebrate Animals; •Debarment and Suspension; •Drug-Free Workplace *(applicable to new [Type 1] or revised [Type 1] applications only)*; •Lobbying; •Delinquent Federal Debt; •Research Misconduct; •Civil Rights (Form HHS 441 or HHS 690); •Handicapped Individuals (Form HHS 641 or HHS 690); •Sex Discrimination (Form HHS 639-A or HHS 690); •Age Discrimination (Form HHS 680 or HHS 690); •Financial Conflict of Interest

2. PROGRAM INCOME *(See instructions, page 20)*

All applications must indicate whether program income is anticipated during the period(s) for which grant support is requested If program income is anticipated, use the format below to reflect the amount and source(s)

Budget Period	Anticipated Amount	Source(s)

3. INDIRECT COSTS

Indicate the applicant organization's most recent indirect cost rate established with the appropriate DHHS Regional Office, or, in the case of forprofit organizations, the rate established with the appropriate PHS Agency Cost Advisory Office If the applicant organization is in the process of initially developing or renegotiating a rate, or has established a rate with another Federal agency, it should, immediately upon notification that an award will be made, develop a tentative indirect cost rate proposal This is to be based on

its most recently completed fiscal year in accordance with the principles set forth in the pertinent *DHHS Guide for Establishing Indirect Cost Rates,* and submitted to the appropriate DHHS Regional Office or PHS Agency Cost Advisory Office Indirect costs will *not* be paid on foreign grants, construction grants, grants to Federal organizations, grants to individuals, and conference grants Follow any additional instructions provided for Research Career Awards, Institutional National Research Service Awards, and specialized grant applications

☐ DHHS Agreement dated: _____

☐ No Indirect Costs Requested

☐ DHHS Agreement being negotiated with _____ Regional Office

☐ No DHHS Agreement, but rate established with _____ Date _____

CALCULATION* *(The entire grant application, including the Checklist, will be reproduced and provided to peer reviewers as confidential information Supplying the following information on indirect costs is optional for forprofit organizations)*

a Initial budget period: Amount of base $ _____ x Rate applied _____ % = Indirect costs (1) $ _____

b Entire proposed project period: Amount of base $ _____ x Rate applied _____ % = Indirect costs (2) $ _____
          (1) Add to total direct costs from form page 4 and enter new total on Face Page, Item 7b
          (2) Add to total direct costs from form page 5 and enter new total on Face Page, Item 8b

*Check appropriate box(es):
☐ Salary and wages base   ☐ Modified total direct cost base   ☐ Other base *(Explain)*
☐ Off-site, other special rate, or more than one rate involved *(Explain)*

Explanation *(Attach separate sheet, if necessary.):*

4. SMOKE-FREE WORKPLACE

Does your organization currently provide a smoke-free workplace and/or promote the nonuse of tobacco products or have plans to do so?
☐ Yes   ☐ No *(The response to this question has no impact on the review or funding of this application)*

JJ   Principal Investigator/Program Director *(Last, first, middle):* _____

Competing Continuation Applications
PERSONNEL REPORT

All Personnel for the Current Budget Period

Name	Degree(s)	SSN	Role on Project (e g PI, Res Assoc)	Date of Birth (MM/DD/YY)	Annual % Effort

PHS 398 (Rev. 5/95)   Page _____   JJ

KK   Principal Investigator/Program Director *(Last, first, middle):* _____

Place this form at the end of the signed original
copy of the application. Do not duplicate

PERSONAL DATA ON
PRINCIPAL INVESTIGATOR/PROGRAM DIRECTOR

The Public Health Service has a continuing commitment to monitor the operation of its review and award processes to detect—and deal appropriately with—any instances of real or apparent inequities with respect to age, sex, race, or ethnicity of the proposed principal investigator/program director.

To provide the PHS with the information it needs for this important task, complete the form below and attach it to the signed original of the application after the Checklist. **Do not attach copies of this form to the duplicated copies of the application.**

Upon receipt of the application by the PHS, this form will be separated from the application. This form will **not** be duplicated, and it will **not** be a part of the review process Data will be confidential, and will be maintained in Privacy Act record system 09-25-0036, "Grants: IMPAC (Grant/Contract Information)." All analyses conducted on the data will report aggregate statistical findings only and will not identify individuals.

If you decline to provide this information, it will in no way affect consideration of your application.

Your cooperation will be appreciated.

DATE OF BIRTH *(MM/DD/YY)*	GENDER
	☐ Female ☐ Male

RACE AND/OR ETHNIC ORIGIN *(check one)*

Note: The category that most closely reflects the individual's recognition in the community should be used when reporting mixed racial and/or ethnic origins.

☐   *American Indian or Alaskan Native.* A person having origins in any of the original peoples of North America, and who maintains a cultural identification through tribal affiliation or community recognition.

☐   *Asian or Pacific Islander.* A person having origins in any of the original peoples of the Far East, Southeast Asia, the Indian subcontinent, or the Pacific Islands This area includes, for example, China, India, Japan, Korea, the Philippine Islands, and Samoa.

☐   *Black, not of Hispanic origin.* A person having origins in any of the black racial groups of Africa.

☐   *Hispanic.* A person of Mexican, Puerto Rican, Cuban, Central or South American, or other Spanish culture or origin, regardless of race

☐   *White, not of Hispanic origin.* A person having origins in any of the original peoples of Europe, North Africa, or the Middle East.

☐   Check here if you do not wish to provide some or all of the above information

PHS 398 (Rev 5/95)   Do not page number this form   KK

Mailing address for application package

Use this label or a facsimile.

**Division of Research Grants
National Institutes of Health
Suite 1040
6701 ROCKLEDGE DR MSC 7710
BETHESDA MD   20892–7710**

Applicants who wish to use express mail or courier
service should change the zipcode to 20817.

C.O.D. applications will *not* be accepted.

For application in response to RFA

Use this label or a facsimile.

IF THIS APPLICATION IS IN RESPONSE TO AN RFA, be sure to put the RFA number in Item 2
of the application face page. In addition, after duplicating copies of the application, cut along the
dotted line below and staple the RFA label to the **bottom** of the face page of the original and
place the original on top of your entire package. Failure to use this RFA label could result in
delayed processing of your application such that it may not reach the review committee on time
for review. *Do not use* the label unless the application is in response to a specific RFA. Also,
application responding to a specific RFA should be sure to follow all special mailing instructions
published in the RFA.

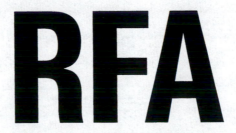

❖

LL

Candidate (Last, first, middle): _____

Use this substitute page for the Table of Contents of Research Career Awards

Type the name of candidate at the top of each printed page and continuation page

RESEARCH CAREER AWARD

TABLE OF CONTENTS

(Substitute Page)

Page Numbers

Section I: Basic Administrative Data

1–3 Face Page, Description and Key Personnel, Table of Contents *(Form pages AA, BB, and this substitute page)* .   ...   1-_____

4 Detailed Budget for Initial Budget Period *(Form page DD)* .   ..   _____

5. Budget for Entire Proposed Period of Support *(Form page EE)* .   .   ..   _____

6. Biographical Sketches *(Candidate and Sponsor[s]*—Form page FF)* .   .   .   _____

7 Other Support *(Candidate and Sponsor[s]*—Format pages GG)* .   .   ..   _____

8. Resources *(Form page HH)*   .   .   ..   _____

Section II: Specialized Information

1. The Candidate

  a Letters of Reference *(Attach to Face Page)*   ..   .   .   _____

  b Candidate's Background   . .   .   .   .   _____

  c Career Goals and Objectives: Scientific Biography . .   .   *(Not to exceed 5 pages)* .   _____

  d Career Development Activities during Award Period   ..   .   _____

2. Statements by Sponsor(s), Consultant(s), and Collaborator(s)*   _____

3. Environment and Institutional Commitment to Candidate

  a. Description of Institutional Environment   . .. .   _____

  b Institutional Commitment to Candidate's Research Career Development   ..   .   _____

4. Research Plan *(Introduction for Revised Application and General Comments)*

  a Statement of Hypothesis and Specific Aims   . .. .   _____

  b Background, Significance, and Rationale   ..   ..   _____

  c Preliminary Studies and Any Results   *(Not to exceed 20 pages)* . ...   _____

  d Research Design and Methods   .. .   .   _____

Section III: Other Information

1. Research Plan Continued *(see pages 17–19)*

  a Minorities and Women*   ..   . .   _____

  b Human Subjects*   .   .   .   . .   _____

  c Vertebrate Animals*   .   .   . .   _____

  d Literature Cited   ..   ..   _____

  e Consortium/Contractual Arrangements* ..   . .   _____

2. Checklist *(Include form pages II–KK)* .. ..   _____

3. Appendix *(Five collated sets. No page numbering necessary.)*

  Number of publications *(not to exceed six)*: _____

  List of key items:

Note: Type density and size for the entire application must conform to the instructions on page 6 of the general instructions.

*Include these items only when applicable

CITIZENSHIP

☐ U S citizen or noncitizen national   ☐ Permanent resident of U.S   ☐ If a permanent resident of the U.S., a notarized statement is included with the application

MM

RESEARCH CAREER AWARD REFERENCE GUIDELINES *(Series K)*

RCA Reference Report   Application Submission Deadline:_____

Title of Award: _____   Type of Award:_____

Name of Candidate *(Last, first, middle):* _____

Name of Respondent *(Last, first, middle):* _____

The candidate is applying to the National Institutes of Health for a Research Career Award (RCA). The purpose of this award is to develop the research capabilities and career of the applicant. These awards provide up to five years of salary support and guarantee them the ability to devote at least 75–80 percent of their time to research for the duration of the award. Many of these awards also provide funds for research and career development costs. The award is available to persons who have demonstrated considerable potential to become independent researchers, but who need additional supervised research experience in a productive scientific setting.

We would appreciate receiving your evaluation of the above candidate with special reference to:

- potential for conducting research;
- evidence of originality;
- adequacy of scientific background;
- quality of research endeavors or publications to date, if any;
- commitment to health-oriented research; and
- need for further research experience and training.

Any related comments that you may wish to provide would be welcomed. These references will be used by PHS committees of consultants in assessing candidates.

Complete the report in English on 8-1/2 x 11" sheets of paper. Return your reference report to the candidate *sealed* in the envelope *as soon as possible* and in sufficient time so that the candidate can meet the application submission deadline. References must be submitted with the application.

We have asked the candidate to provide you with a self-addressed envelope with the following words in the front bottom corner: *"DO NOT OPEN—PHS USE ONLY."* Candidates are not to open the references. Under the Privacy Act of 1974, RCA candidates may request personal information contained in their records, including this reference. Thank you for your assistance.

NN _____ Program Director *(Last, first, middle):* _____

Type the name of the program director at the top of each printed page and each continuation page. (For type specifications, see instructions on page 6.)

INSTITUTIONAL NATIONAL RESEARCH SERVICE AWARD

(Substitute Page)

TABLE OF CONTENTS

Page Numbers

Face Page, Description and Personnel, Table of Contents *(NRSA Substitute Page)* .. ..   1-_____
Detailed Budget for Initial Budget Period *(NRSA Substitute Page)* . ...   _____
Budget for Entire Proposed Period of Support *(NRSA Substitute Page)* . ...   _____
Biographical Sketch-Program Director *(Not to exceed 2 pages)* . . . .   _____
Other Biographical Sketches *(Not to exceed 2 pages for each)* .. . .   _____
Resources .   .. .   _____

Research Training Program Plan

Introduction to Revised Application *(Not to exceed 3 pages)* .. ..   _____
Introduction to Supplemental Application *(Not to exceed 1 page)* . . ..   _____

   a   Background . . . .   _____
   b   Program Plan . .. .   _____
      1   Program Direction . . ..   _____
      2   Program Faculty . . ..   _____
      3   Proposed Training   . . . .   *(Items a–e: not to exceed 25 pages,* _____
      4.   Trainee Candidates . . . .   *excluding tables")* _____
   c   Recruitment of Individuals from Underrepresented Racial/Ethnic Groups . .. .   _____
   d   Responsible Conduct of Research . . . .   _____
   e   Progress Report (Competing Continuation Applications Only) . .. . .   _____
   f   Human Subjects . . . .   _____
   g   Vertebrate Animals . . . .   _____
Checklist . . . .   _____

*Type density and type size of the entire application must conform to limits provided in instructions on page 6

Appendix *(Five collated sets. Pages should be numbered consecutively.)*

OO

Program Director (*Last, first, middle*): _____

DETAILED BUDGET FOR INITIAL BUDGET PERIOD DIRECT COSTS ONLY (NRSA Substitute Page)	FROM	THROUGH

STIPENDS   DOLLAR TOTAL

PREDOCTORAL

                                                                                          No. requested: $

POSTDOCTORAL (*Itemize*)

                                                                                          No. requested: $

OTHER (*Specify*)

                                                                                          No. requested: $

TOTAL STIPENDS ————————————————————————————————→ $

TUITION, FEES, AND INSURANCE (*Itemize*)

                                                                                                                    $

TRAINEE TRAVEL (*Describe*)

                                                                                                                    $

TRAINING-RELATED EXPENSES

                                                                                                                    $

TOTAL DIRECT COSTS FOR INITIAL BUDGET PERIOD (*Also enter on Face Page, Item 7*) ————→ | $ |

PHS 398 (Rev 5/95)   (Form Page 4) Page _____
Number pages consecutively at the bottom throughout the application Do <u>not</u> use suffixes such as 3a, 3b

NRSA Substitute Page
OO

PP   Program Director *(Last, first, middle):* _____

BUDGET FOR ENTIRE PROPOSED PERIOD OF SUPPORT
DIRECT COSTS ONLY (NRSA Substitute Page)

BUDGET CATEGORY TOTALS	INITIAL BUDGET PERIOD *(from Form Page 4)*		ADDITIONAL YEARS OF SUPPORT REQUESTED								
			2nd		3rd		4th		5th		
	No	$	No	$	No	$	No	$	No	$	
PREDOCTORAL STIPENDS											
POSTDOCTORAL STIPENDS											
OTHER STIPENDS											
TOTAL STIPENDS											
TUITION, FEES, AND INSURANCE											
TRAINEE TRAVEL											
TRAINING-RELATED EXPENSES											
TOTAL DIRECT COSTS											

TOTAL DIRECT COSTS FOR ENTIRE PROPOSED PERIOD OF SUPPORT *(Item 8a, Face Page)* → $

JUSTIFICATION For all years, explain the basis for the budget categories requested Follow the instructions for the Initial Budget Period and include anticipated postdoctoral levels. No explanation is required for Training-Related Expenses

APPENDIX 5

Table of random number

Random Numbers

10097	32533	76520	13586	34673	54876	80959	09117	39292	74945
37542	04805	64894	74296	24805	24037	20636	10402	00822	91665
08422	68953	19645	09303	23209	02560	15953	34764	35080	33606
99019	02529	09376	70715	38311	31165	88676	74397	04436	27659
12807	99970	80157	36147	64032	36653	98951	16877	12171	76833
66065	74717	34072	76850	36697	36170	65813	39885	11199	29170
31060	10805	45571	82406	35303	42614	86799	07439	23403	09732
85269	77602	02051	65692	68665	74818	73053	85247	18623	88579
63573	32135	05325	47048	90553	57548	28468	28709	83491	25624
73796	45753	03529	64778	35808	34282	60935	20344	35273	88435
98520	17767	14905	68607	22109	40558	60970	93433	50500	73998
11805	05431	39808	27732	50725	68248	29405	24201	52775	67851
83452	99634	06288	98083	13746	70078	18475	40610	68711	77817
88685	40200	86507	58401	36766	67951	90364	76493	29609	11062
99594	67348	87517	64969	91826	08928	93785	61368	23478	34113
65481	17674	17468	50950	58047	76974	73039	57186	40218	16544
80124	35635	17727	08015	45318	22374	21115	78253	14385	53763
74350	99817	77402	77214	43236	00210	45521	64237	96286	02655
69916	26803	66252	29148	36936	87203	76621	13990	94400	56418
09893	20505	14225	68514	46427	56788	96297	78822	54382	14598
91499	14523	68479	27686	46162	83554	94750	89923	37089	20048
80336	94598	26940	36858	70297	34135	53140	33340	42050	82341
44104	81949	85157	47954	32979	26575	57600	40881	22222	06413
12550	73742	11100	02040	12860	74697	96644	89439	28707	25815
63606	49329	16505	34484	40219	52563	43651	77082	07207	31790
61196	90446	26457	47774	51924	33729	65394	59593	42582	60527
15474	45266	95270	79953	59367	83848	82396	10118	33211	59466
94557	28573	67897	54387	54622	44431	91190	42592	92927	45973
42481	16213	97344	08721	16868	48767	03071	12059	25701	46670
23523	78317	73208	89837	68935	91416	26252	29663	05522	82562
04493	52494	75246	33824	45862	51025	61962	79335	65337	12472
00549	97654	64051	88159	96119	63896	54692	82391	23287	29529
35963	15307	26898	09354	33351	35462	77974	50024	90103	39333
59808	08391	45427	26842	83609	49700	13021	24892	78565	20106
46058	85236	01390	92286	77281	44077	93910	83647	70617	42941
32179	00597	87379	25241	05567	07007	86743	17157	85394	11838
69234	61406	20117	45204	15956	60000	18743	92423	97118	96338
19565	41430	01758	75379	40419	21585	66674	36806	84962	85207
45155	14938	19476	07246	43667	94543	59047	90033	20826	69541
94864	31994	36168	10851	34888	81553	01540	35456	05014	51176
98086	24826	45240	28404	44999	08896	39094	73407	35441	31880
33185	16232	41941	50949	89435	48581	88695	41994	37548	73043
80951	00406	96382	70774	20151	23387	25016	25298	94624	61171
79752	49140	71961	28296	69861	02591	74852	20539	00387	59579
18633	32537	98145	06571	31010	24674	05455	61427	77938	91936
74029	43902	77557	32270	97790	17119	52527	58021	80814	51748
54178	45611	80993	37143	05335	12969	56127	19255	36040	90324
11664	49883	52079	84827	59381	71539	09973	33440	88461	23356
48324	77928	31249	64710	02295	36870	32307	57546	15020	09994
69074	94138	87637	91976	35584	04401	10518	21615	01848	76938
09188	20097	32825	39527	04220	86304	83389	87374	64278	58044
90045	85497	51981	50654	94938	81997	91870	76150	68476	64659
73189	50207	47677	26269	62290	64464	27124	67018	41361	82760
75768	76490	20971	87749	90429	12272	95375	05871	93823	43178
54016	44056	66281	31003	00682	27398	20714	53295	07706	17813

Source: RAND Corporation, 1955. *A Million Random Digits with 100,000 Normal Deviates.* Copyright 1955 and 1983 by the RAND Corporation. Used by permission.

GLOSSARY

The numbers in parentheses refer to chapters in the book.

Acquiescence (13) Acquiescence refers to responses to questions based on respondent's perception of what would be desirable to the interviewer.

Activities of daily living (ADL) (2) ADL are often used to measure functional activity limitations of the elderly and the chronically ill. They include the ability of a person to function independently or with assistance in activities such as bathing, dressing, toileting, transferring in and out of a bed or chair, continence, and feeding. See also *instrumental activities of daily living (IADL).*

Agency relationship (2) Physicians make medical decisions on behalf of patients due to patients' relative ignorance. However, physicians' decisions typically reflect, not only the preferences of their patients, but also their own self-interest, the pressures from professional colleagues and institutions, a sense of medical ethics, and a desire to make good use of available resources.

Analytic research (2) See *explanatory research.*

Applied research (2) Research that focuses on contemporary social problems.

Assumptions (1) Suppositions that are considered true but not tested.

Asymmetrical relationship (1) A form of relationship between two variables in which change in one variable is accompanied by change in the other, but not vice versa.

Attrition (7) A threat to internal validity, attrition refers to the loss of subjects in an experiment. Attrition poses the greatest threat to internal validity when there is differential attrition, that is, when the experimental and control groups have different dropout rates. Invariably, those subjects who drop out differ in important ways from those who remain, so that the experimental conditions are no longer equivalent in composition.

Auspices (13) Auspices refers to responses to questions dictated by the opinion or image of the sponsor, rather than the actual questions.

Basic research (2) See *theoretical research.*

Behavioral risk factors (2) Certain lifestyles deemed harmful to a person's health and predictive of increased risk of certain diseases and mortality. Examples are cigarette smoking, alcohol abuse, lack of exercise, unsafe driving, poor dietary habits, and uncontrolled hypertension.

Biomedical research (1) Research primarily concerned with the conditions, processes, and mechanisms of health and illness at the subindividual level.

Bivariate analysis (14) Bivariate analysis examines the relationship between two variables at a time. Bivariate analysis may be conducted to determine whether there exists a relationship between two variables (i.e., effect) and, if an relationship exists, how much influence one variable has on the other (i.e., magnitude).

Burden of illness (2) Direct and indirect economic costs associated with the use of health care resources and functional restrictions imposed by illness.

Case study (6) A popular qualitative research method, a case study may be defined as an empirical inquiry that uses multiple sources of evidence to investigate a real-life social entity or phenomenon. It is particularly valuable when the research aims to capture individual differences or unique variations from one program setting to another, or from one program experience to another. A case can be a person, an event, a program, an organization, a time period, a critical incident, or a community. Regardless of the unit of analysis, a case study seeks to describe that unit in depth and detail, in context, and holistically.

CATI (13)   Computer-assisted telephone interview system in which survey questions are displayed on computer terminals for interviewers, who type respondents' answers directly into the computer.

Causal modeling (14)   An integral step in path analysis, causal modeling requires the researcher to think causally about the research question and construct an arrow diagram that reflects causal processes. Such a process identifies variables for analysis based on a theoretical framework, literature review, and observations, and the ensuing models are likely to be theory driven.

Causal relationship (1)   A form of relationship between two or more variables in which change in one variable causes change in other variable(s).

Causal research (2)   See *explanatory research*.

Certificate of Need (CON) (2)   A state-based regulatory measure responsible for the planning and diffusion of expensive medical technology. It is a process by which hospitals or other health care providers seeking a substantial expansion of their scope of services or physical facilities seek prior approval from a government-endorsed entity.

Chi-square (14)   A common test for independence. Chi-square (χ^2) is based on a comparison between an observed frequency table with an expected frequency table, or the table the researcher would expect to find if the two variables were statistically independent, that is, unrelated to one another.

Chi-square-based measures (14)   Chi-square-based measures are used to assess the extent of the relationship between two nominal-level variables. These measures modify the chi-square statistics to reduce the influence of sample size and degrees of freedom and to restrict the values between zero and one. Examples include the phi coefficient (ϕ), Pearson's coefficient of contingency (C), and Cramér's V.

Clinical research (1)   Research focusing primarily on studying the efficacy of the preventive, diagnostic, and therapeutic services applied to individual patients.

Cluster sampling (11)   A type of probability sampling method that first breaks population into groups or clusters and then randomly selects a sample of clusters.

Code sheet (13)   A code sheet may be called a data transfer sheet because responses from the instrument are recorded or transferred into the code sheet before being entered into the computer. Code sheets are usually necessary for questionnaires with open-ended questions for which it is impossible to precode.

Code book (13)   A code book is a document that describes the locations allocated to different variables and lists the numerical codes assigned to represent different attributes of variables.

Coding (13)   Coding consists of assigning numbers to questionnaire answer categories and specifying column locations for these numbers in the computer data file.

Cohort (5)   A cohort consists of persons (or other units, such as organizations) that experience the same significant life event within a specified period of time (e.g., a particular illness) or have some characteristic in common (e.g., same date of birth or marriage, membership in the same organization, etc.).

Comparison group (7)   A control group selected by a nonrandom method. The comparison group should be as similar as possible to the experimental group.

Concept (1)   Mental image or perception. Concepts may be impossible to observe directly, such as equity or ethics, or they may have referents that are readily observable, such as a hospital or a clinic.

Conceptual framework (1)   The philosophical concerns, theories, and methodological approaches toward scientific inquiry that characterize a particular discipline.

Conceptualization (2)   The refinement and specification of abstract concepts into concrete terms.

Concurrent validity (12)   A measure of validity, concurrent validity may be tested by comparing results of one measurement with those of a similar measurement administered to the same population at approximately the same time. If both measurements yield similar results, then concurrent validity can be established.

Construct validity (12)   A measure of validity, construct validity refers to the fact that the measure captures the major dimensions of the concept under study.

Contamination (7)   Refers to the phenomenon that the methods or materials of the intervention program are used to some extent by the supposed control group or vice versa.

Content analysis (5)   A research method appropriate for studying human communication and aspects of social or health behavior. The basic goal is to take a verbal, nonquantitative document and transform it into quantitative data. The usual units of analysis in content analysis are words, paragraphs, books, pictures, advertisements, television episodes, and the like.

Content validity (12)   A measure of validity, content validity refers to the representativeness of the response categories used to represent each of the dimensions of a concept.

Control group (7)   Includes those individuals or other units of analysis that do not receive the treatment or program, or receive an alternative treatment or program.

Controlled experiment (7)   See *laboratory experiment.*

Convenience sampling (11)   A type of nonprobability sampling method, convenience sampling relies on available subjects for inclusion as a sample.

Cost–benefit analysis (CBA) (9)   Cost–benefit analysis compares the benefits of a program with its costs. Both direct and indirect benefits and costs are identified, quantified, translated into a common measurement unit (usually a monetary unit), and projected into the future to reflect the lifetime of a program. The net benefits may be used to judge the efficiency level of the program, or they may be compared with those of other competing programs.

Cost-effectiveness analysis (CEA) (9)   Cost-effectiveness analysis compares the benefits of a program with its costs but requires monetizing only the costs of programs and not their benefits. CEA expresses program benefits in outcome units. The efficacy of a program in attaining its goals or in achieving magnitudes of substantive outcomes is assessed in relation to the monetary value of the resources or costs put into the program.

Cross-section data (3)   Data collected at one point in time. Its principal advantage is the relative inexpensiveness to obtain large sample size. Its principal disadvantage is its transitory factor, which makes causal association difficult. See also *time-series data, panel data.*

Cross-sectional survey (8)   In a cross-sectional survey, data on a sample or cross-section of respondents chosen to represent a particular target population are gathered at essentially one point in time, or within a short period of time.

Data cleaning (13)   The process of checking for and correcting errors related to data coding, transferring, and entering.

Deductive process (1)   A process of scientific inquiry that emphasizes theory as guidance for research. Hypotheses are derived from existing theories and serve as guidance for further research.

Demonstration (7)   Interventions carried out primarily to extend or test the applicability of already existing knowledge rather than add to scientific knowledge.

Dependent variable (1)   The variable whose value is dependent upon other variable(s) but which cannot itself affect other variable(s). In a causal relationship, the effect is a dependent variable.

Descriptive research (2)   One of the general purposes of research. Descriptive research is undertaken to describe or portray the characteristics of some phenomenon, such as an individual, group, organization, community, event, or situation, with the purpose of formulating these descriptions into conceptual categories.

Deviant case sampling (6)   See *extreme case sampling.*

Diagnostic-related groups (DRGs) (2)   A prospective payment system for hospital care used by Medicare or other insurances. DRG criteria typically include the patients' age, sex, principal and secondary diagnoses, procedures performed, and discharge status.

Dimension (2)   A specifiable aspect or facet of a concept.

Direct relationship (1)   See *positive relationship.*

Distribution (14)   A distribution organizes the values of a variable into categories. A frequency distribution, also known as a marginal distribution, shows the number of cases that fall into each category. A percentage distribution may be obtained by dividing the number or frequency of cases in the category by the total N.

Double-barreled questions (12)   Double-barreled questions really ask two separate questions in one statement. They are biased because respondents may have different answers toward different questions.

Double-blind experiment (7)   Experiment in which neither the subjects nor the experimenters know which is the experimental group and which is the control group.

Ecological fallacy (5)   Refers to the possibility that patterns found at a group level differ from those that would be found at an individual level. Thus, it may not be appropriate to draw conclusion at the individual level based on analyzing aggregate data.

Effect size (4)   The size or strength of the impact of one factor on another.

Empiricism (1)   An approach used in scientific inquiry to discover the patterns of regularity in life. Such an approach relies on what humans experience through their senses: sight, hearing, taste, smell, and touch.

Environment (2)   Events external to the body over which the individual has little or no control. Environment includes physical and social (including political, economic, cultural, psychological, and demographic) dimensions.

Environmental health research (1)   Research that concentrates on services that attempt to promote the health of populations by treating their environments rather than by treating specific individuals.

Environmental theory (2)   An environment-focused theory of disease causation that identifies environmental risk factors to account for the occurrence of diseases. Traditional environmental factors include sanitation, filth, and pollutants. With increasing industrialization, recent environmental risks include overcrowding, workplace safety and stress, housing, and others.

Epidemiological research (1)   Research that focuses on the population level by studying the frequency, distribution, and determinants of health and diseases.

Ethnographic (6)   A type of qualitative inquiry that describes a culture after extensive field research. The primary method of ethnographers is participant observation through immersing in the culture under study. See also *qualitative research.*

Evaluation research (9)   Evaluation research is the systematic application of scientific research methods for assessing the conceptualization, design, implementation, impact, and/or generalizability of organizational or social (including health services) programs.

Experimental group (7)   Those individuals or other units of analysis that receive the treatment or program.

Experimental research (7)   Experimental research involves planned interventions carried out so that explicit comparisons can be made between or across different intervention conditions to test a scientific hypothesis.

Explanatory research (2)   One of the general purposes of research. Explanatory research is conducted to explain things, test the assumption of a given phenomenon, examine the relationship among variables, answer cause–effect questions, or make projections into the future. It attempts to seek answers to research hypotheses or problems. Explanatory research may be called analytic or causal research.

Exploratory research (2)   One of the general purposes of research. Exploratory research is undertaken when relatively little is known about the phenomenon under investigation. Such an approach often results in meaningful hypotheses about the research problem.

External validity (7)   External validity is related to the generalizability of the experimental results. An experiment is considered externally valid if its effect can be generalized to the population, setting, treatment, and measurement variables of interest.

Extreme case sampling (6)   A qualitative research sampling method, extreme case sampling focuses on cases that are unusual or special in some way. It may distort the manifestation of the phenomenon of interest. It is also called deviant case sampling.

Field experiment (7)   Studies that meet all the requirements of a true experiment but are conducted in a natural setting. The experiment takes place as subjects are going about a common activity, and the manipulations and observations are so subtle and unobtrusive that subjects' normal behavior is not disrupted.

Field research (6)   A term frequently used to denote qualitative research. This is because qualitative researchers observe, describe, and analyze events happening in a natural social setting (i.e., field). Field research implies having direct and personal contact with people under study in their own environments. See also *qualitative research*.

Financing (health services) (1)   Financing is concerned with the magnitude, trend, and sources of medical care spending and consists of both public- and private-sector funding sources.

Fixed-column format (13)   The process of storing information, in the computer data file, for each variable in the same column for all respondents.

Focus group study (6)   A type of focused interview, focus group study is an interview with a small group of people on a specific topic. A focus group typically consists of 6 to 12 people who are brought together in a room to engage in a guided discussion of some topic for one to two hours. Participants for the focus group are selected on the basis of relevancy to the topic under study. See also *focused interview*.

Focused interview (6)   A popular qualitative research method, the focused interview (sometimes called the in-depth interview) is a way of gathering qualitative data by asking respondent(s) questions of interest to the researcher that are unstructured and open-ended, of variable length, and may be extended into additional interviews at later dates.

Germ theory (2)   A popular disease-focused theory that provides the foundation for biomedical research. With germ theory, microorganisms are the causal agent. The source of disease is at the individual level and the disease is communicated from one person to another (referred to as contagion). Strategies to address the disease focus on identification of those people with problems, and follow-up medical treatment.

Grounded theory (1)   Theories created based on observation rather than on deduction from existing theories. A grounded theory may be developed by: (a) entering the fieldwork phase without a hypothesis; (b) describing what happens; and (c) formulating explanations as to why it happens on the basis of observation.

Hawthorne effect (1)   The reactive effect of research on the social phenomena being studied, that is, the attention from the researchers alters the very behavior that the researchers wish to study.

Health services (2)   The total societal effort, whether private or public, to provide, organize, and finance services that promote the health status of the individuals and the community.

Health services research (1)   An applied multidisciplinary field that uses scientific inquiry to produce knowledge about the resources, provisions, organizing, financing, and policies of health services at the population level.

Health status (2)   The state of physical, mental health, and social well-being.

Heuristics (6)   A form of phenomenological inquiry focusing on intense human experience from the point of view of the investigator and co-researchers. It is through the intense personal experience that a sense of connectedness develops between researchers and subjects in their mutual efforts to elucidate the nature, meaning, and essence of a significant human experience. See also *phenomenological inquiry, qualitative research.*

Historical analysis (5)   The attempts to reconstruct past events (descriptive history) and the use of historical evidence to generate and test theories (analytical history).

History (7)   A threat to internal validity, history consists of events in the subjects' environment, other than the manipulated independent variable, that occur during the course of the experiment and may affect the outcome of the experiment.

HMO (health maintenance organizations) (2)   An organization that receives a fixed payment per subscriber to provide all medical care. Employees may pay the premium directly to HMO, or the employer may pay a portion of the premium for the employees as part of the benefits.

Hypothesis (1)   A proposition stated in a testable form and predicting a particular relationship between two or more variables.

Incidence (2)   The number of new cases of a disease in a defined population within a specified period of time.

Independent variable (1)   The variable capable of effecting change in another variable. In a causal relationship, the cause is an independent variable.

Inductive process (1)   A process of scientific inquiry that emphasizes research as impetus for theory. Existing theories are corroborated and modified, and new theories are developed based on the analysis of research data. The resulting corroborated, modified, or reconstructed theories serve as guidance for future research along similar field of inquiry.

Instrumental activities of daily living (IADL) (2)   IADL scales are used to measure less severe functional impairments and to distinguish between more subtle levels of functioning. Compared with ADL, they require a finer level of motor coordination. IADL include the ability to walk a quarter mile, walk up or down a flight of stairs, stand or sit for long periods, use fingers to grasp or handle, and lift or carry a moderately heavy or heavy object. See also *activities of daily living (ADL).*

Instrumentation (7)   A threat to internal validity, instrumentation refers to unwanted changes in characteristics of the measuring instrument or in the measurement procedure. This threat is most likely to occur in experiments when the instrument is a human observer, who may become more skilled, more bored, or more or less observant during the course of the study. Instrumentation effects also may occur when different observers are used to obtain measurements in different conditions or parts of an experiment.

Integrative research review (4)   Integrative research review summarizes past research by drawing conclusions from many separate studies addressing similar or related hypotheses or research questions. The integrative reviewer aims to accomplish the following objectives: present the state of the knowledge concerning the topic under review, highlight issues previous researchers have left unresolved or unstudied, and direct future research so that it is built on cumulative inquiry. See also *research review, theoretical review, methodological review, policy-oriented review*.

Intensity sampling (6)   A qualitative research sampling method, intensity sampling involves the same logic as extreme case sampling but with less emphasis on the extremes. It samples information-rich although not unusual cases that manifest the phenomenon of interest intensely but not extremely. See also *extreme case sampling*.

Interrater reliability (12)   A measure of reliability, interrater reliability involves using different people to conduct the same procedure, such as an interview, observation, coding, rating, and so on, and comparing the results of their work. To the extent that the results are highly similar, interrater reliability has been established.

Internal validity (7)   An experiment is internally valid to the extent that it rules out the possibility that extraneous variables, rather than the manipulated independent variable, are responsible for the observed outcome of the study.

Interval measures (12)   Interval measures refer to those variables whose attributes are not only rank-ordered but are separated by equal distances.

Intervening variable (1)   A variable between the independent and dependent variables. Its identification strengthens the causal inference.

Interview survey (8)   In interview survey, researchers or interviewers ask the questions, provide the response categories (if applicable) orally, and then record the respondents' choices or answers.

Inverse relationship (1)   See *negative relationship*.

Laboratory experiment (7)   Experiments conducted in artificial settings where researchers have complete control over the random allocation of subjects to treatment and control groups and the degree of well-defined intervention.

Leading questions (12)   Leading questions use particular wording to suggest or demand a particular answer. They are biased because they hint at a "desired" answer rather than finding out what the respondent feels.

Lifestyle theory (2)   A popular individual behavior-focused theory of disease causation that tries to isolate specific behaviors (e.g., smoking, lack of exercise) as causes of many health problems. These behaviors are deemed risky and unhealthy. The strategy to improve health status is through changing those behaviors.

Lifestyles (2)   See *behavioral risk factors*.

Linear relationship (1)   A form of relationship between two variables in which the two variables vary at the same rate regardless of whether the values of the variables are low, high, or intermediate.

Loaded questions (12)   Loaded questions use words and phrases that reflect the investigators' perception of a particular issue or event. They are biased because they suggest certain beliefs that could influence respondents' answers.

Logistic regression (14)   Logistic regression is based on the assumption that the logarithm of the odds of belonging to one population is a linear function of several predictors (independent variables) in the model. In logistic regression, the dependent variable is binary or dichotomous (e.g., whether one smokes or not, has health insurance or not).

Longitudinal survey (8)   Longitudinal survey takes a single sample and follows it or another similar sample with repeated (at least two) surveys, over a period of time.

Maturation (7)   A threat to internal validity, maturation refers to any psychological or physical changes taking place within subjects as a result of the passing of time regardless of the experimental intervention.

Mean (14)   As a measure of central tendency, the mean is the arithmetic average computed by adding up all the values and dividing by the total number of cases.

Measurement (12)   The process of specifying and operationalizing a given concept.

Measurement errors (12)   The sources of differences observed in the elements that are not caused by true differences among elements.

Measurement reliability (12)   The extent to which consistent results are obtained when a particular measure is applied to similar elements. A reliable measure will yield the same or a very similar outcome when it is repeated to the same subject or subjects sharing the same characteristics being measured.

Measurement validity (12)   The extent to which important dimensions of a concept and their categories have been taken into account and appropriately operationalized. A valid measure has response categories truly reflecting all important meanings of the concept under consideration.

Measures of central tendency (14)   Summaries of the information about the average value of a variable, some typical value around which all the values cluster. See also the three commonly used measures of central tendency: *mode, median,* and *mean.*

Measures of dispersion (14)   See *measures of variability.*

Measures of variability (14)   The spread or variation of the distribution. See also the commonly used measures of variability: *range, variance,* and *standard deviation.*

Median (14)   As a measure of central tendency, the median is the middle position or midpoint of a distribution. It is computed by first ordering the values of a distribution and then dividing the distribution in half, that is, half the cases fall below the median and the other half are above it.

Medicaid (2)   Joint federal–state medical insurance for the following categories: (a) Aid to Families with Dependent Children (AFDC) families; (b) those covered by Supplemental Security Income (SSI), including the aged, the blind, and the disabled; and (c) state-designated "categorically needy" and/or "medically needy" groups. Every state Medicaid program provides specific basic health services. States may determine the scope of services offered (e.g., limit the days of hospital care or the number of physician visits covered). Payments are made directly to providers of services for care rendered to eligible individuals. Providers must accept the Medicaid reimbursement level as payment in full.

Medicare (2)   Medical insurance that covers hospital, physician, and other medical services for (a) persons 65 and over, (b) disabled individuals who are entitled to Social Security benefits, and (c) end-stage renal disease victims. Part A of Medicare covers hospital insurance. Part B is a supplementary medical insurance, providing payments for physicians, physician-ordered supplies and services, outpatient hospital services, rural health clinic visits, and the like. Until 1992, Medicare has operated primarily on a fee-for-service basis for physicians and related services and, until 1983, on a cost-based retrospective basis for hospital services. Since 1983, the Medicare hospital prospective payment system (PPS) has used diagnosis-related groups (DRGs) to classify cases for payment. Since 1992, the Medicare physician payment system has adopted a resource-based relative value system (RBRVS).

MEDLINE (4)   The world's leading bibliographic database of medical information, covering over 3,500 journals since 1966 and containing information found in the publications *Index Medicus, International Nursing Index,* and *Index to Dental Literature.* MEDLINE contains abstracts of articles published by the most common U.S. and international journals on medicine and health services.

Mental set (13)   The responses to later items of the questionnaire influenced by perceptions based on previous items.

Meta-analysis (4)   A statistical analysis that combines and interprets the results of independent studies of a given scientific issue for the purpose of integrating the findings. It allows the reviewer to synthesize the results of numerous tests so that an overall conclusion can be drawn.

Methodological review (4)   Methodological review summarizes different research designs used to study a particular topic and compares studies with different designs in terms of their findings. The purpose is to identify the strengths and weaknesses of different designs for a particular topic and separate fact from artifact in research results. See also *research review, integrative research review, theoretical review, policy-oriented review.*

Methodology (10)   See *research method.*

Midtests (7)   Measurements made during the time the intervention or program is being implemented; short for midprogram or midexperiment tests.

Mode (14)   As a measure of central tendency, the mode is the value (or category) of a distribution that occurs most frequently.

Model (7)   A representation of a system that specifies its components and the relationships among the components.

Multiple regression (14)   An examination of the impact of two or more independent variables on a dependent variable. Generally, the variables are measured at the interval-ratio level. Multiple regression may be used to examine the relationships among variables or as an inferential method, to test hypotheses about population parameters.

Multivariate analysis (14)   An examination of the relationship among three or more variables at a time. The inclusion of additional variables is based on both theoretical and practical knowledge, which helps specify the direction of influence and test for spuriousness.

Natural experiment (7)   Experiments conducted in real-life settings rather than in laboratories or the controlled environment. Researchers rely on truly naturally occurring events in which people have different exposures that resemble an actual experiment.

Needs assessment (9)   A type of evaluation with the purpose of identifying weaknesses or deficiency areas (i.e., needs) in the current situation that can be remedied or of projecting future conditions to which the program will need to adjust.

Negative relationship (1)   A form of relationship between two variables in which increase (decrease) in one variable is accompanied by decrease (increase) in the other variable.

Nominal definition (12)   A specification of concepts that is built on the consensus or norm over what a particular term should mean.

Nominal measures (12)   Nominal measures classify elements into categories of a variable that are exhaustive and mutually exclusive. There is no rank-order relationship among categories and one cannot measure the distance between categories.

Nonlinear relationship (1)   A form of relationship between two variables in which the rate at which one variable changes in value is different for different values of the second variable.

Nonprobability sampling (11)   In nonprobability sampling, the probability of selecting any sampling unit is not known because units are selected through a nonrandom process. A nonprobability sample may be biased because certain units may be more or less likely included in the sample.

Objectivity (1)   A basic characteristic of scientific inquiry that requires researchers to carry out research related activities unaffected by their emotion, conjecture, or personal biases.

Observation unit (11)   A term used in sampling. The observation unit is the unit from which data are actually collected.

Observational research (6)   A term frequently used to denote qualitative research. The term is used because observation is a primary method of qualitative research. Qualitative researchers observe for the purpose of seeing the world from the subject's own perspective. Qualitative observation emphasizes direct observation, usually with the naked eye, and takes place in the natural setting. Also called participant observation. See also *participant observation, qualitative research.*

Odds ratio (14)   Odds ratio may be defined as the ratio of two odds, that is, the ratio of the probability of occurrence of an event to that of nonoccurrence. See also *relative risk ratio.*

Operational definition (2)   The specification of concepts that is built on a particular observational or data collection strategy. Operational definition spells out precisely how the concept will be measured.

Operationalization (1)   A process that translates general concepts into specific indicators and specifies how a researcher goes about measuring and identifying the variables.

Opportunity costs (9)   A concept used to value costs, opportunity costs reflect alternative ways resources can be utilized.

Ordinal measures (12)   Those indicators or variables whose attributes may be logically rank-ordered along some progression.

Outcome evaluation (9)   A type of evaluation concerned with the accomplishments and the impact of the program and the effectiveness of the program in attaining the intended results.

Panel data (3)   A combination of cross-section and time-series data, surveying the same groups over time. Its principal advantage is its ability to capture trends and causal associations. Its principal disadvantages are attrition rates and its relative expensiveness. See also *cross-section data, time-series data.*

Panel study (5)   A panel study takes as its basis a representative sample of the group of interest, which may be individuals, households, organizations, or any other social unit, and follows the same unit over time with a series of surveys.

Paradigm (1)   A general perspective, a fundamental model or scheme that breaks down the complexity of the real world and organizes our views. Often, a paradigm directs researchers to look for answers and provides them with concepts that are the building blocks of theories.

Parameters (11)   The summary numerical description of variables about the population of interest.

Participant observation (6)   A popular qualitative research method in which the researcher is fully engaged in experiencing the setting under study while at the same time trying to understand that setting through personal experience, observations, and talking with other participants about what is happening. Through direct experience with and observation of programs the researcher can gain information that otherwise would not become available. See also *observational research.*

Path analysis (14)   A procedure that provides the possibility for causal determination among a set of measured variables. It gives a quantitative interpretation of an assumed causal system. Path analysis may consist of a series of regression equations, with many variables in the model taking their places respectively as dependent and independent variables. In other words, most of the variables in the model will be a dependent variable in one equation and an independent variable in one or more different equations.

Pearson product–moment correlation coefficient (14)   The Pearson product–moment correlation coefficient (r) is a measure of association between two interval-ratio level variables.

Phenomenological inquiry (6)   A type of qualitative inquiry focusing on the experience of a phenomenon for particular people. The phenomenon being experienced may be an emotion (e.g., loneliness, satisfaction, anger), a relationship, a marriage, a job, a program, an organization, or a culture. In terms of subject matter, phenomenological inquiry holds that what is important to know is what people experience and how they interpret the world. In terms of research methodology, phenomenological inquiry believes the only way for researchers to really know what another person experiences is to experience it for themselves through participant observation. See also *heuristics, participant observation, qualitative research.*

Policy analysis (9) A type of evaluation with the purpose of laying out goals, using logical processes to evaluate identified alternatives, and exploring the best way to reach these goals.

Policy-oriented review (4) Review summarizing current knowledge of a topic so as to draw out policy implications of study findings. Such review requires knowledge of the major policy issues and debates as well as common research expertise. See also *research review, integrative research review, theoretical review, methodological review.*

Population (11) The target to which investigators generate the study results.

Positive relationship (1) A form of relationship between two variables in which both variables vary in the same direction, that is, an increase in the value of one variable is accompanied by an increase in the value of the second variable, or a decrease in one variable is accompanied by a decrease in the value of the second variable.

Positivism (1) A fundamental assumption of scientific inquiry that holds that life is not totally chaotic or random but has logical and persistent patterns of regularity.

Posttests (7) Tests given at the end of a program or an experiment; short for postprogram or post-experiment tests.

Predictive validity (12) A measure of validity, predictive validity may be examined by comparing the results obtained from the measurement with some actual later-occurring evidence that the measurement aims at predicting. When there is a high degree of correspondence between the prediction and actual event—the predicted event actually takes place—then predictive validity is established.

Prestige (13) Responses to questions intended to improve the image of the respondent in the eyes of the interviewer.

Pretests (7) Tests given before a program or an experiment starts; short for preprogram or preexperiment tests.

Prevalence (2) The number of instances of a given disease in a given population at a designated time.

Primary data source (3) The collection of data by researchers themselves. See also *secondary data source.*

Primary research (5) The analysis of data collected by the researcher firsthand. The data originates with the research; they are not there before the research is undertaken. See also *secondary research.*

Probability sampling (11) In probability sampling, all sampling units in the study population have a known, nonzero probability of being selected in the sample, typically through a random selection process.

Process evaluation (9) A type of evaluation with the purpose of focusing on how a particular program operates. It is concerned with the activities, services, materials, staffing, and administrative arrangements of the program.

Proportional reduction in error (PRE) (14) PRE is a broad framework that helps organize a large number of measures for nominal-, ordinal-, and even interval-ratio-level data. PRE-based measures are typically ratios of a measure of error in predicting the values of one variable based on that variable alone and the same measure of error based on knowledge of an additional variable. The logic behind this framework is that if prior knowledge about another variable improves the knowledge of this variable, then these two variables are related.

Proposition (1) A statement about one or more concepts or variables. Propositions are the building blocks of theories.

Pure research (2)   See *theoretical research*.

Purposive sampling (11)   A type of nonprobability sampling method that selects sampling elements based on expert judgment in terms of the representativeness or typical nature of population elements and the purpose of the study.

Qualitative research (6)   Research methods employed to find out what people do, know, think, and feel by observing, interviewing, and analyzing documents. Specifically, it attempts to gain individuals' own accounts of their attitudes, motivations and behavior. See also *field research, observational research, participant observation, case study, ethnographic, phenomenological inquiry, heuristics, symbolic interactionism*.

Quality of life (2)   Factors that enhance or reduce the meaningfulness of life, including independent functioning, family circumstances, finances, housing, job satisfaction, and so forth.

Quota sampling (11)   A type of nonprobability sampling method that specifies desired characteristics in the population elements and selects appropriate ratios of population elements that fit the characteristics of the sample.

Random sampling (7)   The process of selecting units in an unbiased manner to form a representative sample from a population of interest.

Randomization (7)   The process of taking a set of units and allocating them to an experimental or control group by means of some randomizing procedure.

Randomized clinical trial (1)   A medical experiment in which subjects in a population is randomly allocated into groups, usually called "experiment" and "control" groups, to receive or not receive an experimental procedure. The results are assessed by comparison of outcome measures in the experiment and control groups.

Range (14)   A measure of dispersion, range is the difference between the highest (maximum) and lowest (minimum) values in a distribution.

Rate (14)   A rate is computed by dividing the number of cases or events in a given category by the total number of observations. The resulting proportion is then expressed as any multiple of 10 that clears the decimal, usually 100 or 1,000.

Ratio (14)   A ratio is one number divided by another: the frequency of observations in one category is divided by the frequency in another category of a distribution.

Ratio measures (12)   A measurement similar to interval measures except that ratio measures are based on a nonarbitrary or true-zero point. The true-zero property of ratio measures makes it possible to divide and multiple numbers meaningfully and thereby form ratios. See also *interval measures, ratio*.

Reactive effect (5)   Changes in behavior that occur because subjects are aware they are being studied or observed. This is a potential bias in data collection.

Records (5)   Systematic accounts of regular occurrences.

Regression toward the mean (7)   See *statistical regression*.

Relative risk ratio (14)   A measurement of the strength of association between the presence of a factor (*x*) and the occurrence of an event (*y*). For example, it is the ratio of the incidence of a disease (i.e., lung cancer) among the exposed (i.e., those who smoke) to the incidence of a disease among the unexposed (i.e., those who don't smoke).

Reliability (12)   A reflection of the extent to which the same result occurs from repeated applications of a measure to the same subject. See also *validity*.

Research design (10)   The planning of research. It specifies the questions to be studied, the data to be collected, the methods of data collection, and analysis.

Research method (10)   A body of knowledge that reflects the general philosophy and purpose of the research process, the assumptions and values that serve as a rationale for research, the general approach of data collection and analysis, and the standards used for interpreting data and reaching conclusions.

Research proposal (3) A description of what specific study a researcher intends to accomplish and how. The components of a research proposal generally include the following elements: a title page, a table of contents, an abstract, a detailed project description, references, a detailed budget, a human subjects review, and appendices.

Research review (4) Research review provides a synthesis of existing knowledge on a specific question, based on an assessment of all relevant empirical research that can be found. See also *integrative research review, theoretical review, methodological review, policy-oriented review.*

Resources (health services) (1) Human and nonhuman resources required for the provision of health services. Human resources consist of both physician and nonphysician providers. A major nonhuman health services resource is medical technology.

Sampling (11) The process of selecting a subset of observations from an entire population of interest so that characteristics from the subset can be used to draw conclusions or make inferences about the entire population of interest.

Sampling design (11) The method used to select the sampling units. It may be classified into probability and nonprobability sampling methods. See also *probability sampling, nonprobability sampling.*

Sampling element (11) A term used in sampling. Sampling element refers to the unit of the sample to be collected and provides the information base for analysis.

Sampling frame (11) A term used in sampling. Sampling frame is a list of sampling units from which the sample is actually selected.

Sampling unit (11) A term used in sampling. Sampling unit is the actual unit that is considered for selection.

Scientific inquiry (1) Research by scientists that produces knowledge and improves understanding of particular aspects of the world.

Scientific theory (1) The logical aspect of science. It is used as a framework to guide the understanding and explanation of patterns of regularity in life.

Secondary analysis (5) The reanalysis of data collected by another researcher or organization, including the analysis of data sets collated from a variety of sources to create time-series or area-based data sets. See also *primary research.*

Secondary data source (3) The use of data collected by others. See also *primary data source.*

Selection (7) A threat to internal validity, selection is present whenever there are systematic differences in the selection and composition of the experimental and control groups.

Self-administered survey (8) Questionnaires completed by the respondents themselves complete through reading the questions and entering their own answers.

Simple random sampling (11) A type of probability sampling method, simple random sampling means that every unit in a population has an equal probability of being included in a sample.

Simple regression (14) An examination of the impact of one independent variable on another dependent variable. Generally both variables are measured at the interval-ratio level.

Simulation (7) A special kind of model: a model in motion and operating over a period of time to show, not only the structure of the system (what position each variable or component occupies in the system and the way components are related or connected), but also the way change in one variable or component affects changes in the values of the other variables or components. See also *model.*

Skewedness (14) A distribution of cases that is not symmetric, that is, when more cases are found at one end of the distribution than the other.

Snowball sampling (11)   A type of nonprobability sampling method, snowball sampling relies on informants to identify other relevant subjects for study inclusion.

Social contacts (2)   The number of social activities a person performs within a specified time period. Examples include visits with friends and relatives and participation in social events, such as conferences and workshops. See also *social well-being*.

Social desirability (13)   Responses to questions based on what is perceived as being socially acceptable or respectable, positive or negative.

Social resources (2)   The extent that social contacts such as close friends and relatives can be relied on for tangible and intangible support. Social resources represent personal evaluations of the adequacy of interpersonal relationships. See also *social well-being*.

Social well-being (2)   Social well-being extends beyond the individual to encompass the quantity and quality of social contacts and resources across distinct domains of life, including community, family, and work. See also *social contacts, social resources*.

Socioeconomic status (SES) (2)   An important social measure and a strong and consistent predictor of health status. The major components of SES include income, education, and occupational status.

Sociography (6)   A type of case study, sociography denotes the social mapping of a community's institutions, structure, and patterns of relationships. This type of case study is heavily used in social anthropology for research on nonindustrialized societies, but it is also used to study towns and communities in industrialized societies. See also *case study*.

Spearman's coefficient (14)   Spearman's coefficient of rank correlation (r_s) is a measure of association between two ordinal-level variables.

Split-half reliability (12)   A measure of reliability, split-half reliability involves preparing two sets (or two halves) of a measurement of the same concept, applying them to research subjects at one setting, and comparing the correlation between the two sets of measurement. To the extent the correlation is high, then the measurement is reliable.

Spurious relationship (1)   Spurious relationship exists when two variables appear to be related only because both are caused by a third variable. The variable that causes a spurious relationship is an antecedent variable, which occurs first and is causally related to both the independent and dependent variables.

Standard deviation (14)   A measure of dispersion, the standard deviation is defined as the square root of the variance.

Standard scores (14)   Descriptions of the relative position of an observation within a distribution. For example, the z score uses both the mean and standard deviation to indicate how many standard deviations above or below the mean an observation falls.

Statistical regression (7)   A threat to internal validity, statistical regression is the tendency for extreme subjects to move (regress) closer to the mean or average with the passing of time. This phenomenon is likely to affect experimental results when subjects are selected for an experimental condition because of their extreme conditions or scores. The more deviant the score, the larger the error of measurement it probably contains. On a posttest an invesetigator expects the high scorers to decline somewhat on the average and the low scorers to improve their relative standing regardless of the intervention. Also called regression toward the mean.

Statistics (11)   The summary numerical description of variables about a sample.

straight-line relationship (1)   See *linear relationship*.

Stratified purposeful sampling (6)   A qualitative research sampling method, stratified purposeful sampling is carried out to combine a typical case sampling strategy with others, essentially taking a stratified purposeful sample of above-average, average, and below-average cases.

Stratified sampling (11)   A type of probability sampling method, stratified sampling divides the population into nonoverlapping groups or categories, called strata, and then conducts independent simple random sampling for each stratum.

Suppresser variable (1)   A variable that suppresses the relationship by being positively correlated with one of the variables in the relationship and negatively correlated with the other, with the result that the two variables in the relationship appear to be unrelated. The true relationship between the two variables will reappear when the suppresser variable is controlled for.

Survey research (8)   The use of a systematic method to collect data directly from respondents regarding facts, knowledge, attitudes, beliefs, and behaviors of interest to the researcher, and the analysis of these data using quantitative methods.

Symbolic interactionism (6)   A method of qualitative analysis focusing on a common set of symbols and understanding that have emerged to give meaning to people's interactions. The importance of symbolic interactionism to qualitative research is its distinct emphasis on the importance of symbols and the interpretative processes that undergird interactions as fundamental to understanding human behavior. See also *qualitative research.*

Symmetrical relationship (1)   A form of relationship between two variables in which change in either variable is accompanied by change in the other variable.

Systematic sampling (11)   A type of probability sampling method, systematic sampling selects every *k*th element from the sampling frame after a random start.

Telephone survey (8)   In a telephone survey, researchers or interviewers ask the questions, present the response categories (if applicable) orally via the telephone, and then record the respondents' choices or answers.

Term (2)   Names that represent a collection of apparently related, observed phenomena.

Test–retest reliability (12)   A measure of reliability, test–retest reliability involves administering the same measurement to the same individuals at two different times. If the correlation between the same measures is high (usually above .80), then the measurement is believed to be reliable.

Testing (7)   A threat to internal validity, testing refers to changes in what is being measured brought about by reactions to the process of measurement. Typically, people will score better or give more socially desirable or psychologically healthier responses the second time a test or scale is administered to them.

Theoretical research (2)   Involves testing hypotheses developed from theories that are intellectually interesting to the researcher. Theoretical research is also called basic or pure research.

Theoretical review (4)   Theoretical review summarizes the relevant theories used to explain a particular topic and compares them with regard to accuracy of prediction, consistency, and breadth. Theoretical review contains a description of major findings, assesses which theory is most powerful and consistent with known findings, and refines a theory by reformulating or integrating concepts from existing theories. See also *research review, integrative research review, methodological review, policy-oriented review.*

Time sampling (6)   A qualitative research sampling method that samples periods (e.g., months of the year) or units of time (e.g., hours of the day). It is used when programs are believed to function in different ways at different time periods or units.

Time-series tests (7)   A series of tests or measurements, usually given at equal intervals before and after the program or experiment.

Time-series data (3)   Data that follows the same unit of observation over time. Its principal advantage is its ability to capture historical trends and changes. Its principal disadvantages are limited observations and the relative expensiveness in obtaining large sample size. See also *cross-section data, panel data.*

Trend study (5)   A study with a repeated cross-sectional design in which each survey collects data on the same items or variables with independently selected samples of the same general population of interest.

Triangulation (6)   The combination of several methodologies in the study of the same phenomenon or program.

Typical case sampling (6)   A qualitative research sampling method that provides a qualitative profile of one or more "typical" cases. It is helpful to those not familiar with the program in question.

Unit of analysis (11)   The object about which investigators wish to draw conclusions based on their study.

Unit of observation (3)   The level from which data are actually collected or recorded.

Univariate analysis (14)   An examination of the characteristics of one variable at a time. Descriptive statistics are produced in univariate analysis.

Validity (12)   The validity of a measure is the extent to which it actually assesses what it purports to measure. If a measure is supposed to reflect the quality of care, a researcher would expect improvements in quality to affect the measure positively. See also *reliability*.

Variable (1)   A concept that has more than one measurable value.

Variance (14)   A measure of dispersion that measures the extent to which each of the values of a distribution differs from the mean. It is defined as the average squared deviation from the mean.

INDEX